PHOTODYNAMIC TUMOR THERAPY

PHOTODYNAMIC TUMOR THERAPY

2nd and 3rd Generation Photosensitizers

Edited by

Joerg G. Moser

Institute of Laser Medicine
University of Düsseldorf, Germany

harwood academic publishers
Australia • Canada • China • France • Germany • India
Japan • Luxembourg • Malaysia • The Netherlands • Russia
Singapore • Switzerland • Thailand

Amsteldijk 166
1st Floor
1079 LH Amsterdam
The Netherlands

British Library Cataloguing in Publication Data

Photodynamic tumor therapy: 2nd and 3rd generation photosensitizers
1. Cancer – photochemotherapy 2. Lasers in medicine
I. Moser, Joerg G.
616.9'94'0631

ISBN: 90-5699-139-6

Printed and Bound at Ajanta Offset, New Delhi, India

CONTENTS

PREFACE

This book contains collected answers to the general needs for comprehensive quantitative data on newly developed photosensitizers for photodynamic therapy (PDT) of cancer and other modalities which are widely scattered through sometimes unnoticed literature. The overwhelming statements on these new compounds as being 'good' or 'excellent' sensitizing drugs for PDT without any comparable or just quantifiable data hide the lack of information in physical terms. So, a sieving of these statements was the first crucial aim to bring together the sometimes only small amount of *quantitative* information available. Sometimes published drawings had to be evaluated in terms of physical parameters in order to derive and to generate comparable data.

As expected, this book reflects various very divergent tendencies of PDT research in Europe and in the USA. Our publishers monitored a 'Europe lasting tendency' when presenting the choice of authors of this book. I was brazen-faced enough to answer that we need workers from the lab's bench to write a book on facts and techniques of representative value. Just this collection of meanings is polychromatic enough, by style as well as by ideas, to reflect the tendencies in PDT research on an international scale. All authors were engaged to allow for reproducible and comparable work for a reader working on actual problems in PDT research.

Some chapters could not be written yet. For instance a chapter on *porphycenes* has been wrecked on the rocks of the prospective authors' patent applications. Another chapter concerned with the description of biophysical parameters governing PDT effects on *erythrocytes* will be written in about 10 years when the different authors possibly come to an agreement on what PDT effects have to be measured. Other contributions reached the editor at the last minute. Such circumstances did not make it any easier to present the actual state of the art.

So, the editor thankfully acknowledges the help of all the colleagues who collected and inspired this book. In particular, *Beate Roeder*, *Johan Moan* and *Benjamin Ehrenberg* gave helpful advice on how to complete our vision of the present state. Also *Anja Vervoorts, Petra Plewa*, *Bettina and Dorothee von Albert* were extremely helpful in detailed editorial work. A grant for cooperation between German and Israeli groups given by the *European Commission* was very helpful in completing this book.

So we hope that this book will be able to set some landmarks in the ocean of literature splashing not only over newcomers but also over people longtimes involved in the subject.

PREFACE

CONTRIBUTORS

Ben-Hur, Ehud
New York Blood Center
310 East 67th Street
New York, NY 10021, USA

Berg, Kristian
Department of Physics
Institute of Cancer Research
Montebello
N-0310 Oslo, Norway

Chan, Wai-Shun
New York Blood Center
310 East 67th Street
New York, NY 10021, USA

Chen, Louise
Department of Biological Regulation
The Weizmann Institute of Science
Rehovot 76100, Israel

Ehrenberg, Benjamin
Department of Physics
Bar-llan University
Ramat-Gan 52900, Israel

Fiedor, Leszek
Department of Biochemistry
The Weizmann Institute of Science
Rehovot 76100, Israel

Garbo, Greta M.
GMG Consulting
1953 Elise Way # G
Santa Barbara, CA 93109, USA

Hirth, Andreas
Institute of Organic and
Macromolecular Chemistry
University of Bremen
Leobener Str. NW 2
D-28334 Bremen, Germany

Iani, Vladimir
Department of Physics
The Norwegian Radium Hospital
Institute of Cancer Research
Ullernchauséen
Montebello
N-0310 Oslo, Norway

Jocham, Dieter
Urologische Klinik und Poliklinik
Medizinische Universität
Ratzeburger Allee 160
D-23562 Lübeck, Germany

Kliesch, Holger
Institute of Organic and
Macromolecular Chemistry
University of Bremen
Leobener Str. NW 2
D-28334 Bremen, Germany

Klotz, Markus
Klotz Analytische Meßtechnik
Bad Liebenzell, Germany

Kongshaug, M.
Department of Physics
The Norwegian Radium Hospital
Institute of Cancer Research
Ullernchauséen
Montebello
N-0310 Oslo, Norway

Kostenich, Genady
Plastic Surgery Department
Sheba Medical Center
Tel Hashomer 52621, Israel

Malik, Zvi
Department of Biology
Bar-llan University,
Ramat-Gan 52900, Israel

Melnik, Ivan S.
Kiev Polytechnic Institute
Kiev, Ukraine

Michelsen, Ulrike
Institute of Organic and
Macromolecular Chemistry
University of Bremen
Leobener Str. NW 2
D-28334 Bremen, Germany

Moan, Johan
Department of Biophysics
Institute of Cancer Research
Montebello
N-0310 Oslo, Norway

Moser, Jörg G.
Institute of Laser Medicine
University of Düsseldorf
Universitäts-Str. 1
D-40225 Düsseldorf, Germany

Orenstein, Arie
Plastic Surgery Department
Sheba Medical Center
Tel Hashomer 52621, Israel

Peng, Qian
Department of Physics,
The Norwegian Radium Hospital
Institute of Cancer Research
Ullernchauséen,
Montebello
N-0310 Oslo, Norway

Roeder, Beate
Department of Physics-Photobiophysics
Humboldt University
Invalidenstr. 110
D-10115 Berlin, Germany

Rosenbach-Belkin, Varda
Department of Biochemistry
The Weizmann Institute of Science
Rehovot 76100, Israel

Salomon, Yoram
Department of Biological Regulation
The Weizmann Institute of Science
Rehovot 76100, Israel

Scherz, Avigdor
Department of Biochemistry
The Weizmann Institute of Science
Rehovot 76100, Israel

Shopova, Maria
Institute of Organic Chemistry
Bulgarian Academy of Sciences
1113 Sofia, Bulgaria

Steiner, Rudolph W.
Institut für Laseranwendungen in der
Medizin und Meßtechnik
Universität Ulm, Helmholtzstr. 12
D-89081 Ulm, Germany

Weitemeyer, Andrea
Institute of Organic and
Macromolecular Chemistry
University of Bremen
Leobener Str. NW 2
D-28334 Bremen, Germany

Wöhrle, Dieter
Institute of Organic and
Macromolecular Chemistry
University of Bremen
Leobener Str. NW 2
D-28334 Bremen, Germany

Zilberstein, Judith
Department of Biological Regulation
The Weizmann Institute of Science
Rehovot 76100, Israel

Zuk, Magda
New York Blood Center
310 East 67th Street
New York, NY 10021, USA

1. GENERAL CONSIDERATIONS

1.1. DEFINITIONS AND GENERAL PROPERTIES OF 2nd AND 3rd GENERATION PHOTOSENSITIZERS

JOERG G. MOSER

A photosensitizer is generally defined as a substance inducing light sensitivity to a normally light insensitive chemical or physical process. Examples are e.g. electron transfer reactions greatly enhanced by phthalocyanines (Woehrle *et al.*, 1995).

In a biological sense, photosensitizers induce photosensitivity to whole living cells or their compartments. Photosensitation is possible over the whole spectrum of light, from far UV-C to the far infra-red. Photodynamic 2nd generation photosensitizers induce light sensitivity in the region of 650–850 nm where biological chromophores normally do not absorb light.

Exceptions are plant chlorophylls and bacteriochlorophylls which exert their biologically relevant functional light absorption just on this "photodynamic playground". So, the "photodynamic window" (Fig. 1) is confined by

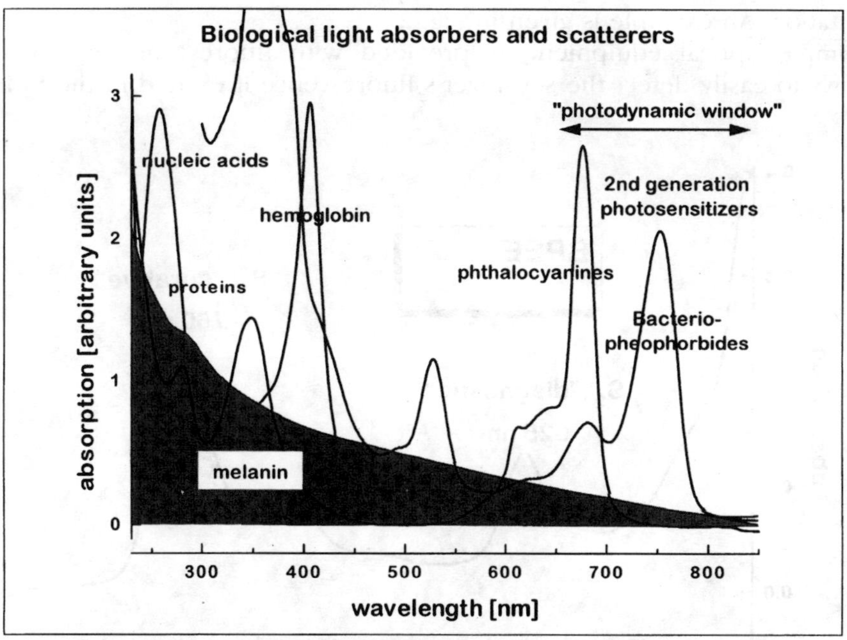

Figure 1 2nd generation photosensitizers absorb light inside the "photodynamic window" of the visible spectrum.

the absorption properties of biological chromophores, e.g. heme in hemoglobin, and light scatterers (e.g. melanin) on its short wavelength side to 650 nm, and on its long wavelength side to 850 nm due to the necessary energy gap between the sensitizer's lowest triplet state, T_1, and the energy acceptor, $^3O_2$, and its activated derivative, $^1O_2$, singlet oxygen. Sensitizers absorbing at longer wavelength show strongly reduced $^1O_2$ yields due to reversibility of energy transfer.

3rd generation photosensitizers are derivatives of 2nd generation photosensitizers attached to or introduced into chemical devices acquiring some biological specificity to deliver or to target such drug to defined kind of living cells. These include e.g. amino acid coupling of sensitizers, polymers coupled to photosensitizers, protein or carbohydrate coupled photosensitizers, and coupling products with antibodies. Recently carrier inclusion complexes and detoxified products were developed and can be comprised into this class of products. Some will be discussed in later chapters of this book.

The spectral properties of 2nd generation photosensitizers can be grouped into those relevant for fluorescence detection of sensitizer distribution ("diagnostic wavelengths") and those relevant for type II photodynamic reactions ("curative wavelengths"). These coincide almost always with the S_2 and the S_1 singlet bands respectively for the sensitizer's light electronic excitation. An example is given in Fig. 2.

Simple optical equipment as provided with fluorescence microscopes allows to easily detect the sensitizer's fluorescence if excited in the S_2 band

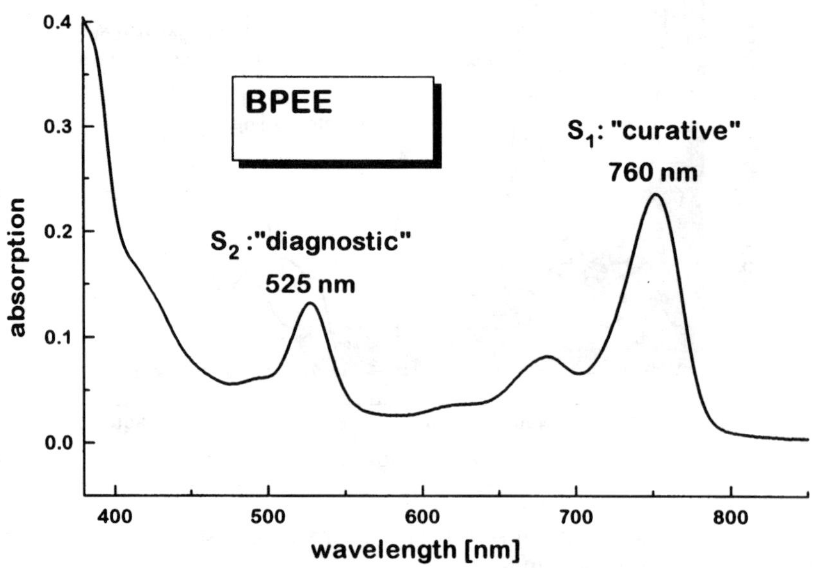

Figure 2 "Diagnostic" and "curative" absorption maxima of a 2nd generation photosensitizer: bacteriopheophorbide ethyl ester.

so far as wide Stokes shifts are possible (e.g. in bacteriopheophorbides). The more effective excitation in the S_1 band needs for more subtle optical equipment to separate excitation and fluorescence spectra. Some sensitizers with high triplet occupation density can be detected only by phosphorescence (e.g. palladium porphyrins) with all the complex equipment of infrared imaging techniques. Table 1 gives an overview of excitation properties of the most commonly used groups of 2nd generation photosensitizers.

2nd generation photosensitizers shift their spectra in biological surroundings due to aggregation and to interaction with lipids or proteins of the biological matrix. So a transfer of data obtained in organic solvents to biological reality is not allowed. In most cases absorption spectroscopy (e.g. Moser *et al.*, 1992) cannot be performed in biological tissue. Fluorescence excitation spectra, therefore, are the tool of choice to obtain indirect information on absorption properties of incorporated sensitizers in biological surroundings (Griffiths *et al.*, 1994). Shifts of more than 20 nm are not uncommon. Apparative equipment has been developed to investigate fluorescence excitation spectra under surgical condition to obtain the optimum therapeutic wavelength (Roeder *et al.*, 1993; Star, 1995).

The absorption of light by the lowest singlet band, S_1, leads either to fluorescence or to population of the lowest triplet band, T_1. The intersystem crossing, ISC, is greatly facilitated in porphyrins and leads to a considerable electron population density at the triplet level. The long triplet lifetimes allow to transfer energy to $^3O_2$ (ground state oxygen) and several other molecules. The proof is the quenching of phosphorescence by the respective species (Wilson and Cerniglia, 1994). The case of triplet quenching by $^3O_2$ leads to the highly reactive species, $^1O_2$ (Type II photoreaction: Foote, 1976). Singlet oxygen undergoes reactions with several organic acceptors (amino acids in proteins, sugar moieties in carbohydrates, unsaturated fatty acids and other molecules). Specific biological and artificial indicators of a direct oxidation by singlet oxygen inside living cells have been described (cholesterol:

Table 1 Excitation Properties of the Most Common Groups of 2nd Generation Photosensitizers

Type of sensitizer	*Fluorescence detection* [nm]	*Curative wavelengths* [nm]
Synthetic porphyrinoids		
Phthalocyanins	610	670–690
Naphthalocyanins	770	740–780
Benzoporphins	530	690
Purpurins	675	640–690
Chlorins	525	680
Porphycenes	645–730	640–720
Natural porphyrinoids		
Pheophorbides	515, 540	680
Bacteriochlorins	530	760
Bacteriopheophorbides	525–530	760

Bachowsky *et al.*, 1992; di-phenyl isobenzofurane: Weishaupt *et al.*, 1976). In the case of cholesterol, the direct oxidation by singlet oxygen leads to a peroxide in position 5 of the ring system. The same molecule shows evidence of secondary reactions of singlet oxygen leading to water-derived radicals oxidizing the position 6 and 7 of the steran skeleton. In the reagent tube, radical reactions can be demonstrated by electron spin resonance in the presence of specific radical indicators. Since those substances cannot pass cell membranes the role of water-derived radicals in photodynamic reactions remains yet unclear. Recently the group of Gal has shown intracellular accumulation of free radical species (Kriska *et al.*, 1996). On the other hand, a direct participation of $^1O_2$ in cell killing could be demonstrated by uptake of diphenyl isobenzofurane into living cells which protected these cells from $^1O_2$ damage and lead to a reduction of death rate (Weishaupt *et al.*, 1976). $^1O_2$ development in photosensitized erythrocyte ghosts has been directly demonstrated by its light emission at 1270 nm by Roeder and coworkers (1994).

Excited sensitizer states may enforce damage of living cells by other energy qualities like X-rays or hyperthermia (Gomer, 1992). We will refer to these topics in later chapters of this book.

3rd generation photosensitizers are designed to induce biological specificity to the biophysically highly effective 2nd generation photosensitizers. It is a *fairy tale* to suppose biological specificity of a porphyrinoid drug as simply demonstrated in jaundice or in porphyria. The way to enrichment of photosensitizers in tumor cells has been described explicitly by two mechanisms: pH dependent dissociation equilibria in the case of polar drugs (Pottier and Kennedy, 1991) and interaction with the lipoprotein system in blood plasma for the more lipophilic drugs (Jori and Reddi, 1992). Ionized species will discharge at the lowered pH of tumor stroma and then taken up by tumor cells. Lipophilic drugs are concentrated in the lipoid cavity of lipoproteins and are taken up via lipoprotein receptors expressed at high density on tumor cell surfaces. So, a certain enrichment *of those drugs in tumors, but never an exclusive specificity of drug uptake* can be achieved. In fact, both mechanisms lead to a nearly statistical distribution of photosensitizing porphyrins in all major organs of a patient or an experimental animal. Impressive pharmacodynamic data concerning e.g. phthalocyanine derivatives were published recently (Dressler *et al.*, 1994). Only brain and muscle tissue take up lower amounts of porphyrinoid sensitizers. Tumors in or of these organs consequently show apparently high sensitizer accumulation (Bonnet, 1994). In general, the absolute amount of a porphyrinoid drug finally accumulated in a tumor does rarely surmount 1% of the drug dose totally applied. Higher accumulations sometimes referred to in the literature should be monitored with skepticism (Grashew *et al.*, 1990).

These handicaps can be surmounted only by 3rd generation photosensitizer designed to introduce real biological specificity into the process of sensitizer targeting. Details on these developments will be given in the later chapter on "Carrier Systems" in this book.

REFERENCES

Bachowsky, G. J., Ben Hur, E., and Girotti, A. W. (1991): Phthalocyanine-sensitized lipid peroxidation in cell membranes: use of cholesterol and azide as probes of primary photochemistry. *J. Photochem. Photobiol.* **9**, 307–321.

Bonnet, R. (1994): Discussion remark. 5th IPA Meeting. Amelia Island FL, USA.

Dressler, C., Ismail, M. S., Nowak, C., Herter, R., Senz, R. G., Hagemann, R., Roeder, B., and Berlien, H. P. (1994): On the pharmacokinetics of the far red absorbing octa-α-butyloxy-zinc-phthalocyanine in *Lewis lung* carcinoma bearing mice. *SPIE Biomed. Optics* **2325**, 220–227.

Foote, C. (1976): Photosensitized oxidation and singlet oxygen: Consequences in biological systems. in: (W. A. Pryor ed.) Free radicals in biology. **2**, 85–133.

Gomer, C. (1991): Laser hyperthermia as an adjunctive treatment for ocular malignancies. *SPIE Conf. Proc. Med-Tech 1991*: Future trends in biomedical applications of Lasers IIIb-1.

Graschew, G. *et al.* (1990) Abstr. 3rd IPA Meeting. Buffalo NY USA.

Griffiths, J., Cruse-Sawyer, J., Wood, S. R., Schofield, J., Brown, S. B., and Dixon, B. (1994): On the photodynamic therapy action spectrum of zinc phthalocyanine tetrasulphonic acid *in vivo*. *J. Photochem. Photobiol.* **24**, 195–199.

Kriska, T., Mal'tseva, E., and Gál, D. (1996): Mechanism and kinetics of photodynamic effect. *SPIE Biomed. Optics* **2924**, -04- (unpublished).

Moser, J. G., Rueck, A., Westphal-Froesch, C., and Schwarzmayer, H. J. (1992): Photodynamic Cancer Therapy: Fluorescence localization and light absorption spectra of chlorophyll-derived photosensitizers inside cancer cells. *Optical Engineering* **31**, 1441–1446.

Oelckers, S., Hanke, T., Moser, J. G., and Roeder, B. (1994): Time resolved detection of singlet oxygen luminiscence in red cell ghosts generated by photosensitizers via excitation in the far red. *SPIE Biomed. Optics* **2325**, 116–120.

Pottier, R. and Kennedy, J. (1990): The possible rôle of ionic species in selective biodistribution of photochemotherapeutic agents toward neoplastic tissue. *J. Photochem. Photobiol.* **8**, 1–16.

Star, W. (1995): *In vivo* action spectra, absorption and fluorescence excitation spectra of photosensitizers for photodynamic therapy. *J. Photochem. Photobiol.* **28**, 101–102.

Weishaupt, K. R., Gomer, C. J., and Dougherty, T. J. (1976): Identification of singlet oxygen as the cytotoxic agent in photo-inactivation of a murine tumor. *Cancer Res.* **36**, 2326–2329.

Wilson, D. F. and Cerniglia, G. J. (1994): Oxygenation of tumors as evaluated by phosphorescence imaging. *Adv. Exp. Med. Biol.* **345**, 539–547.

Woehrle, D., Schlettwein, D., Schnurpfeil, G., Schneider, G., Karmann, E., Yoshida, T., and Kaneko, M. (1995): Phthalocyanines and related macrocycles for multi-electron transfer in catalysis. *Polymer Adv. Technol.* **6**, 118–130.

1.2. PHOTOBIOPHYSICAL PARAMETERS

BEATE ROEDER

For a successful photodynamic therapy, it is important to know the photophysical properties of the photosensitizer molecules. The investigation of these properties has to be carried out at different levels. The first step of characterization is related to the photophysical properties of monomeric dye molecules. Afterwards we have to investigate the hydrophobic properties. That means that one has to study the behaviour of the dyes in water containing environments. These investigations are followed by studies on the sensitizer behaviour in microheterogeneous environment. The aim of these investigations is to clarify whether the dyes deaggregate in such environments or not. On this level we can also answer the question if the dye may generate the phototoxic molecular singlet oxygen in such environments or not. The systems studied under such aspects may be membrane modelling systems (e.g. micelles, liposomes or erythrocyte ghosts) or carrier systems (e.g. cyclodextrins, liposomes, and antibodies). In the next paragraphs we will discuss these questions in greater detail.

1.2.1. PHOTOPHYSICAL CHARACTERIZATION OF SENSITIZER MOLECULES

The pathways of energy dissipation after light absorption of a molecule may be described with the help of the Jablonski-diagram (Fig. 1). Absorbing a light quantum, the molecule is excited to the first or higher excited singlet states. From higher excited singlet states it dissipates very fast (~ps) to the first excited singlet state, which has a lifetime in the range of some ns. The deactivation to the ground singlet state is usually realized by fluorescence or nonradiative deactivation processes. The so-called intersystem crossing (ISC) to the first excited triplet state is forbidden by all known selection rules (Birks, 1973). Only for macrocyclic molecules these rules cannot be exactly applied because of the spin–orbit coupling (Birks, 1973). This is the reason for very high ISC-rates in such molecules, resulting in the population of the long living (from μs to ms) first excited triplet state. This state can be the starting point for different photochemical reactions.

About photosensitization we always discuss two main pathways (Foote, 1968): the radical – or Type-I mechanism and the energy transfer – or Type-II mechanism of sensitizer deactivation.

Type-I mechanism:

$$^3SENS + O_2 \longrightarrow {}^1SENS_{ox} + O_2^-$$

$$^3SENS + SH \xrightarrow{\text{H-transfer}} {}^1SENSH^0 + S^0$$

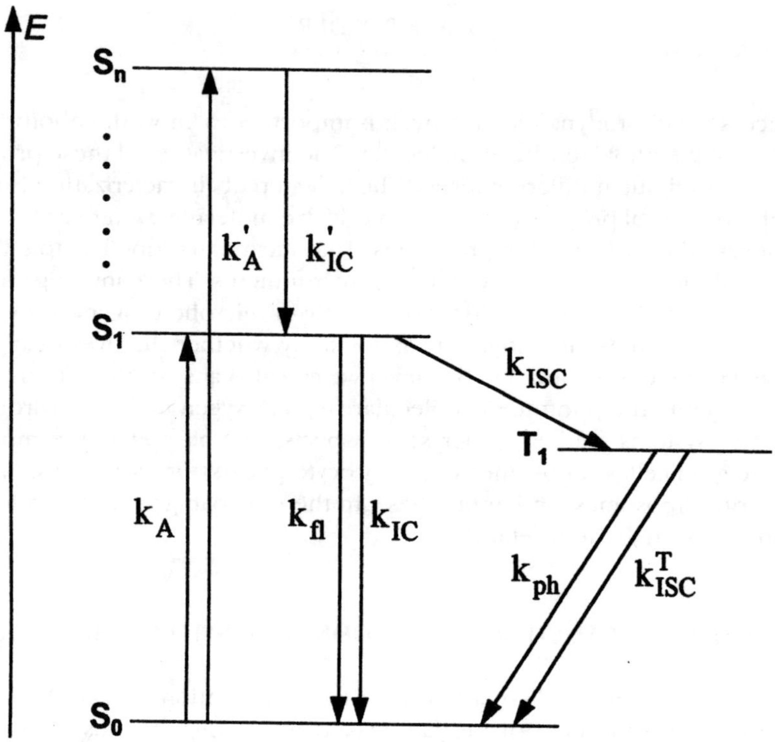

Figure 1 Jablonski-diagram.

$$^3\text{SENS} + \text{S} \xrightarrow{\text{e-transfer}} {}^1\text{SENS}^- + \text{S}^+$$

or

$$^3\text{SENS} + \text{S} \xrightarrow{\text{e-transfer}} {}^1\text{SENS}^+ + \text{S}^-$$

Type-II mechanism:

$$^3\text{SENS} + \text{O}_2 \longrightarrow {}^1\text{SENS} + {}^1\text{O}_2$$

where ^{3}SENS and ^{1}SENS represent the sensitizer molecule in its first excited triplet or singlet state, respectively; S, the substrate molecule; and $^1O_2$, the singlet molecular oxygen.

Both processes are running in competition. Their relative efficiency depends strongly on the surroundings and the nature of the substrate molecules.

In the presence of molecular oxygen, preferably Type-II deactivation of macrocyclic molecules occurs. As it is known, molecular oxygen is an exceptional molecule, which has triplet character in its ground state. Therefore, the energy transfer between excited triplet sensitizer and molecular oxygen may occur without any restrictions. Since the activation energy of singlet molecular oxygen is 0.96 eV, the only condition for such energy transfer is that the energy of the sensitizer's triplet state is in this range. That means that the $S_0 \rightarrow S_1$ absorption transition of the sensitizer must be at wavelengths of no longer than 850 nm.

A full photophysical characterization of dye molecules includes the measurement of the steady-state absorption, fluorescence, and phosphorescence spectra, the determination of the fluorescence lifetime and fluorescence quantum yield, the ISC quantum yield and last but not least the singlet oxygen quantum yield.

The determination of these parameters is possible using different optical-spectroscopic methods. (For more detail, see Lakowicz, 1986 and Bensasson *et al.*, 1993.) The definitions of the different parameters are illustrated in the simplified (without vibrational levels) Jablonski-diagram (see Fig. 1). Then we can write for the fluorescence lifetime (τ_{fl}):

$$\tau_{fl} = \Phi_{fl} \times \tau_0 = \tau_0 \times \left[k_{fl}/\left(k_{fl} + \sum k_{nr}\right)\right],$$

with Φ_{fl} being the fluorescence quantum yield; τ_0, the natural fluorescence lifetime; k_{fl}, the fluorescence rate constant; and $\sum k_{nr}$, the sum of the rate constants of all nonradiative deactivation processes.

The fluorescence lifetime (monoexponential case) can be calculated from the measured time-dependent fluorescence intensity:

$$I(t) = I_0 \times \exp\left[-t/\tau\right].$$

The phosphorescence lifetime can be calculated from the measured time-dependent phosphorescence on the base of a similar algorithm. The ISC-rate constant can be determined from transient absorption measurements.

The most interesting parameter – the singlet oxygen quantum yield (Φ_Δ), can be determined by using different methods. Direct observation of the singlet oxygen luminescence at 1269 nm is the method of choice because no side-effects occur, whereas in photochemical methods the reaction of other activated oxygen species with the monitor molecules may be obtained. For the calculation of this parameter the following equation is used (see Fig. 1):

$$\Phi_\Delta = \Phi_T \times S_\Delta,$$

with

$$\Phi_T = \frac{k_{ISC}}{k_{IC} + k_r + k_{ISC}},$$

$$S_\Delta = \frac{k_{ET} \times [O_2]}{k_{ph} + k_{ISC}^{T} + \{(k_{ET} + k_{pr}) \times [O_2]\}}.$$

In Fig. 2 and Table 1 photophysical parameters for pheophorbide-a monomers (in ethanol) and aggregated pheophorbide-a (in PBS) are summarized. It can be clearly seen that the degree of change in parameters depends on the aggregation state of the dye (Röder, 1986a; Röder *et al.*, 1986b; Marlow, 1986; Röder, 1987). On the one hand, pheophorbide-a obtains very good photophysical parameters in organic solvent, esp. the singlet oxygen quantum yield is about 0.6 (Krasnovsky *et al.*, 1990), but in aqueous environment the energy transfer to molecular oxygen is nearly zero. The question one has to answer now is in what state the sensitizer preferably exists in living cells.

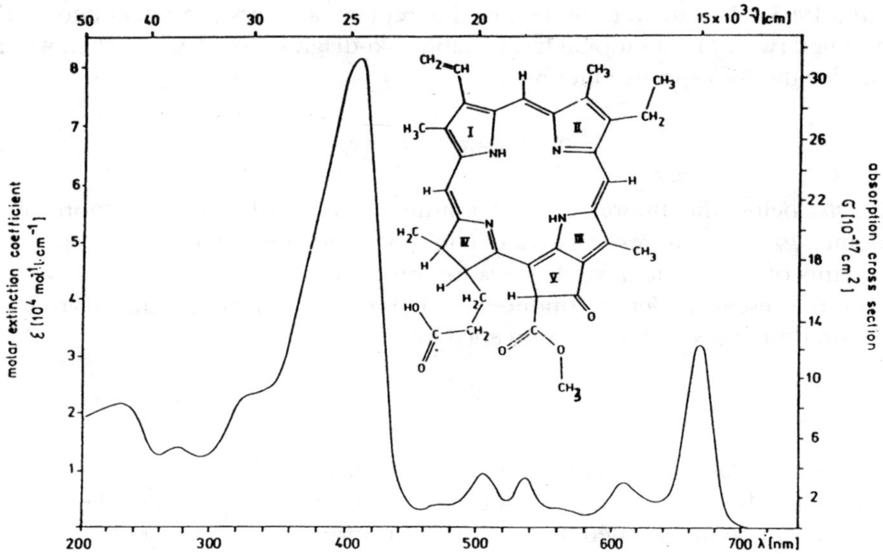

Figure 2 Absorption spectrum of pheophorbide-a in ethanol (inset: structural formula).

Table 1 Photophysical parameters of pheophorbide-a in ethanol and phosphate buffered saline

Photophysical parameter	*Pheophorbide-a*	
	in ethanol	*in PBS*
$\varepsilon_{667\,nm}$ [l/mol × cm]	44,900	not defined
Φ_{fl}	0.3	0.02
τ_{fl} [ns ± 0.1]	5.9	3.7 and 0.9
Φ_{ISC}	~ 0.7	not defined
Φ_{Δ}	0.6	< 0.02*

* In D_2O + 5% ethanol.

1.2.2. INFLUENCE OF MICROHETEROGENEOUS ENVIRONMENT ON THE DEACTIVATION OF EXCITED SENSITIZER MOLECULES

This problem can be studied partly by using membrane-like model systems, such as micelles, liposomes or erythrocyte ghosts. In this chapter we will discuss some possible investigations in micellar systems and erythrocyte ghost suspensions. We will not mention here the liposomal problematic, because liposomes are also possible carrier systems. So it will be discussed in the next paragraph.

Micellar Systems

Micelles are relatively simple models for the simulation of membrane-like structures according to the partition of the solution into hydrophobic and hydrophilic compartments (Tanford, 1982). In such systems the hydrophobicity of potential sensitizer molecules can be studied. Especially the monomerization of hydrophobic dyes can be easily observed by both steady-state absorption and fluorescence spectroscopy and the time-resolved fluorescence measurement.

Besides the above-mentioned parameters, the rotational correlation time (Φ_{rot}) becomes very important. This parameter describes the freedom of molecular movement. It strongly depends on the viscosity of the molecular microenvironment. It also gives us some information about the binding efficiency of the dye to other molecules or assemblies (e.g. liposomes, micelles, cyclodextrins, antibodies). This parameter can be calculated by measuring the time-dependent fluorescence anisotropy of the dye:

$$r(t) = r_0 \times \exp(-t/\Phi_{rot}) + r_\infty,$$

with r_0 being the anisotropy at the time $t = 0$; r_∞, the anisotropy at infinite time; and Φ_{rot} can be calculated from the time-resolved fluorescence measurements as:

$$\Phi_{rot} = \tau_{diff} \times \tau_{total}/(\tau_{total} - \tau_{diff}),$$

τ_{total}, total fluorescence decay time; and τ_{diff}, the difference between the fluorescence decay of the parallel and perpendicular components (concerning the polarization of the exciting laser light).

The value of the residue r_∞ is a direct proof for the amount of rotation hindrance of the dye molecule (Lakowicz, 1986).

Based on these measurements it is possible to calculate the microviscosity near the dye molecules. This parameter is helpful for the definition of the binding site of the sensitizer molecule to the model or carrier system. The calculation can easily be done, using the Einstein-equation:

$$\Phi_{rot} = \rho \times V/(R \times T),$$

where ρ is the viscosity of the microenvironment of the sensitizer in the volume V; T, the temperature; and R, the Boltzmann constant.

From these experiments we can get important information on:

1. the efficacy of monomerization (full or partial monomerization of hydrophobic sensitizers in microheterogeneous environments),
2. efficiency of the photosensitized generation of singlet molecular oxygen in membrane-like environments,
3. information about the incorporation of the sensitizer molecules into the microheterogeneous compartment.

For illustration the results of such investigations, carried out on 13^2-OH-bacteriopheophorbide-a-methylester in different micellar systems, are shown in Table 2. The results of steady-state absorption and fluorescence measurements, and the fluorescence decay times clearly show that the dye undergoes monomerization if detergents to the solution are added. Finding out the value of Φ_{rot}, the microviscosity near the dye molecule can be calculated. The calculated values shown in Table 2 are in good consistency with values figured out by other authors with different methods for unloaded micelles (Tanford, 1980).

Table 2 Fluorescence lifetime (τ_{fl}), rotational correlation time (Φ_{rot}) and calculated microviscosity (η_{exp}) of 13^2-OH-bacterio-pheophorbide-a-methylester in different micellar solutions (Gensch/Röder unpubl. results)

Detergent	λ_{max}^{Abs} [nm]	τ_{fl} [ns] [$\pm$0.01 ns]	Φ_{rot} [ns]	η_{exp} [cP]
Triton X-100	753	2.08	12.0 $\pm$ 1.6	66
Triton X-114	753	2.10	9.2 $\pm$ 1.2	50
Brij 35	752	2.06	5.1 $\pm$ 0.6	28
CTAB	752	1.78	4.8 $\pm$ 0.5	26
CTAC	752	1.98	4.0 $\pm$ 0.3	22
SDS	753	1.91	3.1 $\pm$ 0.2	17

Erythrocyte Ghost Suspensions

Today it is accepted that singlet molecular oxygen is very important in PDT. It is not yet clear if singlet molecular oxygen acts as the most effective phototoxic species, or if it only mediates the photosensitization via radical formation because of the interaction with molecular oxygen or water (Haseloff *et al.*, 1989).

The difficulty of direct singlet oxygen observation in *in vitro* or *in vivo* systems is found in its low excitation energy resulting in a luminescence maximum at 1269 nm. With the very low luminescence quantum yield and the efficient quenching processes in microheterogeneous environment, it will be very difficult to make such observations now and also in the future (Gorman *et al.*, 1992).

One step leading from "simple" lipid bilayer structures like liposomes to living cells may be the use of erythrocyte ghosts or intact erythrocytes. In the last two years a methodology for such investigations was developed in our group (Oelckers *et al.*, 1994). Systematic investigation on the influence of different parameters (e.g. irradiation dose; temperature; dye concentration; buffer composition) were done, using the method of direct time-resolved detection of singlet molecular oxygen luminescence (Oelckers *et al.*, 1997). In Fig. 3 the absorption spectra of pheophorbide in different environments are shown. These spectra clearly demonstrate the deaggregation of pheophorbide-a in the erythrocyte ghost suspensions similar to those observed in liposomal suspensions. The red-shift of the $S_0 \rightarrow S_1$ absorption band indicates the attachment to the ghost membranes suggesting the incorporation of the dye molecules in the ghost membranes. The time-resolved singlet oxygen luminescence measured in a pheophorbide-a containing ghost suspension (in D_2O) after 8 J irradiation of the whole sample at 674 nm is shown in Fig. 4. The decay time was calculated to be around 40 µs. That means the decay time is about 30% shorter than in pure sensitizer/D_2O-solution. It was suggested that this signal is caused by singlet oxygen located near the cell surface in the suspension, and that the decay time is shortened by quenching processes in the suspension (Oelckers, 1994, 1997). All these experimental findings together suggest that the pheophorbide-a is located in, or attached to the cells in a monomerized state, and that it generates singlet molecular oxygen under illumination.

These examples demonstrate that the photophysical characterization of potent hydrophobic photosensitizers in different model systems can be useful to get previous information about their probable behaviour in living cells.

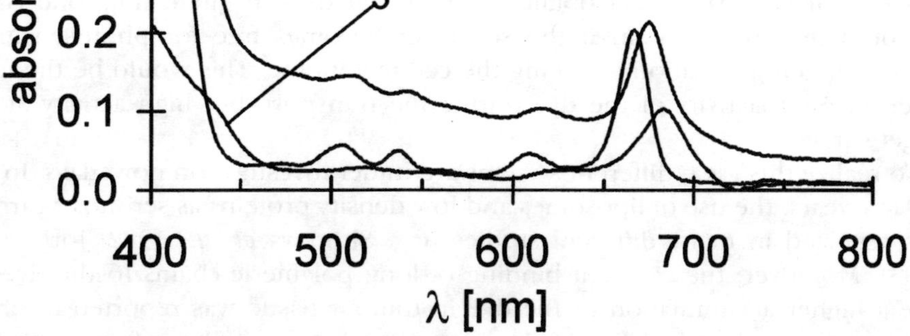

Figure 3 Absorption spectra of pheophorbide-a: (1) in erythrocyte ghost suspension; (2) in ethanol; (3) in PBS (phosphate buffered saline).

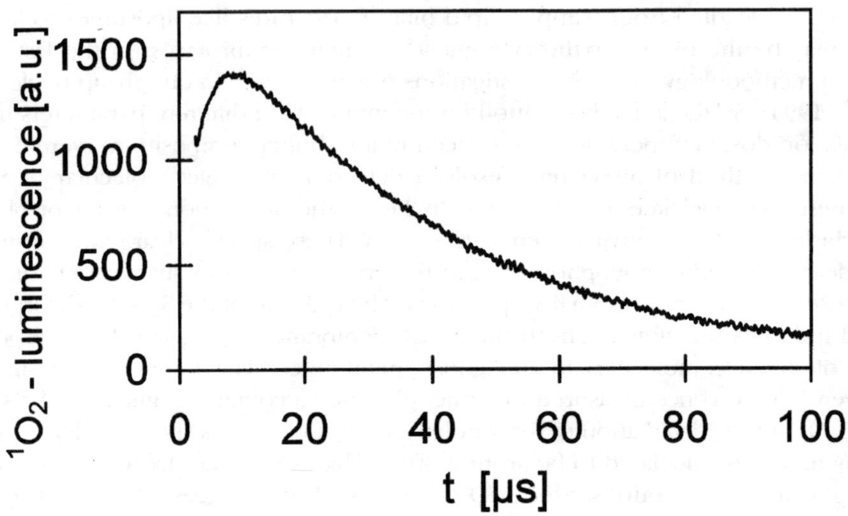

Figure 4 Time-resolved singlet oxygen luminescence photosensitized generated by pheophorbide-a in erythrocyte ghost suspension (irradiation at 674 nm with 8 J).

1.2.3. SENSITIZER-CARRIER COMPLEXES

The existing research indicates that no active accumulations of photosensitizers in tumour tissue occur. Therefore, one has to look for efficient carrier molecules or system, which might transfer the sensitizer to the target cells. The potential carriers must obtain some properties as, e.g. chemical inactivity, and they must be nonexcitable by the used therapeutic light. The most important point is that the singlet molecular oxygen generation must occur in a large amount. That means, the inclusion or binding of the dye to the carrier should not change the deactivation pathways of the sensitizer molecule. However, when one has a very efficient carrier system that obtains high singlet oxygen quenching, one could accept such carrier system if the sensitizer becomes free for photosensitized singlet oxygen generation attaching the cell membrane. This would be the ideal case: no photoactivity of the dye during the transport, but high activity at the target surface.

To realize this idea, different systems are under investigation nowadays. In the last few years, the use of liposomes and low density proteins as sensitizer carriers was reported in many different studies (e.g. Shopova *et al.*, 1992; Jori *et al.*, 1993). Moreover, the covalent binding of long polymeric chains to the dyes to give a higher accumulation of the dye in tumour tissue was reported (Wöhrle, 1992). The covalent binding of dyes to antibodies or antibody-fragments (e.g. Dressler *et al.*, 1992) is also under investigation. The encapsulation of dyes in micelle-like systems like, e.g. cremophors (Kessel, 1991), or the complexation with cyclodextrins (Kessel, 1991) were also proposed. Today the combination of different carrier systems is favoured. The accumulation of dye molecules in liposomes or their complexation with cyclodextrin followed by covalent binding to antibodies is a newer and more interesting concept (Moser *et al.*, 1994).

The introduction of a carrier may, of course, dramatically change the energy dissipation pathways of the dye molecules after light excitation. Therefore, a comparative study of different carrier systems with one photosensitizer can help to get an impression of these processes. Besides the above-discussed photophysical parameters, the rotational diffusion constant can become useful to estimate the sensitizer state in the carrier system. This parameter (D_R) can be calculated in the simplest way by:

$$D_R = (6\Phi_{rot})^{-1}.$$

In Table 3 the results of photophysical investigations on pheophorbide-a in different carrier systems are shown (Röder *et al.*, 1996). One can see that the value of the different photophysical parameters really changes over a wide range. In liposomes the singlet oxygen quantum yield strongly depends on the sensitizer concentration and the content of the liposomes (e.g. the type of fatty acids, the content of cholesterol). At high sensitizer concentrations probably self-quenching processes may occur, which in fact can cause a decreased singlet oxygen signal. In general we can extract the information that particularly this dye will transfer energy to molecular oxygen being located in liposomes or other membranes.

The explanation of the experimental results, obtained on the samples containing the antibody-bound pheophorbide-a, is more difficult. As seen in Table 3, the maximum of the lowest absorption transition is shifted to red wavelengths, suggesting an aggregation of the dye (see also in Table 3 absorption of pheophorbide-a in PBS). The addition of a micelle-forming detergent (here Triton X-100) results in a virtual deaggregation of the dye. Also, the fluorescence spectrum and lifetime suggest the existence of dye monomers. The problem now is how to find out the state of the dye in this system. In general three different cases are possible:

1. the dye molecules are not bound to the antibody and exist in its aggregated form in the surrounding solution;
2. the dye molecules are bound in part to the antibody and another part of free molecules are attached to these molecules;
3. the dye molecules are coupled to the antibody at defined positions very near one to each other, giving the impression of aggregation because of short-distance interactions between the molecules.

The use of the method of dynamic fluorescence anisotropy can help to answer this question. The freedom of mobility is reflected in the parameter of the rotational diffusion constant (see: Lakowicz, 1986).

As you can see in Table 3 this parameter is for pheophorbide-a bound to antibody one order of magnitude lower than in solution with only Triton X-100 or in liposomes and two orders of magnitude lower than in ethanol. These results

Table 3 Photophysical characterization of pheophorbide-a in different environments and carrier systems (CD: cyclodextrin; PAC: pheophorbide-a/antibody-conjugates)

Opt. paramet. *sample*	*Abs. max.* ($Q_{(0,0)}$–$Q_{(1,0)}$) [nm]	*Fluor. maxima* [nm]		*Fluorescence lifetime* τ_{fl} [ns] ±0.1		*Rotat. diff. constant* D[s^{-1}]	*Singl. oxygen quant. yield* Φ_Δ
Ethanol*	667	675	720	5.9		1.2×10^9	0.59
PBS*	683	667	710	3.7	0.9		not detect.
Liposomes							I_Δ/I_Δ (eth.)#
dye* : lipid							
1 : 50	669	680	725	6.2			not detect.
1 : 200	669	680	725	6.2		1.2×10^8	0.23
1 : 500	669	680	725	6.2			0.33
1 : 1.100	669	680	725	6.2			0.51
1 : 1.700	669	680	725	6.2			0.70
Pheo/CD complexes**				λ_{em} = 676 nm	λ_{em} = 726 nm		(Röder, 1994)
c_{CD} = 0.10 M	674	675	725	5.60	5.55		detectable
c_{CD} = 0.20 M	669	675	725	5.65	5.60		not detect.
PAC***							(Röder, 1995)
in PBS	681	675	725	n.d.			not detect.
in PBS + 1% Triton X-100	669	684	725	5.60		1.3×10^7	detectable
Pheo in PBS + Triton X-100 (1%)	669	691	728	5.90		2.8×10^8	detectable

* $c_{(Pheo)} = 1 \times 10^{-5}$ M.
** in PBS (pH = 7.4); $c_{(Pheo)} = 1.5 \times 10^{-5}$ M; T = 348 K.
*** PAC – Pheo-antibody-conjugates in PBS (pH = 7.4); $c_{(Pheo)} = 1.5 \times 10^{-5}$ M.
\# No quantum yield was determined. The ratio between the luminescence intensity of the system liposomes/dye and of the dye in ethanol is shown.

suggest that probably most of the pheophorbide-a are covalently bound to the antibody at positions, which are very near to each other on the antibody allowing short-distance interactions between the macrocyclic ring systems of the dye molecules.

As you can see different carrier systems may have a very strong influence on the photophysical properties of one dye. Depending on the hydrophobicity of the dye, the interaction between the dye and the carrier molecule/systems may also have different strength.

LITERATURE CITED

Bensasson, R. V., Land, E. J., and Truscott, T. G. (1993): Excited States and Free Radicals in Biology and Medicine. Oxford University Press.

Birks, J. B. (1973): Organic Molecular Photophysics, vol. 1. Wiley & Sons, London, New York.

Dressler, C., Möller, U., Lewald, T., Berlien, H. -P., and Röder, B. (1992): Introduction of a simple model for testing immunoconjugates with photosensitizers. In: Photodynamic Therapy and Biomedical Lasers, 164–168, eds.: Spinelli, P., Dal Fante, M., and Marchesini, R., Elsev. Sci. Publ.

Foote, C. S. (1968): Mechanisms of photosensitized oxidation. *Science* **162**, 963–970.

Gensch, Th., Röder, B., Pfeifer, L., and Moser, J. G.: unpubl. results, in prep. for publication in *Biomed. Optics*.

Gorman, A. A. and Rodgers, M. A. J. (1992): Current perspectives of singlet oxygen detection in biological environments. *J. Photochem. Photobiol. B* **14**, 159–176.

Haseloff, R., Ebert, B., and Röder, B. (1989): Generation of free radicals by photoactivation of pheophorbide a, HP and PP. *J. Photochem. Photobiol. B* **3**, 593–602.

Jori, G. and Reddi, E. (1993): The role of lipoproteins in the delivery of tumour-targeting photosensitizers. *Int. J. Biochem.* **25**, 1369–1375.

Kessel, D., Morgan, A., and Garbo, G. (1991): Sites and efficacy of photodamage by tin etiopurpurin in vitro using different delivery systems. *Photochem. Photobiol.* **54**, 193–196.

Krasnovsky, A. A. (jr.), Neverov, K. V., Egorov, S. Yu., Röder, B., and Lewald, T. (1990): *J. Photochem. Photobiol. B* **5**, 245–254.

Lakowicz, J. R. (1986): *Principles of Fluorescence Spectroscopy*. Plenum Press, New York.

Marlow, I., Marlow, F., and Röder, B. (1986): Bestimmung der Aggregationswärme von Pheophorbid a in wäßrigem Milieu. *Z. Chem.* **26**, 338–339.

Moser, J. G., Heuermann, A., Oehr, P., Scheer, H., Vervoorts, A., and Andrees, S. (1994): Carrier systems in PDT: On the way to novel anti-tumor drugs. *SPIE Conf. Proc.* vol. 2325, 92–99.

Oelckers, St., Hanke, Th., Moser, J. G., and Röder, B. (1994): Time-resolved detection of singlet oxygen luminescence in red cell ghosts generated by photosensitizers via excitation in the far red. *SPIE Conf. Proc.* vol. 2325, 339–348.

Oelckers, St., Sczepan, M., Hanke, Th., and Röder, B. (1997): Time-resolved detection of singlet oxygen luminescence in red ghost suspensions. *J. Photochem. Photobiol. B* **39**, 219–223.

Röder, B. (1986a): Pheophorbide a – a new photosensitizer for PDT. *Stud. Biophys.* **144**, 183–186.

Röder, B. and Kricheldorff, K. (1986b): Photodynamic action of pheophorbide a on Tryptophan and Human Serum Albumin. Comparison with HPD. *Stud. Biophys.* **144**, 171–182.

Röder, B. and Wabnitz, H. (1987): Investigation on hematoporphyrin, mesoporphyrin, pheophorbide a and chlorin e6 in ethanol and aqueous solution by time-resolved fluorescence spectroscopy. *J. Photochem. Photobiol. B* **1**, 103–113.

Röder, B., Hackbarth, St., Korth, O., Herter, R., Hanke, Th., and Höhne, W. (1996): Photophysical Properties of Pheophorbide a in Different Carrier-Systems. *SPIE Conf. Proc.* vol. 2625, 179–186.

Shopova, M., Mantareva, V., and Krastev, K. (1992): Comparative pharmacokinetic and photodynamic studies with zinc(II) phthalocyanine in hamster bearing induced or transplanted rhabdomyosarcoma.

Tanford, C. J. (1982): The Hydrophobic Effect. Wiley & Sons. New York.

Wöhrle, D., Ardeschirpur, A., Müller, S., Heuermann, A., Graschew, G., and Schlag, P. (1992): Various reactive Natural Porphyrin Based Sensitizers for Potential Application in PDT. In: Photodynamic Therapy and Biomedical Lasers, eds. P. Spinelli *et al.*, Els. Publ., Amsterdam 1992, 855–860.

1.3. BIOLOGICAL PARAMETERS OF PHOTOSENSITIZATION

JOERG G. MOSER

The uptake and consequent photosensitization of cells by a photosensitizer can be described in physical terms only to a certain degree. A description in terms of subcellular distribution has frequently been tried but touches only main storage compartments without any information upon the primary events of photosensitization. On the other hand the physical description of uptake and resulting phototoxicity is a necessary prerequisite to compare different sensitizers. This necessity has been urgently postulated by Moan *et al.* (1989) without any broader resonance. So up to now there is no or difficult comparability of the results obtained by different laboratories.

In our laboratory a distinct routine has been developed which, after 5 years of consequent application, shows now first comparable results with different sensitizers in *in vitro* experiments in cell cultures. A similar routine is demonstrated in a recent paper by Rosenbach-Belkin *et al.* (1995) dealing with organ distribution and photosensitivity of seryl-chlorophyllides and seryl-bacteriochlorophyllides in mice. We can hope only that a similar or modified scheme will finally be adopted to make results comparable between different laboratories.

1.3.1. SENSITIZER UPTAKE IN CELL SUSPENSIONS

Uptake of sensitizers in tumor cell suspensions has been standardized to a starting concentration of $c_o^0 = 10\,\mu\text{M}$. The sensitizer is pipetted into prewarmed culture medium as a stock solution in ethanol or 2-methoxy ethanol avoiding concentrations of the solvent of more than 2%. At these concentrations no dark toxicity of the solvents was observed. Water-soluble sensitizers can be added to the medium from PBS stock solutions. Incubation in PBS has to be avoided due to extensive cell damage just after 1 h of incubation. Exceptions need for special reference (Schuitmaker *et al.*, 1995).

Incubation time with sensitizers had been standardized to 1 h. Incubation temperature is always 37°C. Incubation media contain always 5–10% fetal calf serum according to culture conditions.

These conditions mimick the dosage of *in vivo* experiments of 5–10 mg/kg. Only the cell number applied (5–10 millions of cells per ml) is much lower as in native tumor tissue.

Samples of these cell suspensions (10–20 millions of cells in 2 ml) are taken in triplicate. To separate effectively the cells from the incubation medium the cell suspensions are layered cautiously onto a step gradient of Percoll® (20% saline isotonic Percoll® solution in culture medium; a brochure on this density gradient medium can be obtained from the producer, Pharmacia, Uppsala, Sweden). The tubes are centrifuged on a swing-out rotor at $800 \times g$ for 5 min. The supernatant is sucked off, and the sediments are frozen at $-20°C$. Extraction of most second generation photosensitizers can be performed with methanol–acetone 1 : 1 (2 ml) by sonicating the cell sediment for 10 s. Under these conditions proteins are precipitated and 98–100% of the sensitizer is recovered in the supernatants. This can easily be checked by reextraction of the sediments. In some cases of incomplete extraction we alternatively used 2% sodium dodecyl sulphate and sonicated the cell sediments in this medium for 20 s. Sonicated samples are centrifuged before measurements at $1000 \times g$ for 5 min. Sometimes the supernatants are somewhat turbid but can be recentrifuged at $2000 \times g$ to obtain fully clear supernatants. which can be read for absorbance in a spectrophotometer at the S_1 maximum. From this the internal concentration parameters are readily calculated.

In general terms, the most adequate expression of uptake is the number of sensitizer molecules inside the cell, n_i^t, at the end of the incubation period. This can be obtained from the moles taken up by a cell using Eq. (1) and (2):

$$m_i^t = \Delta E \cdot V_e / (\varepsilon \cdot 1000 \cdot N_{cells}) \quad [\text{moles/cell}], \tag{1}$$

$$n_i^t = m_i^t \cdot N_A, \tag{2}$$

where ΔE is the difference in absorption at the S_1 maximum with absorption coefficient ε, N_{cell} is the cell number extracted in volume V_e [ml], N_A is Avogadro's number.

Further more speculative data can be derived using m_i^t:

$$c_i^t(\text{av}) = m_i^t / V_{cell}, \tag{3}$$

$$c_o^t(\text{ind}) = c_o^0 - (m_i^t \cdot N_{inc} \cdot 1000), \tag{4}$$

where:

V_{cell} is the cell volume as defined,
N_{inc} is the number of cells per ml during sensitizer incorporation,
c_o^0 is the sensitizer concentration at the beginning of the experiment in the medium,

if c_o^t is not directly determined from the medium. Finally, the quotient

$$f_{i/0} = c_i^t / c_o^t \tag{5}$$

gives the accumulation factor under the relevant conditions of incubation.

Example: Given a sample of 20 millions of OAT SCLC cells, extracted in 2 ml methanol–acetone 1 : 1 for recovery of bacteriopheophorbide ethyl ester ($\varepsilon_{748\,nm}$ in this solvent: 38,200 l/mole · cm).

Measured:

$$\Delta E_{(748\text{–}840\ nm)}: 0.083 - 0.085 - 0.084,$$

$$\text{mean: } 0.084 \pm 0.001,$$

$$V_{cell} = 9.9 \times 10^{-13}\ \text{l/cell}; \qquad N_{inc} = 10^7\ \text{cells/ml}.$$

V_{cell} was determined by microscopic measurements of the diameters of freshly trypsinized cells assuming a globular shape.

Calculations:

according to (1): $m_i^t = 0.084 \cdot 2/38{,}200 \cdot 1000 \cdot 2 \cdot 10^7 = 2.2 \cdot 10^{-16}$ moles/cell,
according to (2): $n_i^t = 2.2 \cdot 10^{-16} \cdot 6.02 \cdot 10^{23} = 1.3 \cdot 10^8$ molecules per cell,
according to (3): $c_i^t(\text{av}) = 2.2 \cdot 10^{-16}/9.9 \cdot 10^{-13} = 2.2 \cdot 10^{-4}$ moles/l,
according to (4): $c_o^t = 10^{-5} - (2.2 \cdot 10^{-16} \cdot 10^7 \cdot 1000) = 7.8\,\mu$M/l,
according to (5): $f_{i/o} = 2.2 \cdot 10^{-4}/7.8 \cdot 10^{-6} = 28.5$.

These data are of practical value in order to compare uptake of sensitizers from culture media. Similar data can be obtained from weighed tissue samples or based on protein determination in the cell or tissue sediments. They have no significance for intracellular distribution of sensitizers which can differ widely just in the same class of sensitizers. Similar methods can be applied for sensitizer uptake kinetics and washout kinetics from cells or tissues. The calculations are in accord to similar data published e.g. by Kessel *et al.* (1995) and several other authors.

1.3.2. DESCRIPTIVE PARAMETERS OF PHOTOTOXICITY IN CELL SUSPENSIONS

Phototoxicity can be described by answering the question, what energy density E (J/cm^2) of a narrow light quality is necessary to reduce a given cell population, F_0, to a fraction F of surviving cells. Other definitions describe the amount of sensitizer (c_o^0 or c_i^t as described in the foregoing paragraph) necessary to reduce F_0 to F at constant light intensity. In our laboratory the former definition was adapted according to West and Moore (1988). Statistic 1 quantum/1 effect-theory predicts an exponential decay of F_0 as dependent on energy E:

$$F/F_0 = \mathrm{e}^{-kE} \tag{6}$$

or in logarithmic form:

$$0.4343 \cdot \ln F/F_0 = {}^{10}\log F/F_0 = -k'E, \tag{7}$$

where k' describes phototoxicity. The diagram of $\log F/F_0$ vs. E results in a straight line with intercept 0 and slope $-\tan\varphi = k'$. An expression familiar to pharmacologists and toxicologists is

$$\mathrm{LD}_{90} = -1/\tan\varphi \quad [\mathrm{J/cm^2}] \tag{8a}$$

or

$$\mathrm{LD}_{50} = -0.3/\tan\varphi \quad [\mathrm{J/cm^2}] \tag{8b}$$

to define the phototoxic effect denoting the energy necessary to kill 90% or 50% resp. of the initial cell population. In biological reality several deviations from this ideal behaviour are observed (Fig. 1).

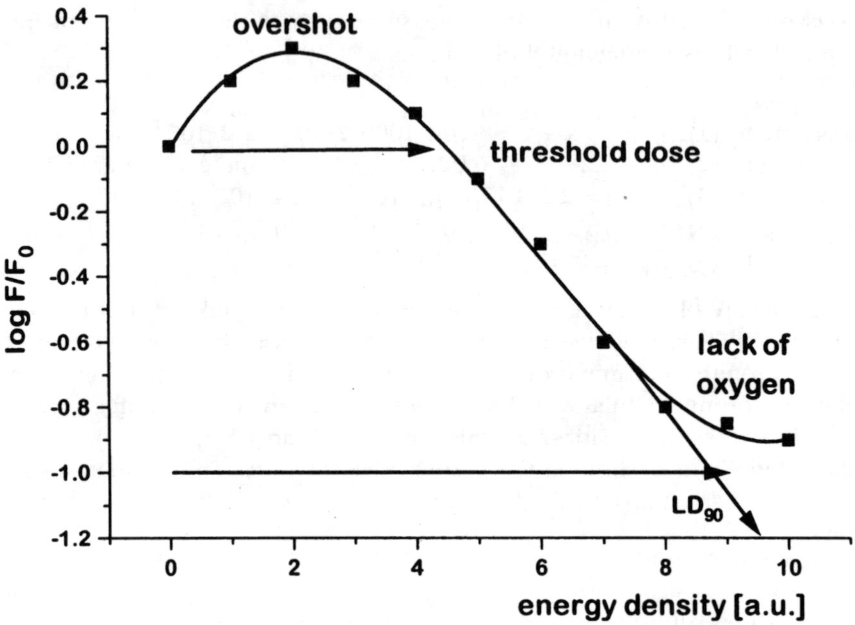

Figure 1 Effects obscuring the dose dependence of photodynamic cell death (from Moser *et al.*, 1994).

Most common deviations are: a minimum energy dose ("threshold dose") at which the photosensitizer begins to become phototoxic, often combined with an overshot signalizing cell proliferation at low *power density* (cf. Moser *et al.*, 1994; Danielowski and Moser, 1995); a flattening of the curve due to lack of oxygen; different steepness in different parts of the curve due to conditioning effects more or less evident at different cell densities; or a combination of these different effects.

To evaluate such complicated functions we correlate values in the steepest part of the function and extrapolate threshold dose and LD_{90} as given above. The definition of LD_{90} can be rewritten as

$$LD_{90} = \text{threshold dose} + (-1/\tan\varphi). \tag{9}$$

The error of LD_{90} can be derived from the 2σ error (=95% confidence interval) of the linear correlation function defining (Campbell, 1974)

$$s^2 = 1/(N-2)\left(\sum YY - \left(\sum XY\right)^2 / \sum XX\right) \tag{10}$$

and

$$2\sigma = \pm {}^{N-2}t_{0.5} \cdot \sqrt{\left(s^2/\sum XX\right)} \tag{11}$$

where ΣXX, ΣYY, and ΣXY are the sums of squared deviations of the individual values from centre coordinates $(\Sigma x_i/N; \Sigma y_i/N)$ and ${}^{N-2}t_{.05}$ the tabulated values of Student's t-function for $(N-2)$ degrees of freedom. As well the extrapolation to the line $\log F/F_0 = 0$ with the different values of the slope $(\pm 2\sigma)$ can be used to define the deviations and the significance of threshold dose.

Threshold doses are of great clinical importance for the application of photosensitizers (Svaasand *et al.*, 1990). Irradiation at power densities higher than threshold are time-additive and lead to tumor destruction. Power densities below threshold have no or adverse effects, i.e. stimulation of tumor growth including the induction of a metastatic potential (Danielowski and Moser, 1995), as demonstrated schematically in Fig. 1 and with a practical example (Fig. 2). So far, we always use power densities in the lowest possible range to describe phototoxicity and to detect thresholds (W/cm^2) and threshold doses (J/cm^2). These values are given in the individual tables and, in part, in Table 2.

How to determine F/F_0 values in practical terms? The most reliable method is FACS analysis of living and dead cells, preferably with the acridine orange/ethidium bromide assay as described by Parks *et al.* (1979). FACS devices are highly expensive, and the method is not applicable to cell clusters frequently obtained in cell suspensions. Optical counting is not applicable in most cases for lack of reliable statistics. Incorporation of radioisotopes (^{3}H-leucine, ^{3}H-thymidine) in chase experiments is as expensive as FACS analysis. Oncogenic cloning is a longterm analytical procedure, and its results often depend on intercellular interactions ("conditioning") as seen from the sometimes steeper slopes of the $\log F/F_0$ vs. E function and enhanced thresholds at low population densities in oncogenic cloning assays. With tumor cell suspensions we can use a metabolic parameter, lactic acid production (Warburg, 1923).

Lactic acid has a pK of 4.7 and is fully dissociated in the biological pH-range (pH 6.8–7.8). We could show that acid production of tumor cell suspensions (OAT 75 SCLC, LoVo) is strictly correlated with the lactic acid found in the culture medium (correlation coefficient $R > 0.95$; slope: 1.00 ± 0.04). Acid production leads to a colour change of the pH indicator dye (in most culture media: phenol red), and this color change is linear over a wide pH range (pH 6.8–7.8) due to the buffer capacity of the serum containing culture media. The decay of absorption at 546 nm (a mercury line isolated by interference filters in most clinical photometers) is linearly dependent on acid added to RPMI or DMEM media (correlation coefficient $R = 0.99\ldots$). In practice, irradiation of 1 million of tumor cells in 1 ml of serum containing medium gives a sample which can be diluted to 5 ml, incubated for 15 h, and centrifuged at $800 \times g$. The supernatant is read at 546 nm to yield the acid production of the surviving cells as compared with the following control values (Moan *et al.*, 1989):

K_A: Untreated cells (no sensitizer, no light),
K_B: Light treated cells (no sensitizer, maximum light dosis),
K_C: sensitizer-treated cells (sensitizer, no light),
K_D: PDT-dead cells (sensitizer + maximum dosis of light),

M: Medium without cells, of the same charge as used in the phototoxicity experiment,

M+: Medium as in *M*+ a defined amount of HCl, e.g. 0.1 ml 0.1 N HCl.

We use all samples as fourfold replicates to obtain reliable statistics. An example is given on the next pages (Table 1 and Fig. 2).

Table 1 Evaluation of an experiment using the lactic acid production assay

Experiment: A 375 (amelanotic human melanoma) cells were incubated with 2-dimethyl amido-3-heptyl chlorin e6 (Montforts *et al.*, 1994); 10 μM, 1 h, 37°C, and irradiated at 670 nm. Each sample containing 1 million of cells was filled up to 5 ml and incubated with slight movement for 12 h. Samples were centrifuged and the supernatants were measured at 546 nm.

Measured values:

Sample	$\Delta E_{546\,nm}$	*Average* [fEq/cell·h]	log F/F_0 [E (J/cm^2)]
M	1.325–1.305–1.295–1.304 (original medium)		
M+	0.697–0.690–0.690–0.691 (medium at 1.961 μEq HCl/ml)		
K_C	0.806–0.865–0.800–0.859	0.833 + 0.022/−0.028/ +0.027/−0.022	
[0]		±0.034	
		[754 ± 49 fEq/cell·h] = F_0	
1	0.857–0.847–0.850–0.845		−0.021/−0.012/ −0.014/−0.010 [0.043 J/cm^2]
2	0.970–0.961–0.955–0.959		−0.133/−0.123/ −0.116/−0.120 [0.086 J/cm^2]
3	1.033–1.019–1.023–1.028		−0.211/−0.192/ −0.197/−0.204 [0.130 J/cm^2]
4	1.078–1.065–1.063–1.103		−0.276/−0.256/ −0.253/−0.318 [0.173 J/cm^2]
K_D	1.335–1.372–1.344–1.358	1.353 ± 0.018	
		[1.85 J/cm^2] = 0 fEq/cell·h	(−∞)

Evaluation:

	R	tan φ	*Intercept*	*Threshold*	*N*

- Correlation calculated for the steepest part of the log F/F_0 vs. E function:

	R	tan φ	*Intercept*	*Threshold*	*N*
3⇒1	−0.992	−2.145.. ±0.195 (=2σ)	0.072	0.034 = 0.6 mW/cm^2; 1 min irradiat.	12
	LD_{90}	0.51 > 0.47 > 0.43 J/cm^2 (according to Eq. (8a))			
	$LD_{90\,(corr)}$	0.55 > 0.51 > 0.47 J/cm^2 (according to Eq. (9))			

- Correlation *M*/*M*+ vs. acid content of the medium:

	R	tan φ	*Intercept*
	−0.9997	−0.3137	1.30725

- Constant for calculation of metabolic activity: $k = -1.44984 \cdot 10^{12}$ Eq/cell to reach an absorption difference of 1.0 at the experimental conditions.

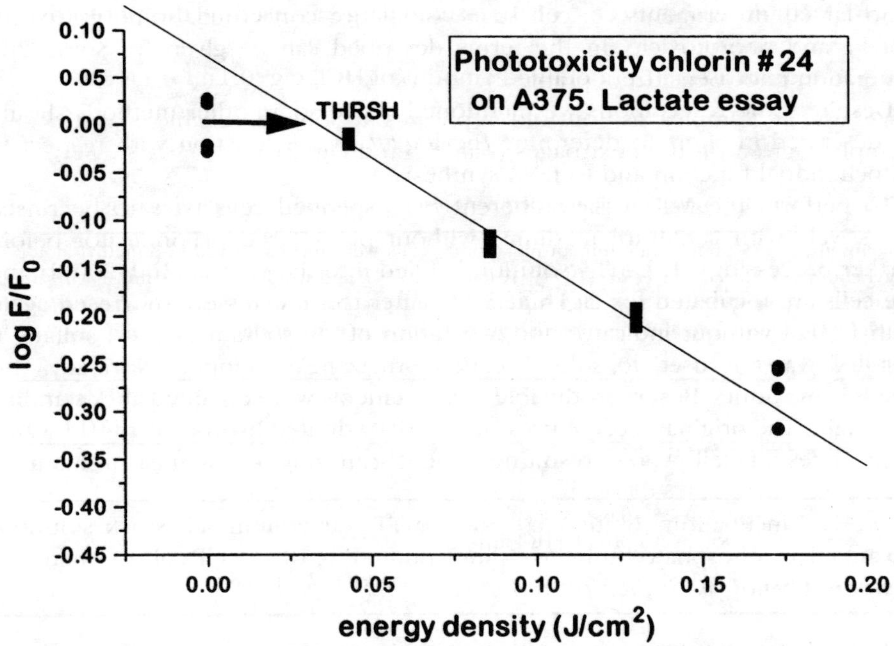

Figure 2 Graphics of the experiment described in Table 1.

For more automatized evaluation several groups use the MTT assay in diverse variants (e.g. Kessel *et al.*, 1995, and the literature cited therein). The MTT assay measures the activity of a mitochondrial enzyme, succinate dehydrogenase, by transformation of a tetrazolium salt to a formazane, which can be quantitated as a solution in diluted HCl or in 2% watery sodium dodecyl sulphate (SDS) with an ELISA reader. In our hands, this test shows sometimes much steeper slopes of the $\log F/F_0$ vs. E function as compared with the lactic acid production test described above. Microscopic controls with the acridine orange/ethidium bromide assay showed high amounts of surviving cells in tumor suspension cultures fully inactivated according to the MTT assay (e.g. with LoVo adenocarcinoma cells). This is due to the fact that mitochondrial energy metabolism can be fully substituted in cancer cells by energy production based on glycolysis. Total inactivation of photosensitized mitochondria is not the limiting factor leading to tumor cell death (Warburg, 1923). With non-malignant cells the use of the MTT assay may be justified (e.g. Placzek *et al.*, 1994).

The calculation of individual $\log F/F_0(i)$ values follows the formula:

$$\log F/F_0(i) = \log\{-k[\Delta E(i) - \Delta E(K_D)]/F_0\}. \qquad (12)$$

These values are correlated to the energy applied. Thresholds are expressed as power densities dividing energy values by 60 indicating the time of irradiation.

So far, as experiments on cell suspensions are concerned, some values for uptake and phototoxicity in the terms described can be given for some 2nd generation photosensitizers (Table 2).

Despite some reservations we mentioned above some other methods should be described in short to determine the $\log F/F_0$ vs. E function with respect to mitochondrial function and to DNA synthesis.

To perform the MTT essay adherent or suspended cells have to be rinsed excessively with a culture medium (without phenol red pH indicator before further processing). The MTT solution is filled into the vessels (100–200 µl) and the cells are incubated for 2–3 h at 37°C. After this the vessels are rinsed again with DMEM without indicator and a solution of 2% sodium dodecyl sulfate in distilled water is used to solubilize the formazane developed. Normally, this needs some hours. Best reproducible measurements were obtained after standing overnight. The original receipe uses sulphuric or diluted hydrochloric acid which precipitates the cell protein resulting in light scattering during measurements.

The MTT incubation solution contains: MTT tetrazolium salt stock solution (5 mg/ml in phosphate buffered saline) diluted 1 : 10 in cell culture medium *without phenol red indicator and only* 1% *calf serum*.

The absorption values can directly be transformed into a logarithmic scale and correlated to the irradiation energy density applied to the vessels. The high scattering of the values needs for 6–8 samples per energy density value.

Besides MTT assay incorporation of fluorescein diacetate into photosensitized tumor cells might be a further possibility to automatize the measurement of F/F_0 vs. E functions for photosensitizer characterization. The fluorescence of the non-esterified dye can be measured by fluorescence ELISA readers. This method is under investigation.

A functional test on DNA synthesis is the *^{3}H-thymidine incorporation* method. The method needs cells during the logarithmic growth phase. We explant in 24-well plates 10^5 cells per well and let them attach and grow overnight. The cells are washed thoroughly before beginning the experiment to remove all free unattached cells and cell debris. The experiment is performed as follows:

To each well of the plate are added exactly 0.5 ml of medium. A stock solution of radioactive thymidine is prepared containing 20 µl of a 1 mCi/ml preparation of (^{3}H-methyl-)thymidine in 2 ml of culture medium. From this stock 50 µl are added per well ($\sim$0.9 Mcpm/sample). After 2 h the wells are rinsed twice with icecold medium, fixed with 2% trichloroacetic acid for 30 min, and rinsed twice with 96% ethanol. 300 µl of 1 N NaOH are added to dissolve the cells. An aliquot of 100 µl is counted by liquid scintillation counting in 5 ml of an adequate water-miscible scintillation cocktail.

Countings with adequate controls can be directly transformed into a log scale and correlated with the energy density applied. As dependent on the sensitizer

Table 2 Uptake and Phototoxicity of Selected 2nd Generation Photosensitizers

Sensitizer	*Cell type*	$n_i^t \times 10^8$ [/cell]	$-k'$ [cm²/J]	LD_{90} [J/cm²]
• Chlorophyll derivatives [1]				
Pheophorbide-a	LoVo, OAT	2	✱ 1–2	0.5–1
13²-Hydroxy pheophorbide-a	LoVo, OAT	5	✱ 1–2	0.5–1
• Bacteriochlorophyll derivatives [2]				
Bacteriopheophorbide ethyl ester	OAT, A375	4–5	✱ 0.24–1.10	0.8–2.6
Bacteriopheophorbide methyl ester	OAT, A375	5–6	✱ 0.16–0.66	1.5–6
Bacteriopheophorbide n-propyl ester	OAT	5	✱ 1	1
Bacteriopheophorbide 2-propyl ester	OAT	1.4	✱ 1	1
Pd-Bacteriopheophorbide ethyl ester	OAT, SkMel	1.6	✱ 1.3–2	0.5–0.8
Bacteriochlorophyllide β-serin ester	OAT, A375	0.5	⊗ 1–2	0.5–1
• Phthalocyanines and Naphthopyrazines [3]				
$Sulfo_{3,4}$ Phthalocyanines	A375	?	✱ (ns)	—
Octahexyloxy phthalocyanine	OAT	<0.1	⊗ (ns)	—
Tetramethoxypyridyloxy phthalocyanine	OAT	<0.1	⊗ (ns)	—
Tri (tert. butylphenoxy) sulfo phthalocyanine	A375	0.2	⊗ 0.03	38
Tri (tert. butylphenoxy) carboxy phthalocyanine	A375	?	⊗ 0.64	1.7
Tri (tert. butylphenoxy) propyl phthalocyanine	A375	?	⊗ 0.06	16
Naphthopyrazine	OAT	<0.1	⊗ (ns)	—
• 3¹-N-diethyl heptyl chlorins [4]				
Chlorin # 18	A375	2–5	⊗ 1.5–2	0.5–0.7
Chlorin # 24	LoVo, OAT, A375	0.02–0.05	✱ ⊗ 2–5	0.2–0.5

✱ laser irradiation; ⊗ halogen lamp + cutoff filter; (ns) not significantly different from 0.
[1] Moser *et al.* (1990); [2] Moser *et al.* (1993); [3] Kliesch *et al.* (this book); [4] Moser *et al.* (1996).

applied sometimes the correlation function gives higher values for k' as found with the lactic acid assay which means that the cells cannot further divide but are metabolically active.

1.3.3: COMMENTS ON *IN VIVO* DATA ON UPTAKE AND PHOTOTOXICITY OF 2nd AND 3rd GENERATION PHOTOSENSITIZERS

Uptake of photosensitizers in intact animals depends on transport mechanisms (Pottier and Kennedy, 1989; Jori and Reddi, 1993; Korbelik and Krosl, 1994) and nonspecific uptake mechanisms involved. A description can follow extraction or fluorescence methods described above or within the following chapters of this book.

Data on phototoxicity suffer from disagreement of most laboratories upon a physical system for its description. The histological measurement of the depth of tissue necrosis is one common means to describe photodynamic effects. In combination with light measurements this method may allow for comparison to results obtained with cell cultures (Svaasand *et al.*, 1990). So far as quantitative data of *in vivo* experiments are available, these will be commented in the individual chapters on sensitizers.

LITERATURE CITED

Campbell, R. C. (1974): Statistics for Biologists. 2nd ed. New York: Cambridge University Press.

Danielowski, T. and Moser, J. G. (1995): Indicators of metastatic potential induced by low power irradiation at photosensitizer threshold dose in mouse melanoma M2R. *SPIE Biomed. Optics* **2625**, 434–439.

Jori, G. and Reddi, E. (1993): The role of lipoproteins in the delivery of tumour-targeting photosensitizers. *Int. J. Biochem.* **25**, 1369–1375.

Junker, R. (1993): Phototoxizitaet von Phaeophorbid-a-Derivaten an Adenocarcinomzellen. MD thesis. University of Duesseldorf.

Kessel, D., Woodburn, K., Gomer, C. J., Jagerovic, N., and Smith, K. M. (1995): Photosensitation with derivatives of chlorin p_6. *J. Photochem. Photobiol.* **28**, 13–18.

Korbelik, M. and Krosl, G. (1994): Tumor associated macrophages (not tumor cells) are the determinants of photosensitizer tumor localization. *SPIE Biomed. Optics* **2371**, 344–346.

Moan, J., Peng, Q., Evensen, J. F., Berg, K., Western, A., and Rimington, C. (1989): Photosensitizing efficiencies, tumor- and cellular uptake of different photosensitizing drugs relevant for photodynamic therapy of cancer. *Photochem. Photobiol.* **46**, 713–721.

Moser, J. G., Ostrowski, A., Gümüsdagli, M., and Kleiber, B. (1993): Bacteriopheophorbide esters: photosensitizers without "threshold dose"? *SPIE Biomed. Optics* **2078**, 193–204.

Moser, J. G., Suchomski, R., Danielowski, T., and Wagner, B. (1994): Significance of threshold doses for photodynamic therapy of melanotic and amelanotic tumors. *SPIE Biomed. Optics* **2371**, 178–186.

Moser, J. G., Montforts, F. P., Kusch, D., Akgün, N., Rueck, A., Andrees, S., and Wagner, B. (1996): How many molecules of a photosensitizer are necessary to photosensitize a tumor cell? *SPIE Biomed. Optics* **2924**, 1–9.

Montforts, F. P., Gerlach, B., Haake, G., Hoeper, F., Kusch, D., Meier, A., Scheurich, G., Brauer, H. D., Schiwon, K., and Schermann, G. (1994): Selective synthesis and photophysical properties of tailor-made chlorins for phòtodynamic therapy. *SPIE Biomed. Optics* **2325**, 29–39.

Parks, D. R., Bryan, V. M., Oi, V. M., Oi, V. T., and Herzenberg, L. A. (1979): Antigen specific identification and cloning of hybridomas with a Fluorescence Activated Cell Sorter. *Proc. Nat. Acad. Sci. USA* **76**, 1962.

Placzek, R., Kempka, G., Ruether, W., and Moser, J. G. (1994): Usefulness of threshold dose to prevent damage of underlying tissue by PDT treatment: an *in vitro* study on chondrocytes. *SPIE Biomed. Optics* **2371**, 526–527.

Pottier, R. and Kennedy, J. C. (1990): The possible role of ionic species in selective biodistribution of photochemotherapeutic agents toward neoplastic tissue. *J. Photochem. Photobiol.* **8**, 1–16.

Rosenbach-Belkin, V., Fiedor, L., Pavlotsky, F., Salomon, Y., and Scherz, A. (1995): Chlorophyll and bacteriochlorophyll derivatives, potentially new photodynamic agents. 1. Tissue distribution in mice bearing melanoma tumors. *Photochem. Photobiol.* **64**, 174–181.

Schuitmaker, J. J., Jannink, J. E., and Dubbelman, T. M. A. R. (1995): Influence of cell culture medium on the photosensitizing effectiveness of bacteriochlorin a. *J. Photochem. Photobiol.* **28**, 143–148.

Svaasand, L. O., Gomer, C. J., and Morinelli, E. (1990): On the physical rationale of photodynamic therapy. In: Future directions and applications of photodynamic therapy (C. J. Gomer ed.). Bellingham WA: SPIE Opt. Eng. Press.

Warburg, O. (1923): Versuche an ueberlebendem Carcinomgewebe. *Biochem. Z.* **142**, 317–333.

West, C. L. M. and Moore, J. V. (1988): Cell survival characteristics of a human adenocarcinoma cell line after photodynamic treatment: a comparison of Photophrin II and TPPS. *Int. J. Radiation Biol.* **54**, 621–634.

2. INDIVIDUAL DATA

2.1. PHEOPHORBIDES

BEATE ROEDER

Pheophorbides are derived from chlorophyll. The absorption spectra of these compounds show an absorption peak at wavelengths near 650–680 nm with a molar absorption coefficient of about 45,000 l/mol cm. The principal structure of pheophorbides is shown in Fig. 1. Beside the strong absorption in the far red region of the spectrum, they obtain triplet quantum yields around 0.7 and singlet oxygen quantum yields of about 0.6. With a relative high photostability and their natural origin, which guarantees their low or non existing cytotoxicity, phorbides are very interesting sensitizers for PDT (Röder, 1990a).

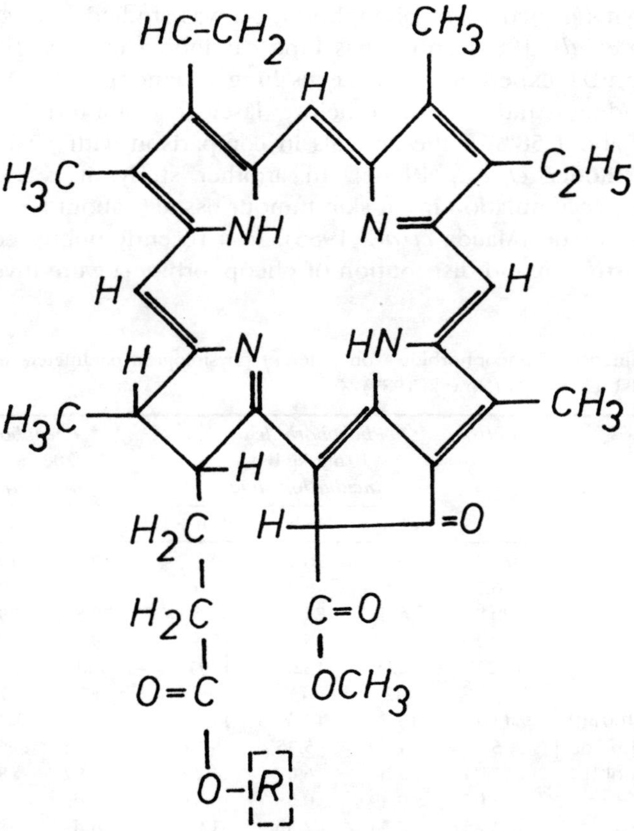

Figure 1 Structural formula of pheophorbides.

2.1.1. PHEOPHORBIDE-a

More than 10 years ago, systematic studies on the photodynamic behaviour of pheophorbide-a began (see review: Röder, 1990b). For this natural occurring dye, no LD50 dose in mice could be determined even if the drug up to 200 mg/(kg body weight) was given. The investigation (Nowak, 1989) of different biochemical parameters also showed no significant changes (Table 1). The observed oscillations of some parameters over time can be interpreted as physiologically caused changes.

It was shown that pheophorbide-a sensitizes cancer cells *in vitro* about 20 times more effectively than HpD (Segelman *et al.*, 1987). In this context, it is interesting to notice, that pheophorbide-b was shown to be much less photoactive than pheophorbide-a (Tapper, 1975). Also the photodynamic activity of a pyropheophorbide dimer (two molecules pyropheophorbide cross-linked with arginine) *in vitro* was studied and shown to be lower than that of the pheophorbide-a (Iwai, 1988).

The photodynamic activity of pheophorbide-a was studied *in vivo* on Ehrlich ascites (Röder *et al.*, 1984) and Lewis lung carcinoma in mice (Röder *et al.*, 1990c). In the PDT experiments on Lewis lung carcinoma (Fig. 2), mice with intratumoral administration 30 min before laser irradiation (670 nm) had a cure figure of about 58% of the animals in comparison with 30% of the HpD treated mice (Röder *et al.*, 1990c). In another study, it was shown that pheophorbide-a accumulation in rat skin tumour tissue is about ten times higher than in normal tissue (Maeda *et al.*, 1985). In a recently published article the *in vivo* administration and distribution of pheophorbide-a were investigated for

Table 1 The influence of pheophorbide-a on different physiological parameters in mice [female BDF_1 mice (C57 B1/6xDBA/2)] (Nowak, 1989)

Parameter	*Control*	*Pheophorbide-a*[1] 10 mg/kg b.w. *incubation time*			*Pheophorbide-a* 200 mg/kg b.w. *incubation time*		
		24 h	48 h	96 h	24 h	48 h	96 h
Body weight [g]	21.3	19.4	20.1	19.2	19.6	19.2	19.9
Leucocytes [G/l]	6.7	7.6	6.2	7.0	6.8	7.9	7.8
Lymphocytes [%]	90.8	n.d.	84.6	84.6	79.8	79.8	84.3
Granulocytes [%]	9.2	n.d.	15.4	15.4	19.6	19.6	15.8
Thrombocytes [G/l]	1267	1223	1328	1294	930	1912	1315
Heamatokrit	47	42	43	45	47	53	47
Heamoglobin [g/100 ml]	13.4	10.7	12.8	11.9	13.4	13.4	12.6
Glucose (blood) [mmol/l]	5.9	4.29	5.75	5.77	4.72	6.22	7.85
Urea (blood) [mmol/l]	7.74	n.d.	6.07	4.29	7.92	8.29	8.53
ALAT[2] [μkat/l]	1.07	0.49	0.58	0.51	n.d.	1.01	1.0
ASAT[3] [μkat/l]	3.25	2.34	2.56	1.97	n.d.	2.13	2.87

[1] The pheophorbide-a was suspended in 10% propylenglykol solution and i.p. administered. Every experimental group and the control group contained 6 animals.

[2] ALAT... alanine aminotransferase.

[3] ASAT... aspartate aminotransferase.

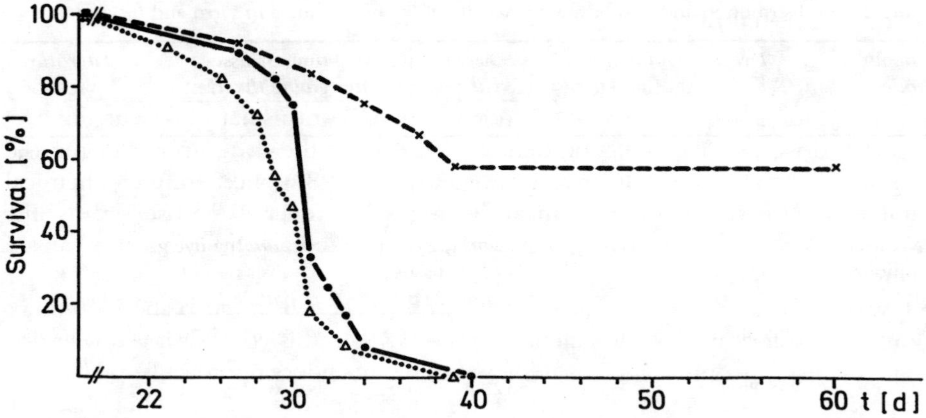

Figure 2 Survival of Lewis lung carcinoma mice (10 mg/kg b.w. pheophorbide-a on day 4 and 6; 30 min before laser irradiation). •—• Pheo-a, $n = 12$, MST = 31.7 days; × --- × Pheo-a + irradiation, $n = 12$, MST = 47.5 days; Δ····Δ saline control, $n = 12$, MST = 29.7 ± 4.4 days.

an acinar pancreatic tumour in Lewis rats (Aprahamian *et al*., 1993). The authors found that the reticulo-endothelial system is the major target for pheophorbide-a, followed by the gut and then the lung and pancreas. They reported a ratio of tumoral to peri-tumoral pancreas pheophorbide-a accumulation of 6.7 : 1, 24 h after i.v. administration of the sensitizer. In context with other authors (Röder *et al*., 1984) they also found only very low pheophorbide-a concentration in skin.

Nishiwaki *et al*. (1989) reported about the possible treatment of liver tumour by PDT usually with pheophorbide-a as the photoactive substance. The pheophorbide-a was dissolved in an oily contrast medium (Lipiodol). Its distribution in rabbits, having the experimental VX-2 liver tumour, was compared after intraarterial and intravenous administration. The authors found that after 24 h incubation time the tumour tissue showed higher values of pheophorbide-a than the liver did. Using a water-soluble pheophorbide-a derivative, they got the reversed picture. In Table 2 the published results of the studies on the biodistribution and photodynamic activity of pheophorbide-a are summarized.

In a preliminary study on seven patients with a chronic-stationary Psoriasis the photodynamic efficacy of pheophorbide-a (Fig. 3) in human was shown (Röder *et al*., 1984). The photosensitizer was topically administered 30 min before illumination in a Biowaschöl®-suspension containing 3.2×10^{-5} M pheophorbide-a and 5% (w/v) salicylic acid. Beside the very good regression of the psoriatic lesions, it was found that the photosensitive side effects were negligible because of the fast retention of the dye. As it is shown in Fig. 3, a normal lamp (Röder *et al*., 1984) can be used for the photodynamic therapy of Psoriasis using pheophorbide-a as the sensitizer.

Table 2 Biodistribution and Photodynamic Activity of Pheophorbide-a *In Vitro* and *In Vivo*

Tumour model	*Dye*	*Adm. dose* [mg/kg]	*Accum.* [μg dye/g tumour tissue] *at time* [h] *after giving the dye* 1 h	24 h	*Literature*
Panc 02 tumour	Pheo a	10	6.3 ± 0.7	n.d.	Kessel, 1989
	Pheo b	10	5.7 ± 0.6	n.d.	
	PT	10	7.2 ± 0.9	4.5 ± 0.3	
VX-2 liver tumour			*Accum.* [μg dye/g tumour tissue] *after* 24 h	*Accum* [μg dye/g liver tissue] *after* 24 h	
•	LPD-Pheo a i.a.	1	84.93 ± 14.09	4.61 ± 0.70	Nishiwaki, 1989
	W-S Pheo i.a.	1	128.77 ± 24.6	6.41 ± 1.11	
	W-S Pheo i.v.	1	5.47 ± 2.68	16.24 ± 1.51	
Acinar pancreatic tumour	Pheo a i.v.	3	*Time* [h] / *Accum.* [μg dye/g tumour tissue]	*Time* [h] / *Accum.* [μg dye/g pancreatic tissue]	Aprahamian, 1993
			1 / 0.98 ± 0.13	1 / 0.57 ± 0.17	
			12 / 0.58 ± 0.07	12 / 0.12 ± 0.02	
			24 / 0.54 ± 0.09	24 / 0.08 ± 0.01	
			48 / 0.39 ± 0.09	48 / 0.05 ± 0.01	

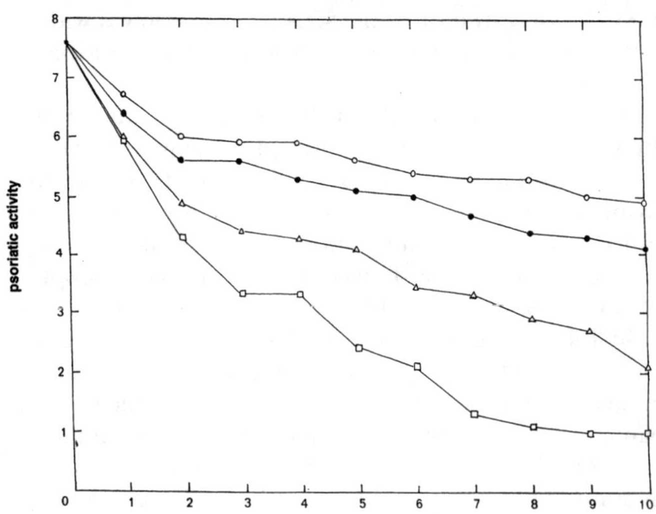

Figure 3 Topical photodynamic treatment of patients with psoriatic lesions (stationary type) with pheophorbide-a (3.2×10^{-5} M in Biowaschöl®), ○—○ Pheo-a, •—• UV-irradiation (NARVA UVS40-2), Δ—Δ Pheo-a + white light (400–800 nm), □—□ Pheo-a + UV, The UV-irradiation started with 0.1 J/cm², the illumination with 1 J/cm². The doses were increased for 10% at every treatment.

2.1.2. PHORBIDES

Beside pheophorbide-a, many other phorbides were found potent photosensitizers (Nakijama *et al.*, 1984). The synthesis of a large variety of phorbides and phorbide dimers has been described. The photodynamic activity and accumulation in tumour tissue *in vitro* and *in vivo* of some of these compounds have also been reported.

Reports on comparative studies on different phorbides and chlorins were given by Kimura (1993) and Pandey *et al.* (1992). In the work of Pandey *et al.* (1992) the antitumour activity *in vivo* of 11 pheophorbide- and bacteriopheophorbide derivatives was investigated in a comparative study in the SMT-F tumour growing subcutaneously in DBA/2 mice. The authors observed in the pyropheophorbide series that by increasing the length of the alkyl ether carbon chain the photosensitizing activity rised. These results are consistent with earlier investigations of these authors on series of alkyl ether derivatives of methyl pheophorbide-a and chlorin-e6 trimethyl ester where they made similar observations (Pandey *et al.*, 1991). However, the hexyl ether derivative of methyl pyropheophorbide was reported (Pandey *et al.*, 1992) to be somewhat superior to the other investigated compounds. It showed promising photodynamic activity even at a dose of 0.3 mg/kg (irradiated after 24 h with 100% tumour response at day 7 and 50% tumour response on day 30).

Table 3 contains the literature data about retention of different phorbides *in vitro* and *in vivo*. The results shown and discussed in this chapter and in

Table 3 Retention and Photodynamic Activity of Different Phorbides *In Vitro* and *In Vivo*

Photosensitizer (i.p.)	*Adm. dose* [mg/kg]	*Time between sens. adm. and illumination* [h]	*Tumour* response* [%] *at days after treatment* 1–2	7	30	*Literature*
Methyl pheophorbide-a	5.0	24	10	10	0	Pandey*, 1991
	1.0	3	100	75	n.d.	
	0.5	3	0	—	—	
Methyl pheophorbide-a phytyl ether	5.0	24	⇓			
	1.0	24	100	100	—	
	0.5	24	100	0	—	
Methyl pheophorbide-a propyl ether	1.0	24	20	0	—	
	0.3	24	0	—	—	
Methyl-pheophorbide-a hexyl ether	1.0	24	100	100	50	Pandey*, 1992
	0.3	24	100	90	0	
	0.3	3	100	100	20	
Methyl pyro-pheophorbide-a hexyl ether	0.3	24	100	100	50	
	0.25	24	100	85	35	
Di-t-butyl aspartyl pyropheophorbide-a hexyl ether	1.0	24	100	100	0	
	0.3	24	100	67	0	

* Tumour model: SMT-F tumour growing subcutaneously in female DBA/2 Ha-DD mice.
⇓ 100% mortality after light exposure.

Chapter 1.2 suggest that phorbides may become important basal compounds for PDT. The reason for this can be summarized in the following points:

- no or very low cytotoxicity;
- relative high photostability;
- cheap and simple preparation;
- high amount of different possible derivatizations;
- excellent photophysical properties in hydrophobic environments;
- uncomplicated coupling to antibodies or antibody fragments;
- the possibility to use all known up to date carrier systems.

The summary shows clearly the excellent behaviour of these dyes. Also, the very broad characterization of pheophorbide-a on different model levels demonstrates its usefulness in comparative studies.

LITERATURE CITED

Aprahamian, M., Evrard, S., Keller, P., Tsuji, M., Balboni, G., Damgé, C., and Marescaux, J. (1993): Distribution of pheoporbide A in normal tissues and in experimental pancreatic cancer in rats. *Anti-Cancer Drug Des.* **8**, 101–114.

Iwai, K. and Kimura, S. (1988): Efficiency of pheophorbide-dimer in photodynamic therapy of mouse tumor. *J. Clin. Biochem. Nutr.* **5**, 145–149.

Kessel, D. and Smith, K. (1989): Photosensitization with derivatives of chlorophyll. *Photochem. Photobiol.* **49**, 157–160.

Kimura, S. (1993): The mechanism of photodynamic action of pheophorbide and its application to cancer-phototherapy and -diagnosis. *Photomed. Photobiol.* **15**, 1–12.

Maeda, N., Ichikawa, K., Kobayishi, T., and Mizuno, N. (1985): Pheophorbide a PDT for chemically induced carcinoma of rat skin. *Clin. Res.* **33**, A633.

Nakijama, S., Samejima, N., Inohara, K., and Takata, H. (1984): Pheophorbide derivatives and pharmaceutical preparations containing them, *European Patent* 0 142 732 A2.

Nishiwaki, Y., Nakamuri, S., and Sakaguchi, S. (1989): New Method of Photosensitizer Accumulation for Photodynamic Therapy in an Experimental Liver Tumor. *Lasers in Surg. Med.* **9**, 254–263.

Nowak, Ch. (1989): Pers. comm., current address: Robert-Roessle-Klinik am Max-Delbrück-Centrum für Molekulare Medizin, Virchow-Klinikum, Medizinische Fakultät der Humboldt-Universität zu Berlin, Lindenberger Weg 80, 13125 Berlin, Germany.

Pandey, R. K., Majchrzycki, D. F., Smith, K. M., and Dougherty, Th. J. (1989): Chemistry of Photofrin II and some new photosensitizers. *SPIE Conf. Proc.* vol. 1065, 164–174.

Pandey, R. K., Bellnier, D. A., Smith, K. M., and Dougherty, Th. J. (1991): Chlorin and Porphyrin Derivatives as Potential Photosensitizers in Photodynamic Therapy, *Photochem. Photobiol.* **53**, 65–72.

Pandey, R. K., Shiau, F. -Y., Sumlin, A. B., Dougherty, Th. J., and Smith, K. M. (1992): Structure/activity relationships among photosensitizers related to pheophorbides and bacteriopheophorbides. *Bioorg. Med. Chem. Lett.* **2**, 491–496.

Poretz, R. D., Vucinek, I., Bergstrom, L., Segelman, A., Sigel, G., (jr.), and Chernomorsky, S. (1989): Intracellular Distribution of Porphyrin-Based photosensitizers in *in vitro* Cultured Human Bladder Tumor Cells. *SPIE Conf. Proc.* vol. 1065, 197–203.

Röder, B., Nicklisch, S., Wischnewsky, G., Slawaticki, E., and Meffert, H. (1984): Mittel zur Behandlung von Hauterkrankungen und Tumoren, Patent from 08.10.1984, WP 248 282.

Röder, B. (1990a): Photosensitizing properties of phorbides. *J. Photochem. Photobiol. B*: **5**, 519–521.

Röder, B. (1990b): Tetrapyrroles: A Chemical Class of Potent Photosensitizers for the Photodynamic Treatment of Tumours. *Lasers Med. Sci.* **5**, 99–106.

Röder, B., Näther, D., Lewald, T., Braune, M., Freyer, W., and Nowak, Ch. (1990c): Photophysical properties and photodynamic activity *in vivo* of some tetrapyrroles. *Biophys. Chem.* **35**, 303–312.

Segelman, A. B., Hagen, I. K., Chernomorsky, S. A., Lee, S.-Y., Gadi, I. K., Weadock, K., and Sigel, G. H. (1987): Highly purified pheophorbide-a as photosensitizer in human blader carcinoma *in vitro*. *SPIE Conf. Proc.* **847**, 205–209.

Tapper, B. A., Lohrey, E., Hove, E., and Allison, R. M. (1975): Photosensitivity from chlorophyll-derived pigments. *J. Sci. Fd. Agric.* **26**, 277–281.

Yamashita, Y., Moriyasu, F., Ono, S., Kimura, T., Kajimura, K., Someda, H., Hamato, N., Nabeshima, M., Sakai, M., and Okuma, M. (1991): Photodynamic therapy using pheophorbide-a and *Q*-switched Nd : YAG laser on implanted hepatocellular carcinoma. *Gastroent. Jap.* **26**, 623–627.

2.2. BACTERIOCHLOROPHYLLIDES, BACTERIOCHLORINS AND BACTERIOPHEOPHORBIDES

JOERG G. MOSER

Bacteriochlorophylls are natural products of several kind of bacteria and algae. The most commonly used product is the bacteriochlorophyll a of the purple bacterium, *Rhodobacter spheroides*. In contrast to artificial photosensitizers, the general advantage of those products and its derivatives is their degradability in the human body limiting its side effects of light sensitization to about 5 days, i.e. the time the patient has to stay in the hospital. So complications of a PDT treatment due to light sensitization can easily be observed and prevented [5].

Bacteriochlorophylls can be prepared in gram amounts with considerable purity [9]. Purity can be demonstrated by HPTLC and by MALDI mass spectroscopy [e.g. 7, 15]. Structural formulae of essential compounds are given in Fig. 1.

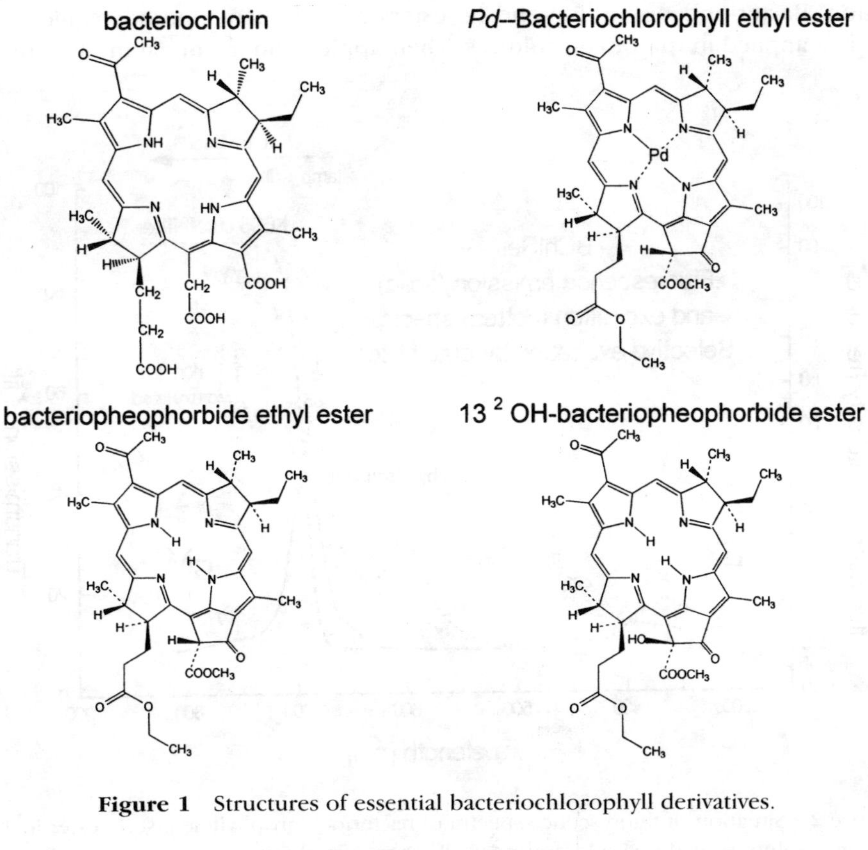

Figure 1 Structures of essential bacteriochlorophyll derivatives.

Bacteriochlorophylls fulfill completely the postulates of PDT with respect to their spectral properties: their major red absorption maximum, S_1, is centred in the "photodynamic window" at about 780 nm, and most of its derivatives show absorption maxima of no less than 760 nm. Figure 2 may demonstrate these features which allow for the use of very cheap diode lasers for photodynamic irradiation.

For photodynamic treatment the bacteriochlorophylls are unsuitable due to their low solubility and nearly no uptake in cancer cells (cf. Henderson *et al.*, 1991). Enzymatic treatment by chlorophyllase (an enzyme found e.g. in green algae, *Chlorella kessleri* and several green plants) leads to the free acids (*Chlorophyllides*) containing the original Mg^{++} central atom [20]. These acids can be esterified to chlorophyllide esters. Some of these esters with hydroxyl functions of amino acids are water soluble (see the chapter by Rosenbach-Belkin). Opening of the ring V leads to formation of bacteriochlorophyllin, and removal of the central Mg^{++} to bacteriochlorin a. Removal of the central metal ion in bacteriochlorophyll a upon acidification yields *bacteriopheophytin*, heating of the acidified acetone solution to *bacteriopheophorbide*, and heating of the acidified alcoholic solutions to the respective *bacteriopheophorbide esters* by transesterification. Bacteriopheophorbide and its esters are excellent photodynamic sensitizers if applied in tumor cell cultures. Their application in animal models and in

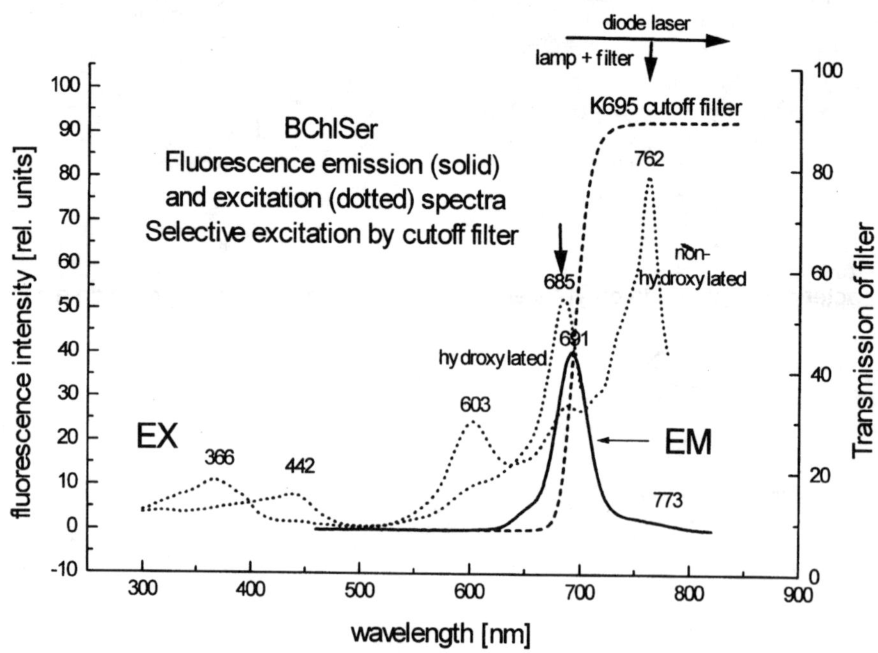

Figure 2 Situation of fluorescence spectra of bacteriochlorophyllide-β-serin ester in 10% albumin solution in the visible and near UV spectrum showing possibilities to irradiate with lasers [↓] or filtered continuous light lamps [→] for PDT.

humans is under investigation. The central metal ion can be exchanged against Cd^{++} and further against Pd^{++}, Zn^{++}, Co^{++}, Ni^{++} and several other divalent cations. This literature is reviewed by Scheer [21].

The most important fact observed with these drugs is the lack of any threshold dose with non-melanotic tumors. The Pd^{++}-derivatives overcome thresholds just in melanotic melanoma [11, 14, 15]. This as combined with biological degradation makes these drugs the most hopeful candidates for tumor PDT at all.

Trials to modify the periphery of Pd-bacteriopheophorbides have recently been published [19]. The intention is to form inclusion complexes of Pd-bacteriopheophorbides with dimeric cyclodextrins [16] in order to target them to tumors over tumor marker antibodies and a biotin-avidin complex system. At the moment the complex binding constants of the modified drug do not yet allow for a targeted application of these sensitizers. Other investigations have been devoted to the inclusion into detergent micelles and lipoid vesicles. Here the drugs remain photophysically active ($^1O_2$ quantum yield between 0.2 and 0.48) while in cyclodextrin inclusion complexes the energy transfer to oxygen is apparently blocked by yet unknown reasons [17]. Inside living cells the quantum yield has not yet been determined. Erythrocyte ghosts serve as a model [17]. The values may be considerable high as judged from the loss of free oxygen in the culture medium of doted cancer cells just at very low irradiation power densities. An application of these sensitizers in therapeutic designs needs for irradiation intervals to restore oxygen partial pressure in tissue as pointed out by Herzog *et al.* [6]. These investigations clearly showed that light transport in tumor tissue is not governed by absorption parameters but by light scattering [13].

Bacteriochlorins have been used immediately after their discovery as well for *in vitro* as for *in vivo* studies which so far are consistently comparable as they were done in the same laboratory [2, 3, 22–26]. As a model for *in vivo* studies a translucent "sandwich" chamber has been implanted into the back skin of hamsters [8, 24, 26]. So the time course of fluorescence after injection of the sensitizer as well as the photodynamic effects after irradiation could be observed continuously, in part under anesthesia.

Bacteriochlorin a and its Mg^{++} complex, bacteriochlorophyllin a, are water soluble and, therefore, penetrate only poorly cell membranes. Both show absorption maxima around 760 nm. The absorption coefficient of bacteriochlorin a with 32,000 [l/mole × cm] and an $\varepsilon_{360}/\varepsilon_{760} = 1.62$ is high enough to surmount significantly the effect of HpD. Absorption values are in an optimal region of the photodynamic window with 10 fold greater light penetration as at 630 nm. In fact the oxygen consumption at the absorption maximum and pH 7.4 is 4 times that of HpD in the presence of $^1O_2$ acceptors like histidine and tryptophane, and the photodynamic effect against L929 cells is at least of the same order as with HpD.

The respective *in vivo* experiments were done at a concentration of 20 mg/kg body weight in rabbits, rats, and hamsters. 24 h after application of the sensitizer a light dose of up to 150 J/cm^2 effected subtotal necrosis of 4–7 mm diameter tumors (green amelanotic melanoma, RMA mammary tumors, rhabdomyosarcoma) and total perfusion stop due to lesions of the vascular endothelial bed and swelling of erythrocytes (as with phthalocyanine polysulfonates). The subtotal necrosis is ascribed to a wash-out of sensitizer in the periphery of tumor vessels 24 h after sensitizer application. This notable effect might be overcome by sensitizer perfusion during irradiation as done by Rosenbach-Belkin *et al.* (cf. the resp. chapter of this book) with seryl bacteriochlorophyllide [20].

Several interesting observations were devoted to the other series of bacteriochlorophyll derivatives containing an intact ring V. For several aliphatic esters of bacteriopheophorbide a the *intracellular* absorption maximum has been determined at 760 nm [e.g. 10]. Uptake and phototoxicity at this wavelength in several cancer cell lines *in vitro* has been determined (Table 2 in the chapter on Biological parameters of photosensitation).

From these data the ethyl ester has been proved to be the most suitable drug.

The very low or neglegible threshold doses in melanotic and amelanotic tumor cells lines are compiled in Table 1.

A dark toxicity has not yet been established. In tumor cell cultures, no significant dark toxicity has been found up to 100 μM which is the highest concentration to be applied without other additives than serum. No or neglegible photobleaching has been observed for bacteriopheophorbide esters in solution [3]. For photobleaching in cells investigations are underway.

The subcellular localization of bacteriopheophorbide methyl and ethyl esters has been investigated [12] and shows about 50% of these drugs in ground cytoplasm and a considerable concentration by a factor of 10 in the Golgi apparatus. The nucleus is free of drug so that genetic damage can be excluded for photodynamic treatment. Semiquantitative data obtained by evaluation of fluorescence intensities are compiled in Table 2. Recently new investigations on this matter are underway [20].

For 13^2-hydroxy bacteriopheophorbide methyl ester pharmacokinetics have been investigated [18]. Dissected organs of nude mice carrying LLC (Lewis Lung Carcinoma) have been extracted, and the concentration of the dye has been estimated by fluorescence photometry. The authors decided 2 h as the best time for tumor irradiation which has to be seen in the frame of the chapters by Moan and by Berg of this book.

Table 1 Threshold doses of bacteriopheophorbide-a ethyl ester (BPEE) and its Pd-derivative in several tumor cell lines (from [11, 14])

Sensitizer	*Concentration* c_o^0 [μM]	*Cell line*	*Threshold* mW/cm^2
For comparison: Pheophorbide-a	6	OAT 75	1.6
BPEE	10–20	A375	0
		Melur SP 18	0.7
		SkAMel	0
		SkMel	2.8
Pd-BPEE	10	SkMel	0

Table 2 Rough estimate of concentration 13^2-hydroxy bacteriopheophorbide ethyl ester in intracellular compartments of OAT75SCLC cells (modified from [12])

Data ascribed to organell	*Estimated number of molecules in compartment* [× 10⁶]	*Volume of compartment* [femtoliters]	*Calculated concentration in compartment* [mM]
Golgi apparatus	19.8	18	1.8
(Undefined)	8.1	20	0.7
Mitochondria	20.4	118	0.3
Basal cytoplasm	52.0	505	0.15
Nucleus	0	330	0
Total		990	overall: $c_i' = 0.17$

Recent developments try to use other bacteriochlorophylls as a source of photosensitizers. A very attractive compound is bacteriochlorophyll *g* from *Heliobacterium chlorum* and its relatives showing an ethylidene group in position C-8^1 combined with a vinyl group in position C-3^1 [1]. Such compounds can peripherally be substituted in a way allowing for formation of inclusion complexes into dimeric cyclodextrins as an inert transport form for the resulting sensitizer to the tumor (see the respective chapter on carrier systems in PDT of this book). These investigations are now underway.

LITERATURE CITED

[1] Amesz, J. (1995): The heliobacteria, a new group of photosynthetic bacteria. *J. Photochem. Photobiol.* **30**, 89–96.

[2] Beems, E. M., Dubbelman, T. M. A. R., Lugtenburg, J., van Best, J. A., Smeets, M. F. M. A., and Boegheim, J. P. J. (1987): Photosensitizing properties of bacterio-chlorophyllin a and bacteriochlorin a, two derivatives of bacteriochlorophyll a. *Photochem. Photobiol.* **46**, 639–643.

[3] van Geel, I. P. J., Oppelaar, H., Oussoren, Y. G., Schuitmaker, J. J., and Stewart, F. A. (1995): Mechanisms for optimising photodynamic therapy: second-generation photosensitisers in combination with mitomycin C. *Br. J. Cancer* **72**, 344–350.

[4] Gensch, T., Röder, B., Pfeifer, L., and Moser, J. (1998): Photophysical properties of 13^2-hydroxy bacteriopheophorbide a methyl ester in ethanol and micellar solutions (to be published).

[5] Henderson, B., Sumlin, A. B., Owczarczak, B. L., and Dougherty, T. J. (1991): Bacteriochlorophyll a as photosensitizer for photodynamic treatment of transplantable murine tumors. *J. Photochem. Photobiol.* **10**, 303–313.

[6] Herzog, M., Moser, J. G., Wagner, B., and Broecker, J. (1994): Shielding effects and hypoxia in Photodynamic Therapy. *J. Oral Maxillo-Facial Surgery* **23**, 406–408.

[7] Kirsch, D., Kaufmann, R., Spengler, B., Heuermann, A., and Moser, J. G. (1995): Cyclodextrin-Chemie: Schnelle Analyse von Reaktionsprodukten durch MALDI-Massenspektroskopie. Abstr. INCOM '95.

[8] van Lengoed, H. L., Schuitmaker, J. J., van der Veen, N., Dubbelman, T. M. A. R., and Star, W. M. (1993): Fluorescence and photodynamic effects of bacteriochlorin a observed *in vivo* in sandwich observation chambers. *Br. J. Cancer* **67**, 898–903.

[9] Mironow, A. F. (1995): Synthesis and properties of new chlorin and bacteriochlorin photosensitizers. *SPIE Biomed. Optics* **2625**, 23–32.

[10] Moser, J. G., Rück, A., Schwarzmaier, H. J., and Westphal-Froesch, C. (1992): Photodynamic cancer therapy: fluorescence localization and light absorption spectra of chlorophyll-derived photosensitizers inside cancer cells. *Optical Engineering* **31**, 1441–1446.

[11] Moser, J. G., Suchomski, R., Danielowski, T., and Wagner, B. (1994): Significance of threshold doses for photodynamic therapy of melanotic and amelanotic tumors. *SPIE Biomed. Optics* **2371**, 178–186.

[12] Moser, J. G., Dembeck, U., Hubert, M., Spengler, B., Bayer, R., and Wagner, B. (1993): Subcellular storage compartments of bacteriopheophorbide sensitizers. *SPIE Biomed. Optics* **2078**, 532–538 (1994).

[13] Moser, J. G., Herzog, M., Broecker, J., and Wagner, B. (1992): Pitfalls in Photodynamic Therapy: "Shielding effects" and hypoxia in photosensitized tumor tissue. An *in vitro* model. Conf. Proc. IPA Meeting Milano.

[14] Moser, J. G., Ostrowsky, A., Gümüsdagli, M., and Kleiber, B. (1993): Bacteriopheophorbide esters: Photosensitizers without "threshold dose"? *SPIE Biomed. Optics* **2078**, 193–204 (1994).

[15] Moser, J. G. (1993): Attempts to treat malignant melanoma by photodynamic therapy using bacteriopheophorbide ester as the sensitizer. *SPIE Biomed. Optics* **1881**, 116–125.

[16] Moser, J. G., Heuermann, A., Oehr, P., Scheer, H., Vervoorts, A., and Andrees, S. (1994): Carrier systems in PDT: On the way to novel anti-tumor drugs. *SPIE Biomed. Optics* **2325**, 90–99.

[17] Oelckers, S., Hanke, T., Moser, J., and Röder, B. (1994): Time resolved detection of singlet oxygen luminescence in red cell ghosts generated by photosensitizers via excitation in the far red. *SPIE Biomed. Optics* **2325**, 116–120.

[18] Roeder, B., Dressler, C., Hagemann, R., Fuchs, B., Berlien, H. P., Nowak, C., and Moser, J. G. (1993): The pharmacokinetics of 13^2-hydroxy-bacteriopheophorbide a methyl ester studied by fluorescence spectroscopy on Lewis Lung Carcinoma bearing mice. *SPIE Biomed. Optics* **2078**, 427–437.

[19] Roehrs, S., Ruebner, A., Hartwich, G., Scheer, H., and Moser, J. G. (1995): Peripheral substitution of pheophorbides and bacteriopheophorbides to promote inclusion into inert carrier systems for PDT. *SPIE Biomed. Optics* **2625**, 333–338.

[20] Rosenbach-Belkin. V., Chen, L., Fiedor, L., Tregub, I., Pavlotsky, F., Brumfeld, V., Salomon, Y., and Scherz, A. (1996): Serine conjugates of chlorophyll and bacteriochlorophyll: Phototoxicity *in vitro* and tissue distribution in mice bearing melanoma tumors. *Photochem. Photobiol.* **64**, 174–181.

[21] Scheer, H. (ed.) (1991): The Chlorophylls. CRC Press, Boca Raton FL (USA).

[22] Schuitmaker, J. J., Jannink, J. E., and Dubbelman, T. M. A. R. (1995): Influence of cell culture medium on the photosensitizing effectiveness of bacteriochlorin a. *J. Photochem. Photobiol.* **28**, 143–148.

[23] Schuitmaker, J. J., Feitsma, R. I. J., Journée-de Korver, J. G., Dubbelman, T. M. A. R., and Pauwels, E. K. J. (1993): Tissue distribution of bacteriochlorin a labelled with ^{99m}Tc-pertechnate in hamster green melanoma. *Int. J. Radiat. Biol.* **64**, 451–458.

[24] Schuitmaker, J. J., van Lengoed, H. L. L. M., van der Veen, N., Dubbelman, T. M. A. R., and Star, W. M. (1993): Laser-induced *in vivo* fluorescence of bacteriochlorin a: preliminary results. *Lasers in Medical Science* **8**, 39–42.
[25] Schuitmaker, J. J., Vrensen, G. F., van Delft, J. L., de Wolff-Rouendaal, D., Dubbelman, T. M. A. R., and de Wolff, A. (1991): Morphologic effects of bacteriochlorin a and light *in vivo* on intraocular melanoma. *Invest. Ophthalmol. a. Visual Sci.* **32**, 2683–2688.
[26] Schuitmaker, J. J., van Best, J. A., van Delft, J. L., Dubbelman, T. M. A. R., Oosterhuis, J. A., and de Wolff-Rouendaal, D. (1990): Bacteriochlorin a, a new photosensitizer in photodynamic therapy. *Ophthalmol. a. Visual Sci.* **31**, 1444–1450.

2.3. PURPURINS AND RELATED CHLORINS

GRETA M. GARBO

Although purpurins have been known since the 1940s as degradation product of chlorophyll, their synthesis was not reported until 1960 (Woodward, 1960). In general the chemistry of purpurins have been ignored, presumably because no biological role has been found for the macrocycle. Morgan and Tertel (1986) reported the synthesis of octaethyl-purpurin, etio purpurin and several metal chelates of these compounds. Our group in Toledo has been involved in testing these and many other similar compounds as photosensitizers for PDT. Figure 1 shows the chemical structure of some of the purpurin and related chlorin derivatives, that were synthesized and tested in Toledo.

Table 1 shows the furthest red absorption band of these compounds. As can be seen in Table 1, these sensitizers absorb further into the red than Photofrin (Morgan and Garbo, 1991).

Emission and absorption maxima of SnET2 were found to be red shifted as the environment changed from polar to non-polar (Sekher and Garbo, 1993).

2.3.1. BIOPHYSICAL AND PHOTOCHEMICAL STUDIES

Table 2 shows the photophysical data that have been collected for various purpurins in benzene (Borland *et al.*, 1988) and in methanol (Macpherson *et al.*, 1990). In general purpurins and related chlorins (e.g. SnNT2H2) have a high triplet quantum yield (ϕ_T) and are efficient generators of singlet oxygen, with

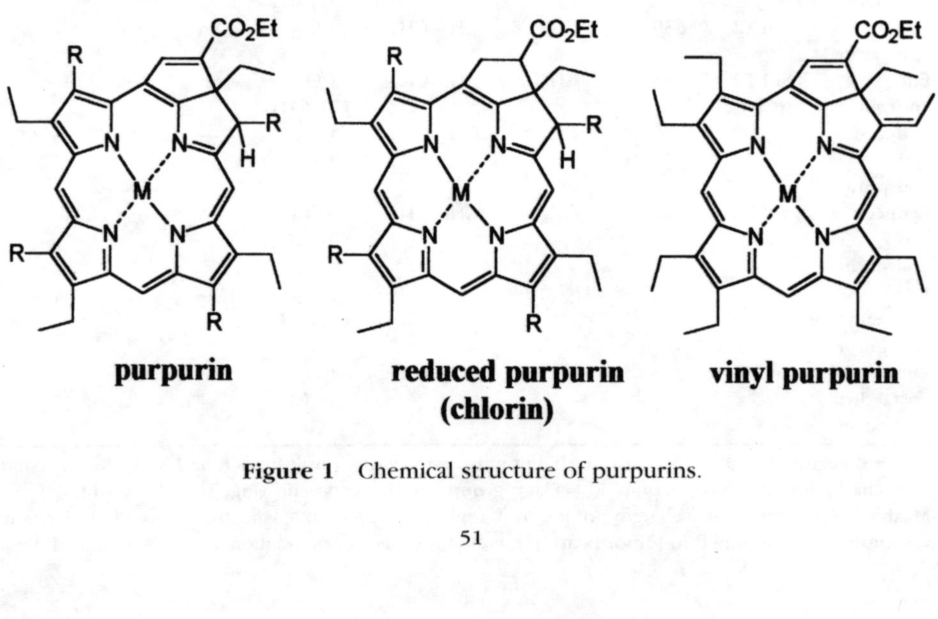

Figure 1 Chemical structure of purpurins.

Table 1 Furthest red absorption band for some purpurins and related chlorin derivatives

Chemical Structure	*Acronym*	MW	R	R_2^*	$R_3^\dagger$	*Metal* M	Q_{max} (NM)	*PDT*[††] *response*
Octaethyl purpurin	NT2	630	CH_2–CH_3	CH_2–CH_3	CO_2–CH_2CH_3	—	690	+
Oxidized octaethyl purpurin	NT2O2	662	CH_2–CH_3	CH_2–CH_3	CO_2–CH_2CH_3	—	680	+
Octaethyl purpurin	ZnNT2	695	CH_2–CH_3	CH_2–CH_3	CO_2–CH_2CH_3	Zn	656	++
Octaethyl purpurin	SnNT2 (Cl_2)	819	CH_2–CH_3	CH_2–CH_3	CO_2–CH_2CH_3	Sn	660	++
Octaethyl purpurin	GG1	616	CH_2–CH_3	CH_2–CH_3	CO_2–CH_3	—	695	NONE
Copro purpurin	JP1	806	CH_3	CH_2CH_2–CO_2CH_3	CO_2–CH_2CH_3	—	695	NONE
Copro purpurin	ZnJP1	871	CH_3	CH_2CH_2–CO_2CH_3	CO_2–CH_2CH_3	Zn	655	NONE
Reduced octaethyl purpurin	NT2H2	632	CH_2–CH_3	CH_2–CH_3	CO_2–CH_2CH_3	—	665	++
Reduced octaethyl purpurin	NiNT2H2	691	CH_2–CH_3	CH_2–CH_3	CO_2–CH_2CH_3	Ni	623	NONE
Reduced octaethyl purpurin	AgNT2H2	740	CH_2–CH_3	CH_2–CH_3	CO_2–CH_2CH_3	Ag	620	NONE
Reduced octaethyl purpurin	SnNT2H2 (Cl_2)	822	CH_2–CH_3	CH_2–CH_3	CO_2–CH_2CH_3	Sn	638	+++
Etio purpurin	ET2	574	CH_3	CH_2–CH_3	CO_2–CH_2CH_3	—	690	++
Etio purpurin	ZnET2	639	CH_3	CH_2–CH_3	CO_2–CH_2CH_3	Zn	656	++
Etio purpurin	SnET2 (Cl_2)	764	CH_3	CH_2–CH_3	CO_2–CH_2CH_3	Sn	660	+++
Reduced etio purpurin	ET2H2	576	CH_3	CH_2–CH_3	CO_2–CH_2CH_3	—	665	++
Reduced etio purpurin	SnET2H2 (Cl_2)	766	CH_3	CH_2–CH_3	CO_2–CH_2CH_3	Sn	638	+++
Vinyl octaethyl purpurin	NT1	658	CH_2–CH_3	CH_2–CH_3	CO_2–CH_2CH_3	—	715	++
Vinyl octaethyl purpurin	ZnNT1	723	CH_2–CH_3	CH_2–CH_3	CO_2–CH_2CH_3	Zn	677	++

MW = Molecular Weight; R = First side chain on the pyrrole ring (indicate as R on Fig. 1); R_2^* = Second side chains on the pyrrole ring; $R_3^\dagger$ = Ester group on the exocyclic ring, usually CO_2Et; Q_{max} = Maximum absorption wavelength in the red region of the visible spectrum; [††] = Photodynamic response was determined in tumor bearing rats by histological examination 4 and 24 h after PDT.

Table 2 Photophysical data for various purpurins in benzene and methanol

*Sensitizer**	ϕ_T	ϕ_Δ	S_Δ
NT2	0.82	0.68	0.83
NT2H2	0.86	0.71	0.83
SnNT2H2	0.96	0.82	0.85
NTW	0.08	0.08	*ca.*1
NT2O2	0.6	0.4	0.7
ZnNT2**	1.0	0.54	0.54

* in methanol; ** in benzene; ϕ_T = Triplet quantum yield; ϕ_Δ = Oxygen quantum yield; $S_\Delta = \phi_T/\phi_\Delta$ efficiency of quenching of the sensitizer triplet state by singlet oxygen.

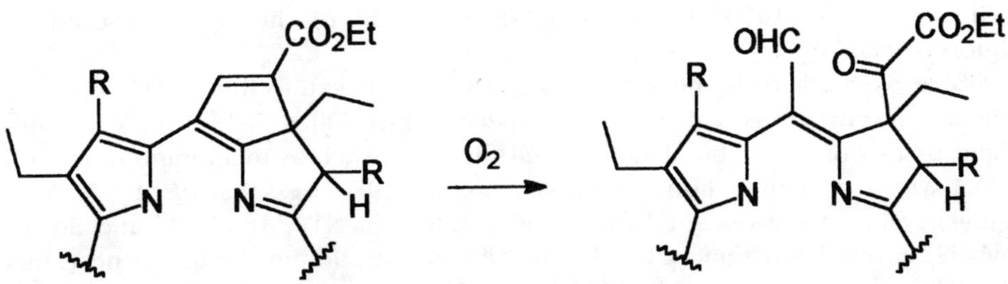

Figure 2 Purpurin photo-oxidation by light.

high singlet oxygen quantum yields (ϕ_Δ). In deoxygenated solvents the triplet lifetimes are *ca.* 100 μs.

Fluorescence lifetimes of purpurins are short and their fluorescence yields are low despite the much greater intensity of the Q band absorption band when compared to porphyrins (Kessel, 1989; Macpherson *et al.*, 1990).

Irradiation of octaethyl and etio purpurins with light leads to oxidative cleavage of the isocyclic ring to form the corresponding formyl chlorins (Morgan *et al.*, 1988c), as shown in Fig. 2.

In aqueous solutions it appears that this species undergoes hydration with a corresponding blue shift in the absorption of the Q band. For example, if NT2 ($R = CH_2{-}CH_3$) is oxidized by light: NT2O2 will form in organic solvents, the methyl acetal of NT2O2 will form in methanol, while in aqueous environment the hydrate derivative/s will result. The oxidized purpurin/s are still active generators of singlet oxygen (Macpherson *et al.*, 1990) and so they could still be involved in the overall PDT effect, if formed *in vivo*. SnET2 photobleaching studies showed photoproducts similar to those obtained from NT2 and ET2 (Sekher and Garbo, 1993). The photobleaching constants varied, depending on the environment in which the dye was located: SnET2 appeared to photo-oxidize faster in polar environments compared to non-polar solvents (Sekher and Garbo, 1993). On the contrary, the chlorin SnNT2H2 is very stable and does not photobleach under steady state irradiation (Macpherson *et al.*, 1990).

2.3.2. *IN VITRO* TESTING

Several purpurins and related chlorins have been tested *in vitro*, using L1210 leukemia cells in suspension (Kessel, 1989; Kessel *et al.*, 1991). Cells (3×10^6) were incubated in growth medium containing various concentration of sensitizers in various carriers. After thirty minutes incubation a steady state was reached, cells were collected by centrifugation, washed and resuspended in fresh media for the light experiment (1200 mJ/cm^2 red light from a non-coherent source). To measure cellular uptake, the cell pellet was treated with detergent (10 μM CTAB) and concentration of the dye measured by fluorescence.

Table 3 summarizes the intracellular (IC_{50}) and extracellular (EC_{50}) micromolar concentrations (μM) of the sensitizers, which killed 50% of the cells after light treatment or inhibited various cell functions such as membrane transport, DNA synthesis or mitochondrial activity (Kessel, 1989; Kessel *et al.*, 1991). Very similar values were obtained for the IC_{50} values of NT2, SnNT2H2 and SnET2 when delivered by Cremophor EI, but the concentration in the media necessary to achieve them were quite different. SnET2 needed 10 and 75 times lower concentration in the media (EC_{50}) than SnNT2H2 and NT2, to kill 50% of the cells. It is interesting that the same μM concentration of SnNT2H2 caused 50% cell killing and 50% inhibition of the cycloleucin transport, while for SnET2 the concentration necessary to inhibit the transport of this aminoacid was higher than the IC_{50}. Fluorescence microscopy studies with fluorescent probes, specific for various cell sites, showed membrane and lysosomes damage after SnET2 and light (Kessel, 1993).

Gomer demonstrated *in vitro* gene induction of stress proteins after SnET2 and light. He also showed that the expression pattern of stress proteins varied with different sensitizers (Gomer, 1994).

The effects of SnET2 and light on erythrocytes membranes were investigated with assays for acyl hydroperoxides and thiobarbituric acid. A linear dependence of the lipid peroxidation and light fluence was observed in photosensitized membranes. The concentration of phospholipids decreased in the photo-activated membranes, while lipid fluorescence increased (Morgan *et al.*, 1990b).

Sodium azide was able to inhibit lipid peroxidation by SnET2 and light, in sensitized membranes, while superoxide dismutase (SOD) and catalase showed no effect. Since the quenching of singlet oxygen by sodium azide did not completely inhibit lipid peroxidation, other processes may be involved (Morgan *et al.*, 1990b).

Table 3 Concentration of sensitizers which killed or Inhibited 50% of cells or cell functions

Measurement	NT2 CRM	SnNT2H2 CRM	SnET2 EtOH	SnET2 CRM	SnET2 Mol	SnET2 γ cycl.
EC_{50}	15.0	2.1	0.6	0.2	0.3	0.2
IC_{50}	0.75	1.05	25.3	1.2	4.3	2.6
DR	0.05	0.5	43.0	6.2	15.2	13.3
Transport	nd	1.1	22.5	1.4	4.6	4.7
Mitochondrial	nr	nr	112.6	5.9	8.6	8.2
Localization of PDT damage	damage to DNA synthesis	membrane	membrane lysosomes	membrane lysosomes	membrane lysosomes	membrane lysosomes

EtOH = in ethanol; CRM = in Cremophor El; Mol = in Molecusol Pharmatec; γ cycl = in gamma cyclodextrins; nd = not detectable; nr = not reported; EC_{50} = Extracellular concentration of the purpurin that killed 50% of the cells after 30 min incubation and light treatment; IC_{50} = Intracellular concentration of the purpurin that killed 50% of the cells after 30 min incubation and light treatment; DR = Distribution Ratio (IC_{50}/EC_{50}); Transport = Intracellular dye concentration required to inhibit cycloleucin accumulation by 50% upon light treatment; Mitochondrial = Intracellular dye concentration required to inhibit 50% of mitochondrial function upon light treatment.

2.3.3. PDT EXPERIMENTS IN ANIMALS BEARING TRANSPLANTED TUMORS

In vivo experiments were performed using the FANFT (N-[4-{5-nitro-2-furyl}-2-thiazolyl]formamide) induced urothelial cell carcinoma transplanted into Fischer CDF(F-344) rats (Morgan *et al.*, 1987; Selman *et al.*, 1987; Morgan *et al.*, 1988a,b).

As a light source, both a Kodak slide projector, a xenon arc lamp, or tuned dye laser have been used (Morgan and Selman, 1988). Typical power densities range from 50 to 200 mW/cm^2 with total energy output ranging from 50–360 J/cm^2. In the case of broad-band light sources, the energy actually absorbed by the sensitizer depends on the absorption characteristics of the molecules.

Histological sections of treated tumors 4 and 24 h after PDT were examined with all the compounds. The first screening examined the presence of disruption of tumor vasculature and cell necrosis after PDT (see Table 1). The majority of these compounds showed *in vivo* photodynamic activity at doses ranging from 15.9 μM/kg b.w. (micromoles per kg body weight) for the octaethyl purpurin (NT2) to 0.61 μM/kg b.w. for the tin octaethyl-reduced purpurin SnNT2H2. To quantify the effect of the sensitizers on this tumor model, both 12-days tumor dry weight studies and tumor cure rates (30 days survival study) were performed (Selman *et al.*, 1987).

The etio purpurin derivative appeared to be more active compared to the octaethyl purpurin (Fig. 3). Insertion of metal increased the photosensitizer activity *in vivo*, with tin superior to zinc: complete tumor cure in the rat tumor model was obtained at doses of 1.3 μM/kg for SnET2 and 0.61 μM/kg for SnNT2H2 (Morgan and Selman, 1988) (Fig. 4).

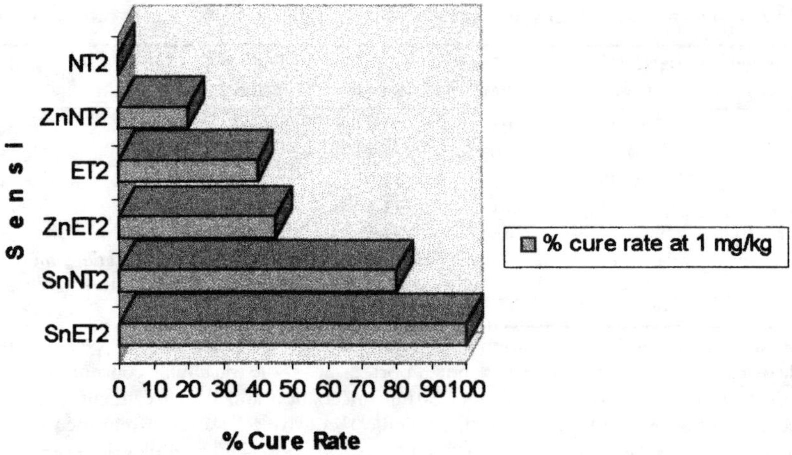

Figure 3 PDT tumor response in rats (dose = 1 mg/kg b.w.).

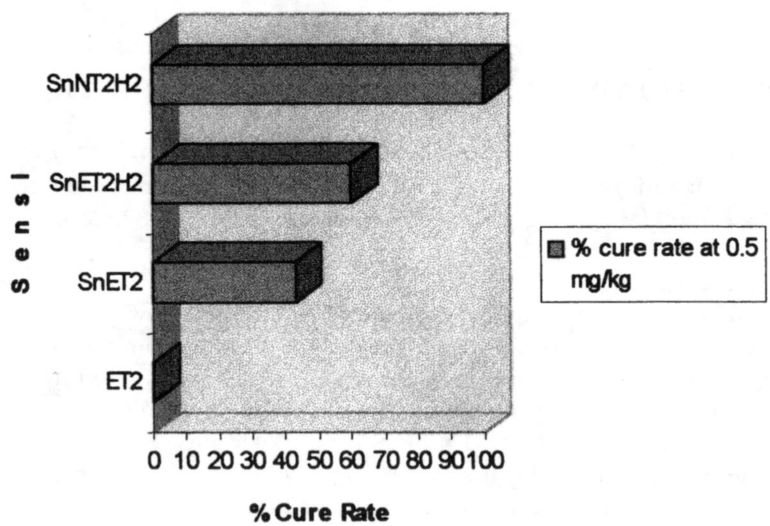

Figure 4 PDT tumor response with purpurins (dose = 0.5 mg/kg b.w.).

The effect of therapeutic light doses on normal tissues has been studied using the rat foot-pad model. This involves treating non-tumor bearing animals with the photosensitizer and 24 h after administration, irradiating one foot-pad with the light dose used for PDT. The thickness of the foot-pad is compared to that of the untreated foot-pad, which thus serves as internal control. The octaethyl derivative with or without metal produced higher normal skin photosensitivity in the rat foot-pad model (Morgan *et al.*, 1989b).

The sensitivity of normal tissue to sunlight after injection of SnET2, has been studied using the protocol described by Manyak *et al.* (1988). This protocol involves the use of hairless mice and a Solar Simulator. Minimal skin reaction were seen at SnET2 therapeutical dose (Morgan *et al.*, 1990a).

2.3.4. *IN VIVO* VASCULAR PHOTODAMAGE AFTER PURPURIN AND LIGHT

Changes in blood flow to transplantable bladder tumor in rats after purpurin-PDT has been reported using a radioactive microsphere technique (Selman *et al.*, 1987, 1990). The decrease in blood flow occurred whether the vehicle for delivery of the sensitizer was an emulsion or a liposome formulation. Systemic heparinization of the animals prior to light treatment did not alter the changes in tumor blood flow (Selman *et al.*, 1990).

Intravital microscopy studies in the rat cremaster muscle, after administration of SnET2 and light treatment, showed absence of platelet aggregation, increased leakage from venules and dilation of arterioles (Fingar *et al.*, 1992). Blood flow stasis was observed only much later than previously observed for Photofrin in the same model. The same authors reported increased release of thromboxane after PDT experiments with Photofrin and demonstrated that this change caused arterioles constriction (Fingar *et al.*, 1990, 1993). After SnET2-PDT they measured much higher release than normal of both prostacyclins and thromboxane. The increased release of both these cyclooxygenase products, allowed to maintain the normal equilibrium between them and avoid vessel constriction (Fingar *et al.*, 1992).

In vitro–in vivo assays of SnET2-PDT in rat aorta demonstrated that this purpurin directly damages the endothelial lining of the rat aorta (He *et al.*, 1991). When animals were treated *in vivo* with light, sacrificed immediately and the aorta placed in an explant culture for 24 h, only 0.3% of the endothelial lining remained. Similarly when the aorta was irradiated *in vitro* and maintained in culture for 24 h, 0.4% of the endothelial lining remained. Minimal or no changes were seen in the endothelial lining of the control aorta maintained in explant culture for 24 h (He *et al.*, 1991).

2.3.5. EFFECT OF DELIVERY SYSTEMS: PHARMACOKINETICS AND LIPOPROTEINS BINDING PATTERNS

Various delivery systems were examined as carriers for SnET2: emulsions, cyclodextrins and liposomes containing various phospholipids were prepared using different encapsulation methods (Garbo, 1990; Sekher and Garbo, 1993).

SnET2 tissue distribution studies were performed both in C3H-HeJ mice bearing the RIF tumor system and in 344 Fisher rats with a transplantable urothelial tumor (Morgan *et al.*, 1991; Kessel *et al.*, 1993). In the rodents this sensitizer reached highest tumor level 24 h after injection with a tumor/normal tissue ratio close to 4 : 1. As with many other sensitizers, SnET2 had very high uptake levels in liver, kidneys and spleen and a multiphasic serum clearance (Morgan *et al.*, 1991).

The PDT tumor response data seemed to suggest that the affinity of the carrier to the tumor influenced the distribution and selectivity of the sensitizer. Selective tumor localization can be explained by elevated levels of Low Density Lipoproteins (LDL) receptors in neoplastic cells (Gal *et al.*, 1981; Vitolis *et al.*, 1990). Since binding of photosensitizers to LDL has been previously demonstrated by many other groups (Barel *et al.*, 1986; Candide *et al.*, 1986; Kessel, 1986), *in vitro* and *in vivo* studies were performed to analyze the binding affinity of the SnET2-delivery system complexes with serum proteins (Garbo, 1990; Kessel *et al.*, 1991; Polo *et al.*, 1992; Kongshaw *et al.*, 1993; Kessel *et al.*, 1993). Initially it appeared that Cremophor El exerted some LDL orientating action (Garbo, 1990; Kessel *et al.*, 1991; Polo *et al.*, 1992). Later it was published that this surfactant actually modifies the density of the High Density Lipoproteins (HDL), so that this fraction runs in the density gradient at the same level where the LDL are usually separated (Kongshaug *et al.*, 1991; Woodburn and Kessel, 1994). Studies with octabutoxy-phthalocyanines demonstrated that sensitizers delivered by Cremophor El remained longer in the circulation and this permits a higher accumulation in the target site (Soncin *et al.*, 1994).

2.3.6. CONCLUSIONS

PDT Inc. in Santa Barbara has recently reported promising preliminary Phase I/II clinical results for SnET2 for the treatment of some skin malignancies and AIDS-related Kaposi's sarcoma (PDT Inc. Press Release, Dec. 11, 1995).

More studies should be performed with the reduced purpurin SnNT2H2. This chlorin appears to be even more interesting than SnET2, since it is stable to light, does not photobleach and achieves complete tumor regression in the rat model at doses quite lower than SnET2.

ACKNOWLEDGMENTS

This review summarizes the experimental work performed with purpurin and related chlorins by various laboratories: Dr. Morgan and his group at the University of Toledo, Dr. Selman and his group at the Medical College of Ohio, Dr. Kessel and his group at Wayne State University, Dr. Truscott and his group at Paisley College, Dr. Fingar and his group at the University of Louisville and many others.

LITERATURE CITED

Barel, A., Jori, G., Peron, A., Romandini, P., Pagnan, A., and Biffanti, S. (1986): Role of high-, low-, and very low-density lipoproteins in the transport and tumor delivery of hematoporphyrin *in vivo*. *Cancer Lett.* **32**, 145–150.

Borland, C. F., McGarvey, D., Truscott, T. G., and Morgan, A. R. (1988): Laser flash photolysis of purpurins: novel potential photosensitizers of interest for photodynamic therapy of cancer. *J. Photochem. Photobiol. B Biol.* **2**, 427–434.

Candide, C., Maziere, J. C., Goldstein, S., Santus, R., Dubertret, L., Reyftmann, J. P., and Polonovsky, J. (1986): *In vitro* interaction of the photoactive porphyrin derivative Photofrin II with low density lipoprotein, and its delivery to cultured human fibroblasts. *FEBS Lett.* **207**, 133–138.

Dougherty, T. J. (1993): Photodynamic therapy. *Photochem. Photobiol.* **58**, 895–900.

Fingar, V. H., Wieman, T. J., and Weber Doak, K. (1990): Role of thromboxane and prostacyclin release on photodynamic therapy-induced destruction. *Cancer Res.* **50**, 2599–2603.

Fingar, V. H., Wieman, T. J., Wiele, S. A., and Siegel, K. A. (1992): Effect of PDT using tin etiopurpurin on tissue microvasculature. (abstract) *Photochem. Photobiol.* **55**, 55S.

Fingar, V. H., Siegel, K. A., Wieman, T. J., and Weber Doak, K. (1993): The effects of thromboxane inhibitors on the microvascular and tumor response to photodynamic therapy. *Photochem. Photobiol.* **58**, 393–399.

Gal, D., McDonald, P. C., Porter, J. C., and Simpson, E. R. (1981): Cholesterol metabolism in cancer cells in monolayer culture-II. Low density lipoprotein metabolism. *Int. J. Cancer* **28**, 315–319.

Garbo, G. M. (1990): The use of liposomes, emulsions or inclusion complexes may potentiate *in vivo* effects of SnET2. *SPIE Conf. Proc.* **203**, 118–125.

Gomer, C. J. (1994): Does gene induction following photodynamic therapy alter cell sensitivity? (abstract) *Photochem. Photobiol.* **59**, 14S.

He, D. P., Hampton, J. A., Keck, R., and Selman, S. H. (1991): Photodynamic therapy: Effect on the endothelial cell of the rat aorta. *Photochem. Photobiol.* **54**, 801–804.

Kessel, D. (1986): Porphyrin–lipoprotein association as a factor in porphyrin localization. *Cancer Lett.* **33**, 183–188.

Kessel, D. (1989): Determinants of photosensitization by purpurins. *Photochem. Photobiol.* **50**, 169–174.

Kessel, D., Morgan, A. R., and Garbo G. M. (1991): Sites and Efficacy of photodamage by tin etiopurpurin *in vitro* using different delivery systems. *Photochem. Photobiol.* **54**, 193–196.

Kessel, D., Garbo, G. M., and Hampton, J. A. (1993): The role of lipoproteins in the distribution of tin etiopurpurin (SnET2) in the tumor-bearing rat. *Photochem. Photobiol.* **57**, 298–301.

Kessel, D. (1993): Use of fluorescent probes for characterizing sites of photodamage. *The Spectrum* **6**(2), 1–6.

Kongshaug, M., Cheng, L. S., Moan, J., and Rimington, C. (1991): Interactions of Cremophor El with human plasma. *Int. J. Biochem.* **23**, 473–478.

Kongshaug, M., Moan, J., Cheng, L. S., Garbo, G. M., Kolbe, S., Morgan, A. R., and Rimington, C. (1993): Binding of drugs to human plasma proteins, exemplified by Sn(IV)-etiopurpurin dichloride delivered in Cremophor and DMSO. *Int. J. Biochem.* **25**, 739–760.

Macpherson, A. N., Kessel, D., Morgan, A. R., Munro, I., and Truscott, T. G. (1990): A photophysical study of some purpurins. *J. Chem. Soc. Faraday Trans.* **86**, 3081–3085.

Manyak, M. J., Smith, P. D., Harrington, F. S. I., Steinberg, S. M., Glatstein, E., and Russo, A. (1988): Protection against dihematoporphyrin ether photosensitivity. *Photochem. Photobiol.* **47**, 823–830.

Morgan, A. R. and Tertel, N. C. (1986): Observations on the synthesis and spectroscopic characteristics of purpurins. *J. Org. Chem.* **51**, 1347–1350.

Morgan, A. R., Garbo, G. M., Kreimer-Birnbaum, M., Keck, R. W., Chaudhuri, K., and Selman, S. H. (1987): Morphologic studies of the combined effect of purpurin derivatives and light on transplanted bladder tumors. *Cancer Res.* **47**, 496–499.

Morgan, A. R., Garbo, G. M., Keck, R. W., and Selman, S. H. (1988a): New photosensitizers for photodynamic therapy: Combined effect of metallopurpurin derivatives and light on transplantable bladder tumors. *Cancer Res.* **48**, 194–198.

Morgan, A. R., Kreimer-Birnbaum, M., Garbo, G. M., Keck, R. W., and Selman, S. H. (1988b): Purpurins: improved photosensitizers for photodynamic therapy. *SPIE Conf. Proc.* **847**, 29–35.

Morgan, A. R., Garbo, G. M., and Truscott, T. G. (1988c): Photophysical and photochemical properties of purpurins. *SPIE Conf. Proc.* **997**, 139–144.

Morgan, A. R. and Selman, S. H. (1988): New photosensitizers for photodynamic therapy of tumor. *Drugs of the Future* **12**, 1073–1082.

Morgan, A. R., Rampersaud, A., Garbo, G. M., Keck, R. W., and Selman, S. H. (1989): New sensitizers for photodynamic therapy: controlled synthesis of purpurins and their effects on normal tissue. *J. Med. Chem.* **32**, 904–908.

Morgan, A. R., Garbo, G. M., Keck, R. W., Eriksen, L. D., and Selman, S. H. (1990a): Metallopurpurins and light: Effect on transplantable rat bladder tumors and murine skin. *Photochem. Photobiol.* **51**, 589–592.

Morgan, A. R., Cheng, L. S., Skalkos D., and Garbo, G. M. (1990b): Tin etiopurpurin dichloride-sensitized lipid photooxidation of erythrocyte membranes. *Photochem. Photobiol.* **52**, 987–991.

Morgan, A. R., Garbo, G. M., Krivak, T., Mastroianni, M., Petousis, N., St. Clair, T., Wiesenberger, M., and van Lier, J. E. (1991): New sensitizers for PDT. *SPIE Conf. Proc.* **1426**, 350–355.

Morgan, A. R. and Garbo, G. M. (1991): Biomedical application of porphyrin photosensitizers. *Trends Photochem. Photobiol.* **2**, 229–236.

Polo, L., Reddi, E., Garbo, G. M., Morgan, A. R., and Jori, G. (1992): The distribution of the tumour photosensitizers Zn(II)-phthalocyanine and Sn(IV)-etiopurpurin among rabbit plasma proteins. *Cancer Lett.* **66**, 217–223.

Sekher, P. and Garbo, G. M. (1993): Spectroscopic studies of tin ethyl etiopurpurin in homogeneous and heterogeneous systems. *J. Photochem. Photobiol. B Biol.* **20**, 117–125.

Selman, S. H., Garbo, G. M., Keck, R. W., Chaudhuri, K., and Morgan, A. R. (1987): A dose response analysis of purpurin derivatives used as photosensitizers for the photodynamic treatment of transplantable FANFT induced urothelial tumors. *J. Urol.* **137**, 1255–1257.

Selman, S. H., Qin, B., James, H. R., Keck, R. W., Garbo, G. M., and Morgan, A. R. (1990): Hemodynamic effect of the metallopurpurin SnET2 and light on transplantable FANFT induced bladder tumor. *J. Urol.* **143**, 630–633.

Soncin, M., Polo, L., Reddi, E., Jori, G., Kenney, M. E., Cheng, G., and Rodgers, M. A. J. (1995): Effect of delivery system on the distribution of Ge(IV)-octabutoxy-phthalocyanine in tumor bearing mice. *Cancer Lett.* **89**, 101–106.

Vitolis, S., Angelin, B., Erickson, S., Gahrton, G., Juliusson, G., Masquelier, M., Paul, C., Peterson, C., Rudling, C., Söderbery-Reid, K., and Tidefelt, U. (1990): Uptake of low density lipoproteins by human leukemia cells *in vivo*: relation to plasma lipoprotein levels and possible relevance for selective chemotherapy. *Proc. Natl. Acad. Sci. USA* **87**, 2598–2602.

Woodburn, K. and Kessel, D. (1994): The alteration of plasma lipoprotein by Cremophor El. *J. Photochem. Photobiol. B Biol.* **22**, 197–201.

Woodward, R. B. (1960): Totalsynthese des Chlorophylls. *Angew Chem.* **72**, 651–751.

2.4. PHTHALOCYANINES

WAI-SHUN CHAN, MAGDA ZUK and EHUD BEN-HUR

INTRODUCTION

Phthalocyanines (Pc's) are synthetic, porphyrin-like dyes, whose pyrrole moieties are bridged by aza nitrogens and with benzene rings fused onto the pyrroles (Fig. 1). The phthalocyanine macrocycle can chelate with many metals and these can carry axial ligands. The benzene rings can be substituted with diverse substituents. Their attraction for photodynamic therapy (PDT) derives from the ability of many Pc's to serve as efficient photosensitizers and their prominent absorption ($>10^5 M^{-1}cm^{-1}$) in the far red (660–700 nm) region of the light spectrum. Moreover, Pc's are stable, non-toxic and tend to localize in tumor tissues. The Pc's were first suggested for use in PDT by Ben-Hur and Rosenthal (1985) and since then have been extensively studied for this purpose. Currently, three Pc's are either in, or about to enter, clinical trials. They are the sulfonated aluminum phthalocyanine (either the disulfonated analog, $AlPcS_2$, in the UK, or a mixture of sulfonates, $AlPcS_n$, in Russia); ZnPc in liposomal formulation (Ciba-Geigy, Switzerland); and the SiPc (Pc 4, Oleinick *et al.*, 1993) in the USA. This chapter will focus on these three Pc's.

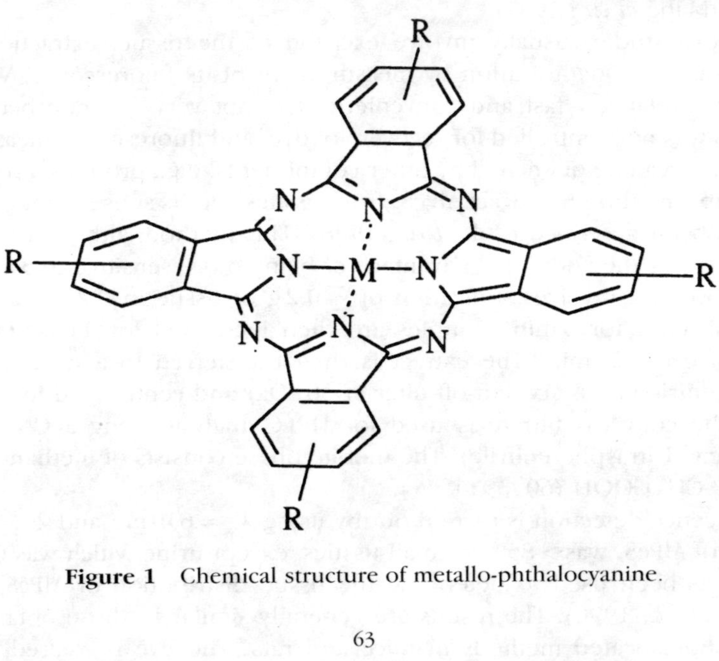

Figure 1 Chemical structure of metallo-phthalocyanine.

SULFONATED ALUMINUM PHTHALOCYANINE ($AlPcS_2$ AND $AlPcS_n$)

This was the first Pc to be used *in vivo* for the treatment of experimental rat tumor (Selman *et al*., 1986). It has been studied in many experimental animals for the quantitative response of both tumor (Anholt *et al*., 1994; Chan *et al*., 1987, 1991; Peng *et al*., 1990; Roberts *et al*., 1991) and normal tissues (Chatlani *et al*., 1991; Leach *et al*., 1993). The toxicity and tissue distribution of $AlPcS_n$ have been studied in detail in various species (Leach and Peaston, 1994; Peavy *et al*., 1995; Weintraub *et al*., 1988). The relative magnitude of $AlPcS_n$ retention by tissues was found to be liver > spleen > small intestine > kidney ⩾ lung ⩾ heart ⩾ urinary bladder > stomach ⩾ colon > brain (Chan *et al*., 1988). Preferential retention of $AlPcS_n$ in tumors versus surrounding normal tissue can be found in many cases. However this ratio may vary dramatically dependent on the tissue origin of the tumor and the location of tumor growth (Chan *et al*., 1988, 1989).

An unusual selective effect of $AlPcS_n$-PDT can be seen in pancreatic tumors. This is based not on selective accumulation of the sensitizer in tumor tissue, which was only 2-fold higher than in normal tissue. But, the photodynamic threshold dose which was 7 times as high for normal pancreas as for pancreatic cancer (Chatlani *et al*., 1992). Such selectivity was not found for other tissues, e.g., colon (Barr *et al*., 1990). It was postulated that normal pancreas cells contain higher levels of scavengers of reactive oxygen species and are thus protected better from PDT damage than tumor cells. Indeed, dihematoporphyrin ether was found to undergo photobleaching faster in pancreatic tumors than in normal pancreas (Mang *et al*., 1987).

The above studies usually involve excision of the tissue, extraction of the dye in alkali and quantification by measurement of its fluorescence. While this approach is relatively fast and convenient, it is not very accurate because the extraction was not controlled for recovery of dye, and fluorescence measurement in the extract can be quenched by other components, e.g., proteins. An accurate, reproducible method to extract $AlPcS_n$ from tissues and its subsequent analysis by HPLC has been described (Zuk *et al*., 1988). This method, although more time consuming, has the additional advantage of being more sensitive (0.5 ng/ml).

The procedure involves sonication of ~0.2 g of tissue in 0.2 M NaOH (total volume of 1 ml) for 5 min. Samples are then incubated for 1 h at 60°C with sonication every 20 min. The extract is then transferred to a microseparation system (Centricon 30, MW cut-off filter at 30 kDa) and centrifuged for 30 min at 4000 g. The colorless filtrate is used for HPLC analysis using a CN analytical column (e.g. Ultraspherenitrile). The mobile phase consists of methanol: 0.05 M $NaH_2PO_4 : CH_3COOH$ (60 : 39 : 1, v/v).

Fluorescence detection is carried out by using $\lambda_{ex} = 610$ nm and $\lambda_{em} = 685$ nm. Recovery of $AlPcS_n$ was > 85% from all tissues, except urine which was 60%. This method has been used to determine the tissue distribution of $AlPcS_n$ in dogs (Ben-Hur *et al*., 1990). The results are generally similar to those obtained with the less sophisticated methods in mice and rats. The dye is cleared from the circulation within 24 h, primarily via the kidneys, and is accumulated mainly in the reticuloendothelial system (liver, spleen and bone marrow). Interestingly, clearance is faster in males than in females and there are tissue distribution differences between the genders.

$AlPcS_n$ can be measured non-invasively *in vivo* in superficial tissues based on its fluorescence (Chen *et al.*, 1993). This technique has the advantage of being rapid and convenient and the results agree qualitatively with the extraction technique. It is limited, however, to superficial tissues, is not as sensitive and is not quantitative.

Good Pc retention by the tissue, however, does not necessarily correlate with PDT efficacy. Chan *et al.* (1991) demonstrated that, while the $AlPcS_{3-4}$ were accumulated in tumor tissue in much greater extent than the $AlPcS_2$, the latter mediated PDT was far more effective in eradicating tumor. Using a cooled CCD (charge-coupled device) camera to detect Pc fluorescence on cryosections (Peng and Moan, 1995), it was found that $AlPcS_2$ is mainly localized in the interstitium and in the neoplastic cells of the tumor, whereas $AlPcS_4$ is located only in the stroma of the tumor but none in tumor cells. Such difference in localization in tumor thus explains the differences in PDT efficacy of these dyes.

Other sensitive devices have been used to detect photosensitizer localization in tissues, e.g. confocal microscopy (Peng *et al.*, 1990). However, the cooled CCD camera appears to be the choice for quantitative measurement. Apart from the high sensitivity over a wide range of the spectrum, it possesses an extremely wide dynamic range and high geometric rigidity which assures photometry linearity over a signal range of 10^4 magnitude (Hiraoka, 1987). A detailed CCD camera equipped fluorescence microscopic set up has been described (Pope *et al.*, 1991). In this system, an 8 mW helium–neon laser was used to generate excitation light (632.8 nm). Apart from its spectral purity, such long wavelength light substantially reduces tissue auto-fluorescence which is often problematic for low fluorescence signal detection.

An early photodynamic effect of $AlPcS_n$ is blood flow stasis (Selman *et al.*, 1986). This effect on the vasculature can be demonstrated dramatically by visual observations of the chicken comb, a highly vascularized tissue (Ben-Hur *et al.*, 1990). Immediately after treatment the irradiated area becomes darker because of vasodilation. This is followed by hematoma due to extensive hemorrhage and finally blanching as a result of vascular destruction. This effect is highly specific to the blood vessels, other tissue components are not affected, and the effect is maximal 1 h after i.v. administration of $AlPcS_n$. Similar vascular effects can be observed histologically in Pc treated tumor (Nelson *et al.*, 1988).

While obvious damage to the vasculature occurs early after $AlPcS_n$ PDT, it was not certain whether tumor necrosis is the result of the direct tumor cell cytotoxicity or is the consequence of an indirect mechanism. A clonogenicity assay which is a classical method for determining radiosensitivity of neoplastic cells in tumor has been used to quantify tumor cell survival following PDT (Henderson *et al.*, 1985; van Bruggen *et al.*, 1992). A modified method which we found to produce higher tumor cell yield is described here. Various times after PDT, animals are killed and the PDT treated tumors (10–30 mg) are excised and weighed. Tumor tissue is minced with a scalpel and is then disaggregated in 5–10 ml serum freed medium containing enzyme cocktail (0.05% collagenase type I, 0.015% pronase and 0.01% DNase, w/v). Tissue is kept at 37°C in a CO_2 incubator with continuous magnetical stirring at low speed for 1.5 h. Cells are washed with medium, diluted and plated in a Petri dish. Cell colonies are fixed 1–2 weeks after plating and stained with 0.5% crystal violet in methanol. Each colony represents a single surviving cell. Using this method, it was found that loss of tumor cell viability occurs considerable time after $AlPcS_n$ mediated PDT. This delayed cell death phenomenon reflects the occurrence of the indirect mechanism that is responsible for tumor cell killing (van Bruggen *et al*., 1992). In contrast, $AlPcS_2$ mediated PDT brought about a substantial reduction in tumor cell clonogenicity ($\sim$70%) immediately after photoirradiation (Chan *et al*., 1996). These results suggest the difference in action mechanisms between the mixed $AlPcS_n$ and the purified $AlPcS_2$.

Various methods have been employed to improve $AlPcS_n$ targetability. One approach is the use of antibody. Morgan *et al*. (1994) compared the direct and liposomal antibody conjugates of $AlPcS_n$ for selective photoimmuno-destruction of tumor cells *in vitro*. At the equimolar Pc dose the photocytotoxicity produced by both conjugates are similar. However, at the equimolar antibody, immunoliposomes possess greater efficacy (up to 13-fold) in killing tumor cells than the Pc-antibody conjugates. The *in vivo* activity of these conjugates remains to be determined.

Pc-antibody conjugate is prepared by mixing 3 mg of monoclonal antibody (in 2 ml carbonate buffer, 0.1 M at pH 9.6) and 2.5 mg of Pc (dissolved in 200 μl of dimethylsulfoxide). The mixture is stirred and incubated at room temperature for 2 h, then overnight at 4°C, to allow the formation of sulfonamide bonds between the chloride group of Pc and the free amino groups of the antibody. Unbound Pc can be separated on a Sepharose 6B-CL column (1.5 cm × 30 cm) previously equilibrated with buffer containing 10 mM Hepes and 145 mM NaCl at pH 7.3. The quantities of antibody and the Pc are estimated by absorbance at 280 nm and 675 nm, respectively. This procedure, as suggested, can couple an average of 10 molecules of Pc onto each antibody molecule. The conjugates which are Millipore-filtered (0.2 μm) and stored at 4°C in dark appear to be stable for at least 6 months.

Pc immunoliposomes are formed by 2 steps: the initial formation of Pc liposome and the subsequent antibody coupling. The lipid composition of liposome used is Lα-dipalmitoyl phosphatidylcholine (DPPC), dipalmitoyl phospatidylethanolamine-pyridyldithiopropionate (DPPE-DTP) and cholesterol (66 : 1 : 33 molar ratio). 100 μmol of total lipids are dissolved and mixed in chloroform. Following rotary evaporation, the dried film of lipids is suspended with 3 ml of Pc (1 mM) in Hepes/NaCl buffer, vortex mixed at 50°C, and passed through an extruder with 2 lot of 2 stacked polycarbonate membranes (0.2 and 0.1 μm) at 50°C under high pressure of N_2. Pc liposomes and free-Pc are separated on a Sephadex G50 column. *N*-hydroxysuccinimidyl 3-(2-pyridyldithio) propionate

(SPDP) is used as a linking agent for antibody and DPPE-DTP. Basically, 3 mg of antibody in 1 ml phosphate-buffered saline (PBS) and 1.7×10^{-7} mol SPDP (50 times molar excess) in 4.3 µl methanol are mixed and incubated at room temperature for 30 min. This mixture is titrated to pH 4.0 and is then added with dithiothreitol (0.5 M in water) to 50 mM final concentration. 1 ml of Pc liposome (containing 3 mM DPPC) is mixed with antibodies and allowed to incubate for at least 24 h at room temperature in the dark. Unbound antibody is removed by separation in a Spharose 6B-CL column. The authors estimated that the immunoliposome produced are in average of 100 nm diameter in size with a bilayer of 4 nm depth and each entraps ~250 molecules of Pc and couples with ~2.5 molecules of antibody.

ZINC PHTHALOCYANINE (ZnPc)

ZnPc because of hydrophobicity is insoluble in aqueous solution for intravenous delivery *in vivo*. Most studies on ZnPc/PDT utilize liposomes as Pc carrier. Previously, ZnPc liposomes were prepared by slow injection of solvent dissolved ZnPc and DPPC into aqueous phase (Valduga *et al.*, 1987). This method can only produce very diluted liposome suspension. An additional drawback is the toxicity of pyridine which is used as a solvent for ZnPc. The optimal method for manufacturing liposomes containing monomeric ZnPc in large scale has been developed (Isele *et al.*, 1994). Such procedure can be adopted to prepare small quantity of ZnPc liposome for laboratory investigation (Isele *et al.*, 1995) which is described below.

The lipid composition used here and the method for formation of liposomes are somewhat different than that for preparing immunoliposome described previously. In brief, 2 mg/ml of ZnPc dissolved in *N*-methylpyrrolidone is combined with 200 mg/2 ml of phospholipids (1-palmitoyl-2-oleoylphosphatidylcholine and 1,2-dioleoyl-phosphatidylserine; 9 : 1 w/w) in *tert*-butyl alcohol. ZnPc-liposome is formed by slowly diluting the preheated (50°C) organic phase into an excess (16- fold volume) of aqueous solution (4°C) containing 9.45% lactose and 0.027% NaCl, w/v, with vigorous magnetical stirring. The liposomal suspension is concentrated 10-fold at room temperature using stirred cells (Filtron) with a polyether sulfone membrane (MW 100-kDa cutoff). The suspension is then dialyzed (membrane MW cutoff of 6000–8000 Da) against 3 × 1 l of lactose/NaCl buffer to remove the remaining NMP and alcohol. Liposomes are sterilized by filtration through a 0.22 µm Millipore filter and are lyophilized for storage. Under these conditions, the liposomes formed are expected to be mainly unilamellar with 50–150 nm mean size and the incorporated ZnPc is in a monomeric state. The lyophilizates are stable for at least 6 months and the reconstituted liposomes should be physically unchanged for at least 24 h at room temperature.

The photodynamic efficacy of liposome-delivered ZnPc both *in vitro* and *in vivo* have been subjected for intensive studies. Extensive tumor necrosis that is comparable to that induced by Photofrin II (PII) can be generated by ZnPc mediated PDT at a drug dose > 20-fold lower than that used for PII (Reddi *et al*., 1990). The action mechanism of ZnPc induced necrosis was suggested to be predominantly the result of direct tumor cell cytotoxicity. Ultrastructural study on the treated tumor showed that damage to mitochondria and rough endoplasmic reticulum of the neoplastic cells are apparent early (3 h) after ZnPc/PDT, prior to any obvious histopathological changes in tumor associated capillaries (Milanesi *et al*., 1990). Re-implantation of tumor into the animal immediately after PDT, however, always produces tumor regrowth suggesting the presence of surviving tumor cells (van Lengoed *et al*., 1994). An additional mechanism, e.g., vascular damage, therefore contributes to the complete tumor regression observed with ZnPc/PDT. The exact extent of tumor cell killing induced by ZnPc-PDT whether it is via direct or/and indirect mechanism can be quantified using the clonogenic assay described previously.

Tissue uptake and retention of ZnPc can be determined using sodium dodecyl sulfate (SDS) extraction method (Reddi *et al*., 1987). This involves homogenizing excised tissues (~200 mg) in 4 ml of 2% SDS, followed by magnetic stirring for 1 h. Clear supernatant obtained by centrifugation (3000 rpm, 10 min) is measured spectrofluorimetricaly ($\lambda_{ex} = 610$ nm and $\lambda_{em} = 630$–740 nm) for determination of ZnPc content. It was found that tumors reach the maximum ZnPc retention (~$0.6\,\mu g\,g^{-1}$) at 18–24 h following drug administration ($0.5\,mg\,kg^{-1}$ b.w.). By that time there is little drug remaining in most normal tissues, which results in high drug content in tumor versus adjacent muscle as well as liver tissue (Shopova *et al*., 1992).

After administration of liposomal ZnPc, the drug was shown to be rapidly transferred to serum proteins where it binds almost exclusively to VLDL, LDL and HDL (Ginevra *et al*., 1990; Rensen *et al*., 1994). However, *in vitro* assays showed that only the presence of LDL can enhance ZnPc mediated photo-killing of cultured cells although the gross drug uptake in cells do not increase (Obochi *et al*., 1993). It was therefore postulated that, *in vivo*, ZnPc is largely transported into the cells via LDL receptor-mediated endocytosis where the subcellular targets are both susceptible to PDT damage and vital to cell survival. Attachment of LDL to photosensitizers thus seems worthwhile exploring for effective delivery of the sensitizers and enhancement of PDT efficacy.

Recently colloidal particles have been used as vehicles for delivering ZnPc derivatives to enhance tumor targeting. Such an approach should be suitable for delivering other types of metallo-Pc's with both hydrophilic and hydrophobic properties. In one system, Pc was encapsulated in nanocapsules formed by the interfacial polymerization of isohexylcyanoacrylate with poloxamer coating (Lenaerts *et al*., 1995). In another system poly (D, L-lactic acid) formulated nanoparticles containing polyethylene glycol coating (PEG, MW 20000) was employed (Allémann *et al*., 1995). These colloidal particles are biodegradable and possess low systemic toxicity. Both poloxamer and PEG coatings appear to play an important role in lowering hepatic uptake, as they provide a hydrophilic uncharged surface on the particles which protect against phagocytes and hence increase drug availability in tumor.

SILICON Pc (Pc 4)

Pc 4 [$HOSiPcOSi(CH_3)_2$-$(CH_2)_3N(CH_3)_2$] is the most potent SiPc derivative that has been tested for photoinactivation of cultured cells and was found to be more photo-potent than $AlPcS_n$ both in cells (Oleinick *et al.*, 1993) and in model membranes (Zaidi *et al.*, 1993). This increased activity of Pc 4 was suggested to be, in part, attributed by the presence of its axial ligand carrying an amine function. Pc 4, at the dose of 20 nM and 20 J/cm^2 red light, produced 6 $\log_{10}$ killing of breast cancer cells and HL-60 leukemia cells but no cytotoxicity to bone marrow progenitors (CFU-GM) (Pretti *et al.*, 1995) thus suggesting its potential for photolytic purging of cancer cells for autologous transplantation of bone marrow.

The use of Pc's for sterilization of infectious contaminants in red blood cell concentrate (RBCC) has been of major interest because of the intense absorption of red light where hemoglobin absorption is minimal. For this purpose, Pc 4 is particularly promising. It is not only highly potent in virus killing, but also effectively inactivates *Trypanosoma cruzi* and *Plasmodium falciparum* (the parasites that cause Chagas disease and malaria, respectively) in RBCC (Ben-Hur and Horowitz, 1995). Human immunodeficiency viruses (HIV) in all forms (cell free, cell associated, and latent) can be photoinactivated by Pc 4 ($\geqslant 5.5$, $\geqslant 6.5$ and $\geqslant 5.5 \log_{10}$ kill, respectively, at 2 μM drug dose and 90 J/cm^2 red light) (Margolis-Nunno *et al.*, 1996). However the mechanisms of inactivation appear to be different. In case of cell-free HIV, the lipid envelope is targeted; whereas latent HIV in infected cells is found to be susceptible to the loss of viral PCR signal, implicating destruction of viral genome, probably due to apoptosis (Ben-Hur *et al.*, 1997).

Following phototreatment, some RBC damage do occur which can be explained by binding of Pc 4 to RBC membrane. A sensitive, reproducible method has been developed for measuring Pc 4 content in RBC and plasma (Zuk *et al.*, 1995). Pc 4 treated RBCC is centrifuged at 2500 rpm (1300 g) for 15 min to separate plasma and RBC. Aliquot of 0.6 ml plasma, RBC or RBCC, is mixed with 0.1 ml of 8 M guanidine-HCl (aminomethaneguanidine hydrochloride). The mixture is incubated for 15 min at room temperature. Pc 4 is then extracted with 2.5 ml of acetonitrile by vortexing for 1 min and ultrasonication for another 10 min. Following centrifugation (2500 rpm), the acetonitrile layer is isolated and the residue is extracted once more and pooled. The extract is then dried by evaporation under N_2 stream at 45–50°C. The dried material is dissolved in 0.1 ml of 5% Cetrimide (hexadecyltrimethylammonium bromide), vortex-mixed, further diluted with 3 ml water and is then transferred to a C_{18} Sep-Pak reversed-phase cartridge (Waters). Pc 4 is eluted with 18 ml methanol and the eluant is dried by vacuum. The residue is dissolved in 1 ml methanol, filtered through a 0.45 μm filter, and is then analyzed in an HPLC system using C_{18} column. The mobile phase consists of 10% H_2O and 1% CH_3COOH in methanol. Fluorescence detection is set at $\lambda_{ex} = 610$ nm and $\lambda_{em} = 670$ nm. The detection limit is ~ 2 ng/ml. Recovery of Pc 4 in plasma was 100% and in RBCC was $> 80\%$. When incubation of Pc 4 in RBCC at 2 μM concentration, it was found that 42% were associated with plasma whereas 58% of drug were associated with RBC of which 97% of Pc 4 were membrane associated.

To reduce Pc 4 binding on, or, induced damage to RBC without reducing the virucidal effect, some physical and chemical parameters have been employed. One approach is to use highlight fluence rate (Ben-Hur *et al*., 1995a). Although the phenomenon is not readily explainable, it was found that RBC was less susceptible to sensitizer mediated photodamage at 80 mW/cm^2 than at 5 mW/cm^2 while virus killing was not affected by such changes.

Other approaches involve the use of quenchers. RBC photodamage is suggested to be caused by both type I and type II energy transfer reaction whereas virus killing is mainly caused by type II reaction. Therefore addition of agents, such as mannitol and GSH (reduced glutathione), that specifically quench radicals generated by type I reaction, prior to photoirradiation, can effectively reduce RBC damage but without reducing anti-viral activity (Rywkin *et al*., 1992, 1995). GSH also prevents Pc-sensitized IgG binding to RBCs. Trolox, a water soluble vitamin E analogue, was shown to be able to reduce RBC potassium leakage and to prevent Pc-induced reduction of negative charge on RBCs following photosensitization. The optimal concentrations of these quenchers in RBCC are set out to be 4, 4 and 5 mM, for mannitol, GSH and Trolox, respectively (Margolis-Nunno *et al*., 1996). These quenchers should be added to RBCC prior to photoirradiation.

Delivery vehicle can also have influence on the integrity of RBC following Pc photosensitization. In the earlier studies, SiPc derivatives were delivered in DMSO because of their insolubility in aqueous solution. Recently, using cremophor EL (CRM, polyoxyethylene glycol triricinoleate) for formulation, despite the fact that a slight increase of Pc 4 was found to bind on RBC versus that formulated with DMSO, there was a significant reduction in RBC hemolysis but without affecting virucidal activity. It was postulated that Pc 4 formulated in CRM may bind on RBC at the site which is less sensitive to photodamage and/or may be in an aggregated form upon binding which is photochemically inactive (Ben-Hur *et al*., 1995b). Pc 4 in CRM solution is prepared by dissolving Pc 4 (3 mg) in 2 ml methanol. 1 ml of prewarmed (45°C) CRM is dropped slowly into the methanol solution with vigorous mixing. Methanol is evaporated and 9 ml of PBS is added to obtain final concentration of 10% CRM and 0.4 mM Pc 4.

REFERENCES

Allémann, E., Brasseur, N., Benrezzak, O., Rousseau, J., Kudrevich, S. V., Boyle, R. W., Leroux, J.-C., Gurny, R., and van Lier, J. E. (1995): PEG-coated poly(lactic acid) nanoparticles for the delivery of hexadecafluoro zinc phthalocyanine to EMT-6 mouse mammary tumours. *J. Pharm. Pharmacol.* **47**, 382–387.

Anholt, H., Peng, Q., and Moan, J. (1994): Uptake, localization and effect of laser treatment on CaD2 tumors sensitized with aluminum phthalocyanine tetrasulfonate. *Lasers Med. Sci.* **9**, 111–118.

Barr, H., Tralau, C. J., Boulos, P. B., Mac Robert, A. J., Krasner, N., Phillips, D., and Bown, S. G. (1990): Selective necrosis in dimethylhydrazine-induced rat colon tumours using phthalocyanine photodynamic therapy. *Gastroenterology* **98**, 1532–1537.

Ben-Hur, E., Geacintov, N. E., Studamire, B., Kenney, M. E., and Horowitz, B. (1995a): The effect of irradiance on virus sterilization and photodynamic damage in red blood cells sensitized by phthalocyanines. *Photochem. Photobiol.* **61**, 190–195.

Ben-Hur, E. and Horowitz, B. (1995): Advances in photochemical approaches for blood sterilization. *Photochem. Photobiol.* **62**, 102–108.

Ben-Hur, E., Oetjen, J., and Horowitz, B. (1997): Silicon pthalocyanine Pc4 and red light causes apoptosis in HIV-infected cells. *Photochem. Photobiol.* **65**, 456–460.

Ben-Hur, E. and Rosenthal, I. (1985): The phthalocyanines: a new class of mammalian cells photosensitizers with a potential for cancer phototherapy. *Int. J. Radiat. Biol.* **47**, 145–147.

Ben-Hur, E., Zuk, M. M., Chin, S., Banerjee, D., Kenney, M. E., and Horowitz, B. (1995b): Biodistribution and virus inactivation efficacy of a silicon phthalocyanine in red blood cell concentrates as a function of delivery vehicle. *Photochem. Photobiol.* **62**, 575–579.

Ben-Hur, E., Zuk, M. M., Orenstein, A., Rosenthal, I., and Crane, S. W. (1990): Mechanism and relevance to photodynamic therapy of chloroaluminum sulfonated phthalocyanine tissue distribution in dogs. *Lasers Life Sci.* **3**, 255–262.

Chan, W. S., Brasseur, N., La Madeleine, C., and van Lier, J. E. (1996): Evidence for different mechanisms of EMT-6 tumor necrosis by photodynamic therapy with disulfonated aluminium phthalocyanine or photofrin: tumor cell survival and blood flow. *Anticancer Res.* **16**, 1887–1892.

Chan, W. S., Marshall, J. F., and Hart, I. R. (1987): Photodynamic therapy of a murine tumor following sensitisation with chloro aluminum sulfonated phthalocyanine. *Photochem. Photobiol.* **46**, 867–871.

Chan, W. S., Marshall, J. F., and Hart, I. R. (1989): Effect of tumour location on selective uptake and retention of phthalocyanines. *Cancer Lett.* **44**, 73–77.

Chan, W. S., Marshall, J. F., Lam, G. Y. F., and Hart, I. R. (1988): Tissue uptake, distribution, and potency of the photoactivable dye chloroaluminium sulfonated phthalocyanine in mice bearing transplantable tumors. *Cancer Res.* **48**, 3040–3044.

Chan, W. S., West, C. M. L., Moore, J. V., and Hart, I. R. (1991): Photocytotoxic efficacy of sulphonated species of aluminium phthalocyanine against cell monolayers, multicellular spheroids and *in vivo* tumors. *Br. J. Cancer* **64**, 827–832.

Chatlani, P. T., Bedwell, J., MacRobert, A. J., Barr, H., Boulos, P. B., Krasner, N., Phillips, D., and Bown, S. G. (1991): Comparisons of distribution and photodynamic effects of di- and tetra-sulphonated aluminum phthalocyanine in normal rat colon. *Photochem. Photobiol.* **53**, 745–751.

Chatlani, P. T., Nuutinen, P. J. O., Toda, N., Barr, H., MacRobert, A. J., Bedwell, J., and Bown, S. G. (1992): Selective necrosis in hamster pancreatic tumours using photodynamic therapy with phthalocyanine photosensitization. *Brit. J. Surg.* **79**, 786–790.

Chen, J. Y., Chen, W., and Cai, H. X. (1993): Studies on pharmacokinetics of sulfonated aluminum phthalocyanine in a transplantable mouse tumor by *in vivo* fluorescence. *J. Photochem. Photobiol. B: Biol.* **18**, 233–237.

Ginevra, F., Biffanti, S., Pagnan, A., Biolo, R., Reddi, E., and Jori, G. (1990): Delivery of the tumour photosensitizer zinc(II)-phthalocyanine to serum proteins by different liposomes: studies *in vitro* and *in vivo*. *Cancer Lett.* **49**, 59–65.

Henderson, B. W., Waldow, S. M., Mang, T. S., Potter, W. R., Malone, P. B., and Dougherty, T. J. (1985): Tumor destruction and kinetics of tumor cell death in two experimental mouse tumors following photodynamic therapy. *Cancer Res.* **45**, 572–576.

Hiraoka, Y., Sedat, J. W., and Argad, D. A. (1987): The use of a charge-coupled device for quantitative optical microscopy of biological structures, *Science* **238**, 36–41.

Isele, U., Schieweck, K., Kessler, R., van Hoogevest, P., and Capraro, H.-G. (1994): Pharmacokinetics and body distribution of liposomal zinc phthalocyanine in tumor-bearing mice: Influence of aggregation state, particle size, and composition. *J. Pharm. Sci.* **84**, 166–173.

Isele, U., van Hoogevest, P., Hilfiker, R., Capraro, H.-G., Schieweck, K., and Leuenberger, H. (1994): Large-scale production of liposomes containing monomeric zinc phthalocyanine by controlled dilution of organic solvents. *J. Pharm. Sci.* **83**, 1608–1616.

Leach, M. W., Khoshyomn, S., Bringus, J., Autry, S. A., and Boggan, J. E. (1993): Normal brain tissue response to photodynamic therapy using aluminum phthalocyanine tetrasulfonate in the rat. *Photochem. Photobiol.* **57**, 842–845.

Leach, M. W. and Peaston, A. E. (1994): Adverse drug reaction attributable to aluminum phthalocyanine tetrasulfonate administration in domestic cats. *Vet. Pathol.* **31**, 283–287.

Lenaerts, V., Labib, A., Chouinard, F., Rousseau, F., Ali, H., and van Lier, J. E. (1995): Nanocapsules with a reduced liver uptake: Targeting of phthalocyanines to EMT-6 mouse mammary tumour *in vivo*. *Eur. J. Pharm. Biopharm.* **41**, 38–43.

Mang, T. S., Dougherty, T. J., Potter, W. R., Boyle, D. G., Sommer, S., and Moan, J. (1987): Photobleaching of porphyrins used in photodynamic therapy and implications for therapy. *Photochem. Photobiol.* **45**, 501–507.

Margolis-Nunno, H., Ben-Hur, E., Gottlieb, P., Robinson, R., Oetjen, J., and Horowitz, B. (1996): Inactivation of multiple forms of human immunodeficiency virus in red cell concentrates by phthalocyanine photosensitization. *Transfusion*, **36**, 743–750.

Milanesi, C., Zhou, C., Biolo, R., and Jori, G. (1990): Zn(II)-phthalocyanine as a photodynamic agent for tumours. II. Studies on the mechanism of photosensitised tumour necrosis. *Br. J. Cancer* **61**, 846–850.

Morgan, J., Lottman, H., Abbou, C. C., and Chopin, D. K. (1994): A comparison of direct and liposomal antibody conjugates of sulfonated aluminum phthalocyanines for selective photoimmunotherapy of human bladder carcinoma. *Photochem. Photobiol.* **60**, 486–496.

Nelson, J. S., Liaw, L.-H., Orenstein, A., Roberts, W. G., and Berns, M. W. (1988): Mechanism of tumor destruction following photodynamic therapy with hematoporphyrin derivative, chlorin, and phthalocyanine. *J. Natl. Cancer Inst.* **80**, 1599–1605.

Obochi, M. O. K., Boyle, R. W., and van Lier, J. E. (1993): Biological activities of phthalocyanines. XIII. The effects of human serum components on the *in vitro* uptake and photodynamic activity of zinc phthalocyanine. *Photochem. Photobiol.* **57**, 634–640.

Oleinick, N. L., Antunez, A. R., Clay, M. E., Rihter, B. D., and Kenney, M. E. (1993): New phthalocyanine photosensitizers for photodynamic therapy. *Photochem. Photobiol.* **57**, 242–247.

Peavy, G. M., Krasieva, T. B., Tromberg, B. J., Eusantos, E. D., and Berns, M. W. (1995): Variations in the distribution of a phthalocyanine photosensitizer in naturally occurring tumors of animals. *J. Photochem. Photobiol. B: Biol.* **27**, 271–277.

Peng, Q. and Moan, J. (1995): Correlation of distribution of sulphonated aluminium phthalocyanines with their photodynamic effect in tumour and skin of mice bearing CaD2 mammary carcinoma. *Brit. J. Cancer* **72**, 565–574.

Peng, Q., Moan, J., Nesland, J. M., and Rimington, C. (1990): Aluminum phthalocyanines with asymmetrical lower sulfonation and with symmetrical higher sulfonation: a comparison of localizing and photosensitizing mechanism in human tumor LOX xenografts. *Int. J. Cancer* **46**, 719–726.

Pope, A. J., MacRobert, A. J., Phillips, D., and Bown, S. G. (1991): The detection of phthalocyanine fluorescence in normal rat bladder wall using sensitive digital imaging microscopy. *Br. J. Cancer* **64**, 875–879.

Pretti, R., Fitzgerald, M., Keij, J. F., Visser, J. W. M., and Ben-Hur, E. (1995): Photolytic purging of SK-BR3 and HL-60 tumor cells with the phthalocyanine Pc 4. *J. Hematotherapy* **4**, 246 (abstract).

Reddi, E., Lo Castro, G., Biolo, R., and Jori, G. (1987): Pharmacokinetic studies with zinc(II)-phthalocyanine in tumour-bearing mice. *Br. J. Cancer* **56**, 597–600.

Reddi, E., Zhou, C., Biolo, R., Menegaldo, E., and Jori, G. (1990): Zn(II)-phthalocyanine as a photodynamic agent for tumours. I. Pharmacokinetic properties and phototherapeutic efficiency. *Br. J. Cancer* **61**, 407–411.

Rensen, P. C. N., Love, W. G., and Taylor, P. W. (1994): *In vitro* interaction of zinc(II)-phthalocyanine-containing liposomes and plasma lipoproteins. *J. Photochem. Photobiol. B: Biol.* **26**, 29–35.

Roberts, W. G., Klein, M. K., and Loomis, M. (1991): Photodynamic therapy of spontaneous cancers in felines, canines and snakes with chloroaluminum sulfonated phthalocyanine. *J. Natl. Cancer Inst.* **83**, 18–23.

Rywkin, S., Ben-Hur, E., Reid, M. E., Oyen, R., Ralph, H., and Horowitz, B. (1995): Selective protection against IgG binding to red cells treated with phthalocyanines and red light for virus inactivation. *Transfusion* **35**, 414–420.

Rywkin, S., Lenny, L., Goldstein, J., Geacintov, N., Margolis-Nunno, H., and Horowitz, B. (1992): Importance of type I and type II mechanisms in the photodynamic inactivation of viruses in blood with aluminum phthalocyanine derivatives. *Photochem. Photobiol.* **56**, 463–469.

Selman, S. H., Kreimer-Birnbaum, M., Chaudhuri, K., Garbo, G. M., Seaman, D. A., Keck, R. W., Ben-Hur, E., and Rosenthal, I. (1986): Photodynamic treatment of transplantable bladder tumors in rodents after pretreatment with chloroaluminum tetrasulfophthalocyanine. *J. Urol.* **136**, 141–145.

Shopova, M., Mantareva, V., Krastev, K., Hadjiolov, D., Milev, A., Spirov, K., Jori, G., and Ricchelli, F. (1992): Comparative pharmacokinetic and photodynamic studies with zinc(II)-phthalocyanine in hamsters bearing an induced or transplanted rhabdomyosarcoma. *J. Photochem. Photobiol. B: Biol.* **16**, 83–89.

Valduga, G., Reddi, E., and Jori, G. (1987): Spectroscopic studies on Zn(II)-phthalocyanine in homogeneous and microheterogeneous systems. *J. Inorg. Biochem.* **25**, 59–65.

van Bruggen, N., Chan, W. S., Syha, J., Marshall, J. F., Proctor, E., Williams, S. R., Gadian, D. G., and Hart, I. R. (1992): Cell and tissue responses of a murine tumour to phthalocyanine-mediated photodynamic therapy. *Eur. J. Cancer* **28**, 42–46.

van Lengoed, H. L. L. M., Cuomo, V., Versteeg, A. A. C., van der Veen, N., Jori, G., and Star, W. M. (1994): *In vivo* fluorescence and photodynamic activity of zinc phthalocyanine administered in liposomes. *Br. J. Cancer* **69**, 640–845.

Weintraub, H., Abramovici, A., Altman, A., Ben-Hur, E., and Rosenthal, I. (1988): Toxicity, tissue distribution and excretion studies of aluminum phthalocyanine tetrasulfonate in mice. *Lasers Life Sci.* **2**, 185–196.

Zaidi, S. I. A., Agrawal, R., Eichler, G., Rihter, B. D., Kenney, M. E., and Mukhtar, H. (1993): Photodynamic effects of new silicon phthalocyanines: *In vitro* studies utilizing rat hepatic microsomes and human erythrocyte ghosts as model membrane sources. *Photochem. Photobiol.* **58**, 204–210.

Zuk, M. M., Kenney, M. E., Horowitz, B., and Ben-Hur, E. (1995): High-performance liquid chromatographic determination of the silicon phthalocyanine Pc 4 in human blood. *J. Chromatogr. B* **673**, 320–324.

Zuk, M. M., Tyczkowska, K., Ben-Hur, E., Newman, H. C., Rosenthal, I., and Crane, S. W. (1988): Reversed-phase liquid chromatographic determination of chloroaluminum phthalocyanine tetrasulfonate in canine tissues and fluids. *J. Chromat. Biomed. Appl.* **433**, 367–372.

2.5. NAPHTHALOCYANINES AS PHOTOSENSITIZERS FOR PDT

H. KLIESCH, ANDREA WEITEMEYER, ULRIKE MICHELSEN, MARIA SHOPOVA, and DIETER WÖHRLE

2.5.1. INTRODUCTION

The interest for long wavelength absorbing photosensitizers directed the research of scientists to new classes of dyes. Recently 2,3-naphthalocyanines (Nc) (Fig. 1), the tetrabenzo-annelated phthalocyanines, have been proposed as PDT photosensitizers (Cuomo *et al.*, 1990; Yates *et al.*, 1990; Paquette *et al.*, 1990; Ho *et al.*, 1990; Sounik, 1990), because these compounds show intense absorption between 750–850 nm (extinction coefficient greater than $10^5\,L\,mol^{-1}\,cm^{-1}$). In this spectral region the light penetration through skin and tissue is substantially higher than that at 630 nm (λ_{max} of HpD) (Svaasand *et al.*, 1990; see also Chapter 3.2.1) which allows the treatment of larger and deeper lying tumors. The penetration depth of light below 700 nm in heavily pigmented tumors (like pigmented melanoma) is lower than in normal tissue (Svaasand *et al.*, 1990) due to the absorption and light scattering properties of melanin. Whereas HpD and Photofrin are not suitable for the treatment of such tumors (Dougherty, 1987; Zhou, 1989), naphthalocyanines are a very promising alternative (Biolo *et al.*, 1994).

2.5.2. OVERVIEW ON 2,3-NAPHTHALOCYANINES

In the following chapter an overview about the synthesis, some general properties and some results on the photodynamic activity of 2,3-naphthalocyanines is given. Then for *in vivo* experiments, the photodynamic activity of differently substituted naphthalocyanines using liposomes as delivery systems is shown in more detail in order to demonstrate the excellent properties of these compounds for the treatment of tumors. The final discussion will critically reveal the liposome delivery method and show possibilities to improve the selectivity of tumor accumulation of such photosensitizers.

a. Synthesis of Naphthalocyanines

2,3-Naphthalocyanines were synthesized first by Bradbrook and Linstead (Bradbrook *et al.*, 1936). Today various 2,3-naphthalocyanines with different substituents and different central metal ions are known. For the syntheses naphthalene-2,3-dicarboxylic acid derivatives are employed as starting compounds. In most cases naphthalene-2,3-dicarbonitriles (e.g. Mikhalenko *et al.*,

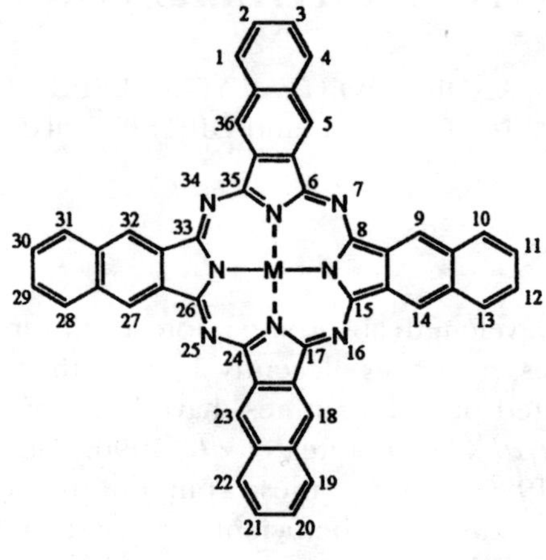

2,3-naphthalocyanine (Nc)
tetranaphtho[2,3-b:2,3-g:2,3,3-l:2,3-q]porphyrazine

Substituents	M	λ_{max} *in* nm (ε *between* 2 *and* 5×10^5 L $mol^{-1}cm^{-1}$)	*Ref.*
Unsubstituted, 2,11,20,30-tetraalkyl substituted	2 H(I)	~ 780/750	a
Unsubstituted, 2,11,20,30-tetraalkyl substituted	Zn(II), Al(III)X	~ 765–775	a, b
1–4 Sulfonic acid groups by statistical substitution	Zn(II), Al(II)X	~ 760–770	c
2,11,20,30-tetraalkoxy,-amino, -amido substituted	Zn(II)	~ 770/780	d
2,3,11,12,20,21,29,30-octaalkoxy substituted or octaalkylthio substituted	Zn(II) Cu(II)	~ 800	e
1,4,9,14,18,23,27,32-octaalkyloxy substituted	—	—	f
Unsubstituted	Si (OSialkyl, aryl)$_4$	~ 770–780	g

[a] Lukyanets *et al.*, 1989; [b] Wöhrle *et al.*, 1992; [c] Paquette *et al.*, 1990; [d] Wöhrle *et al.*, 1993; Müller *et al.*, 1996; [e] Kitahara *et al.*, 1990; [f] Cook *et al.*, 1988; [g] Firey *et al.*, 1987; Ford *et al.*, 1988.

Figure 1 Structures of 2,3-naphthalocyanines and their Q-band transitions.

1969; Kovshev *et al.*, 1972; Paquette *et al.*, 1990) or their diiminoisoindolenines (e.g. Brach *et al.*, 1970; Kitahara *et al.*, 1990; Wheeler *et al.*, 1984) were used.

Also syntheses starting from naphthalene-2,3-dicarboxylic acid (Vogeler *et al.*, 1980), their imides and anhydrides (Goncharova *et al.*, 1982) are known. In general the employed compounds were heated in bulk (Mikhalenko *et al.*, 1969; Wöhrle *et al.*, 1993) or in high boiling solvents (e.g. chinoline, chlornaphthalene

(Kovshev *et al.*, 1972) or urea (Kovshev *et al.*, 1972b)) up to temperatures of around 200°C. Another possibility is the cyclotetramerisation in pentanol in the presence of the strong base DBU (Wöhrle *et al.*, 1992). If the syntheses are carried out in the presence of metal salts, the corresponding metal complexes are obtained. The metal free Ncs can be synthesized also by reacting dinitriles with lithium in pentanol (Cook *et al.*, 1988). The dilithium(I)-naphthalocyanines were obtained which can be converted easily into the metal free compounds by strong acids and then metalated with various metal salts in polar organic solvents like DMF. In contrast, Al(III)- or Si(IV)naphthalocyanines are synthesized only when $AlCl_3$ (Paquette *et al.*, 1990) or $SiCl_4$ (Wheeler *et al.*, 1984) are present during the cyclotetramerization of the dinitriles.

Substituents at the naphthalene units are introduced by employing substituted naphthalene carboxylic acid derivatives (Kovshev *et al.*, 1972b) or by reacting unsubstituted Nc's with sulfuric acid (Paquette *et al.*, 1990). Further reactions at these substituents can be carried out afterwards (Wöhrle *et al.*, 1993; Müller *et al.*, 1996). Si(Cl_2)Nc's can be modified by exchanging the chlorine with other substituents like alcohols.

Very essential for the use of Ncs is their purification. A general method uses at first treatment with solvents in a Soxhlet-apparatus followed by e.g. flash chromatography. The yields of Nc's in dependence on the method and kind of substituents are in the order of 10–60%. No general rule which method results in higher yields can be given.

b. General Properties of Naphthalocyanines

The solubility of Nc's depends on the kind of substituent at the ligand. Some substituted naphthalocyanines are good soluble in various organic solvents, whereas unsubstituted Ncs are only slightly soluble in DMF and chloronaphthalene. Substituted as well as unsubstituted naphthalocyanines can be solubilized monomeric in aqueous solution in the presence of liposome forming materials.

The UV/Vis-spectra of naphthalocyanines are characterized by major absorptions in the Soret-band region at around 350 nm and with higher intensity in the Q-band region at 750–850 nm with their detailed positions in dependence on the ligand, substituents and solvent (Figs. 1 and 2). The central metal ion has only a limited effect on the absorption wavelength, but the metal ion strongly influences other photophysical properties. High values of the product of triplet quantum yield and triplet lifetime lead to high singlet oxygen quantum yields. Porphyrazine dyes with Zn(II), Al(III) and Si(IV) as central ions show good values in contrast to those with Cu(II), Fe(II) or metal free compounds (Röder *et al.*, 1991). Despite of the fact that energy transfer from the triplet state of Si(IV)-naphthalocyanine to $^3O_2$ is slightly endergonic, the process has a high efficiency ($\Phi_\Delta = 0.19 \pm 0.02$) (Firey *et al.*, 1987; Ford *et al.*, 1988). Singlet oxygen quantum yields of Zn(II)-naphthalocyanines are higher with values of around 0.4 (Michelsen *et al.*, 1996; Müller *et al.*, 1996), and naphthalocyanines absorbing above 800 nm also produce $^1O_2$ in satisfactory amounts (Wöhrle *et al.*, 1994).

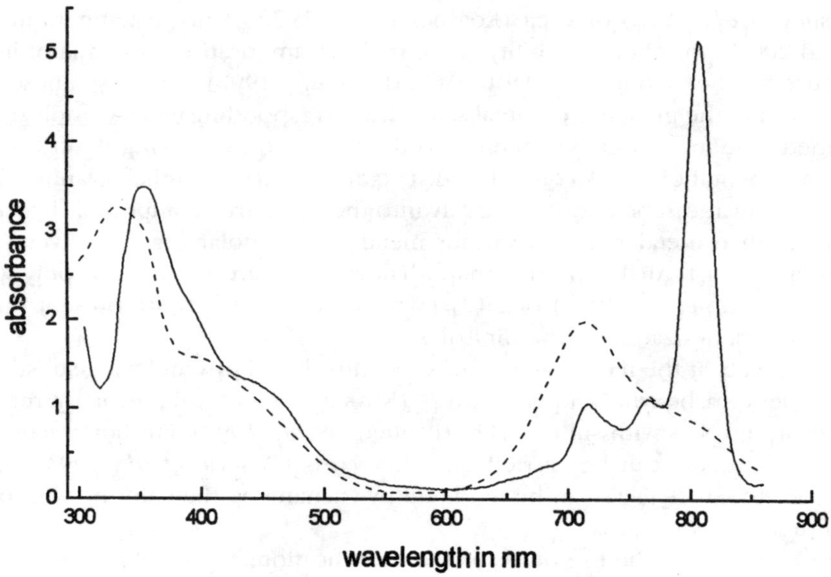

Figure 2 UV/Vis-spectra of aggregated (in hexane----) and monomeric (in DMF——) 1,4,9,14,18,23,27,32-octaoctylthio-zinc(II)-2,3-naphthalocyanine.

These values were determined for the monomeric naphthalocyanines in polar solvents DMF. Because Nc's are large planar aromatic systems, they have a strong tendency to form aggregates, which can be seen in the Vis-spectra (Fig. 2). This tendency is more pronounced compared to phthalocyanines (e.g. aluminum(III)-phthalocyanine-tetrasulfonic acid is monomeric in water, whereas the analogue naphthalocyanine is also water soluble but aggregated). The aggregated forms of porphyrazines produce little or no singlet oxygen (Daraio *et al.*, 1991).

Another important property of Nc's that may influence the photodynamic activity is the photooxidative stability. Compared to phthalocyanines, Nc's are less stable when exposed to light in the presence of oxygen (Schnurpfeil *et al.*, 1997; see Chapter 3.2.3). Too fast photobleaching of the dyes in the tumor under irradiation may lead to a reduced PDT effect. Because bleaching of the photosensitizers in upper cellular layers increases the therapeutical depth of the light (Dougherty *et al.*, 1991), limited photostability can also have positive influences (see also Mang *et al.*, 1987).

c. Naphthalocyanines in PDT

Several Nc's were tested as PDT photosensitizers. They contain Al(III), Si(IV) or Zn(II) as central metal ions. Since sulfonated phthalocyanines show very promising results (Berg *et al.*, 1989; Paquette *et al.*, 1990), similar good properties were expected for analogous Nc's. But sulfonated Zn(II)- and Al(III)-naphthalocyanines exhibit only poor photodynamic effects after in *in vitro* cell experiments compared to phthalocyanines (Paquette *et al.*, 1990; Yates *et al.*, 1990). It was found that the investigated compounds are strongly aggregated in the examined cell lines (Yates *et al.*, 1990). In addition it was shown that the monomeric Nc's were photobleached rapidly (Yates *et al.*, 1990), whereas the inactive aggregated naphthalocyanines were relatively photostable (Paquette *et al.*, 1990; Yates *et al.*, 1990).

Therefore other authors used Si(IV)-naphthalocyanines (Biolo *et al.*, 1994; Cuomo *et al.*, 1990), which are more photostable (Schnurpfeil *et al.*, 1997) and exhibit a lower tendency to form aggregates (Zuk *et al.*, 1994). Incorporation of the naphthalocyanines into liposomes reduces the degree of aggregation and delivers the compounds in a monomeric form to the cells. The experiments with liposome delivered Si(IV)-Ncs showed a satisfactory phototoxic effect (Biolo *et al.*, 1994) but low accumulation of the sensitizer in the tumor tissue in comparison to the surrounding tissue.

2.5.3. LIPOSOME DELIVERED Zn(II)-2,3-NAPHTHALOCYANINES

A number of investigations showed that hydrophobic Zn(II)-Nc's incorporated into unilamellar liposomes of DL-α-dipalmitoylphosphatidylcholine (DPPC) are after *in vivo* experiments active photosensitizers for PDT. By these investigations the influence of different substituents at the naphthalene units on the photodynamic efficiency for the treatment of the agressive Lewis lung carcinoma was studied (Wöhrle *et al.*, 1993; Shopova *et al.*, 1994; Mantareva *et al.*, 1994; Müller *et al.*, 1996). As additional tumor model a pigmented melanoma was selected in order to compare the photodynamic activity of photosensitizers absorbing at different wavelength (Shopova *et al.*, 1996).

a. Materials and Methods

The following Zn(II)-Nc's with four substituents in the positions 2,11,20,29 (and structural isomers) (see. Fig. 1) were synthesized starting from substituted 2,3-naphthalenedicarbonitriles (Mantareva *et al.*, 1994; Müller *et al.*, 1996): ZnNc1, unsubstituted; ZnNc2, $-NHCOCH_3$; ZnNc3, $-NH_2$; ZnNc4, $-NHCOC_6H_5$; ZnNc5, $-NHCOC_6H_4OCH_3$; ZnNc6, $-NHCOC_5H_{11}$; ZnNc7, $-NHCOC_{11}H_{23}$. After the UV/Vis-spectra the ZnNcs are incorporated monomeric into the liposome vesicles in aqueous solution.

Two tumor models in the right kind leg of male C57Bl/6 mice were used: Lewis lung carcinoma (LLC) (external diameter 3–5 mm) and B 16 pigmented melanoma (external diameter 3–4 mm). Twenty-four hours after intraperitoneal liposome-incorporated drug injection (ZnNc concentrations of only 0.3–0.5 mg kg^{-1} b.w. compared to Photofrin with around 3–5 mg kg^{-1} b.w.) irradiation in the absorption maximum of the photosensitizer by an Argon-dye laser connected with a laser fibre was carried out with a fluence of 350–450 J cm^{-2} (power at the end of the fiber around 40 mW to avoid temperature increase; see Reddi *et al.*, 1990).

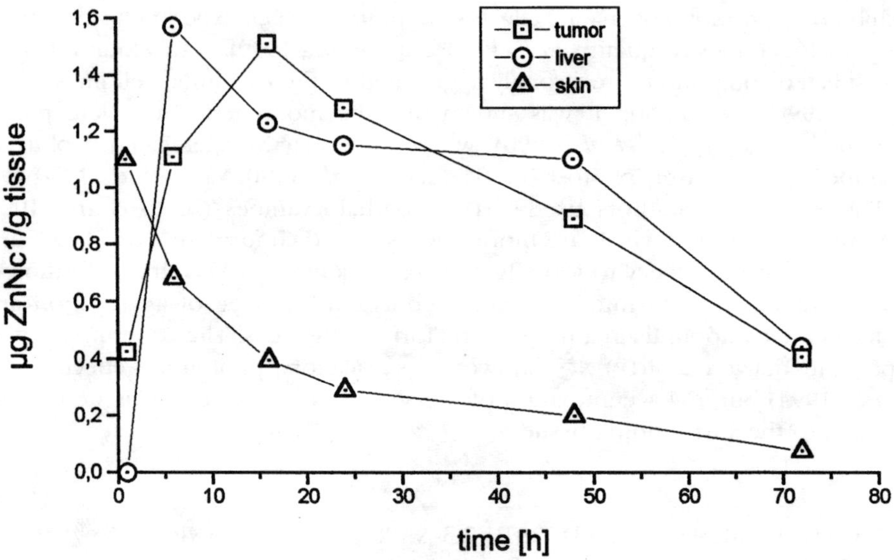

Figure 3 Pharmacokinetic of ZnNc1 in different tissues.

b. Results

The pharmacokinetic studies showed similar results for all examined photosensitizers. For the LLC tumor model the concentration of the ZnNc's in the tumor reached 16–20 h after injection around 1.5 µg per gram tissue (Fig. 3). At this time the concentration of the ZnNc's in skin was around 0.4 µg per gram (tumor/surrounding tissue (here skin) ratios around 4 : 1). The amount of dyes in skin dropped below 0.1 µg per gram at 72 h after injection (with further falling tendency) making a long term skin sensibilization unlikely. Since liposomes were used as delivery system, the photosensitizers accumulate also in inner organs like liver. But after *in vitro* experiments no dark toxicity was observed (M. Peeva, H. Diddens, D. Wöhrle, manuscript in preparation). After photodynamic treatment three main parameters were observed: the tumor regrowth, the average surviving time and the formation of metastasis.

Surprisingly, the very low concentrations of photosensitizers used led to a significant delay in the tumor regrowth. Tumor growth was inhibited in the following decreasing order:

ZnNc4 (▲) > ZnNc6 (□) > ZnNc2 (◆) > ZnNc1 (●) ≫ ZnNc5 (Δ) > ZnNc3 (◊) > ZnNc7 (○) ≫ control, without ZnNc (■).

In addition it is important to mention that with the aggressive LLC tumor the number of metastases after PDT was also reduced; e.g. only 25% of the animals treated with ZnNc4 developed lung metastasis 14 days after tumor implantation (mean 7 days after PDT treatment) compared to 75% of the untreated control group. The total volume of the metastasis was 4.5 times lower than that of the control animals (Mantareva *et al.*, 1994).

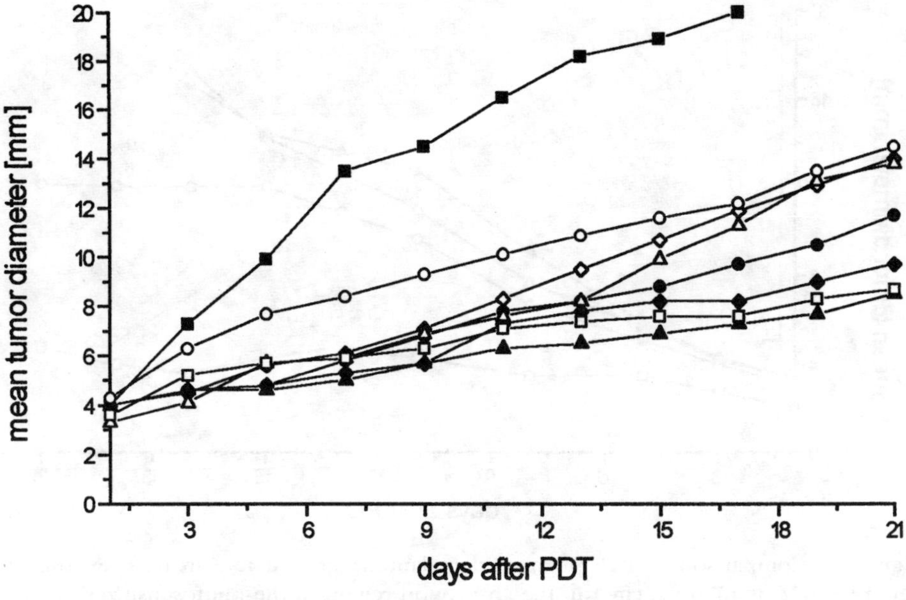

Figure 4 Comparison of the tumor growth (mean tumor diameter of LLC versus time) for the control group and the PDT treated mice employing ZnNc1–7 (symbols see text) incorporated into liposomes.

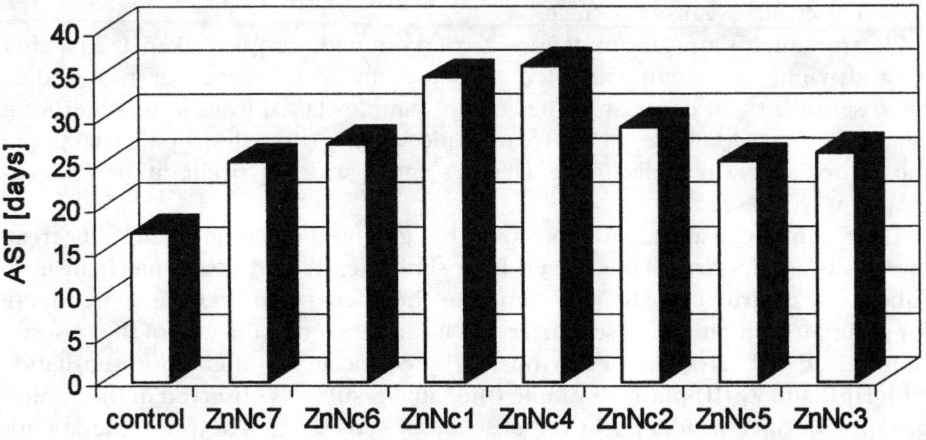

Figure 5 Average survival time of mice bearing LLC after PDT treatment using ZnNc1–7.

Following the lethality of the animals up to the end of the observation period (a month after tumor implantation and 25 days after PDT) a statistically reliable increase in the average survival time was established for the treated compared with the untreated (control) animals (Fig. 5). The AST was prolonged by the

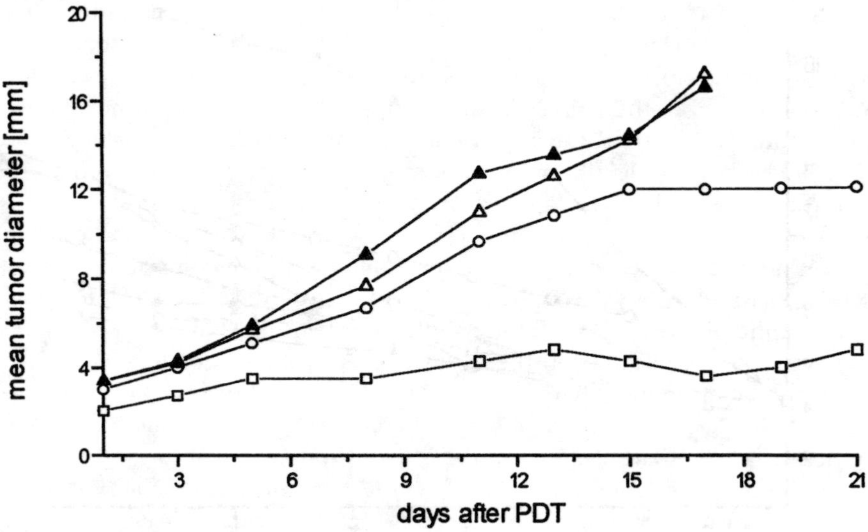

Figure 6 Comparison of B16 pigmented melanoma growth rate in mice exposed to light of 360 J cm^2 (370 mW cm^2) in the absorption region of the photosensitizer. Δ: HpD (5 mg kg^{-1} b.w., irradiation at 630 nm). ▲: ZnPc (0.3 mg kg^{-1} b.w., irradiation at 673 nm). ○: ZnNc1 (0.3 mg kg^{-1} b.w., irradiation at 756 nm). □: ZnNc4 (0.5 mg kg^{-1} b.w., irradiation at 774 nm).

sensitizers with the following declining efficiency: ZnNc4 > ZnNc1 > ZnNc2 > ZnNc6 ≫ ZnNc3 > ZnNc5 > ZnNc7.

Electron-microscopic examinations carried out with samples taken at 24 h after photodynamic treatment exhibited one and the same trend for the studied photosensitizers. In contrast to the control samples taken from untreated tumor bearing mice, the samples of the treated mice clearly show dystrophic changes in the cytoplasmic organelles. The changes most strongly occur at the tumors treated with ZnNc4.

The morphological examinations of B16 pigmented melanoma cells after treatment with ZnNcs are characterized by a similar early and direct mechanism of subcellular destruction. Figure 6 compares the effect of photodynamic treatment for different generations of sensitizers. As it can be seen at the end of the observation period (21 days after PDT) no PDT-effect occurred after photosensitation with HpD and Zn(II)-phthalocyanine (the same result was observed in the control group with mice irradiated in the absence of sensitizer). The phototherapeutic effect is however pronounced with ZnNcs, especially with the ZnNc4.

c. Discussion

In contrast to Si(IV)Nc's (Biolo *et al.*, 1994) the pharmacokinetic studies show that zinc(II)-naphthalocyanines incorporated into liposomes accumulate in the tumor. Zn(II)Nc's delivered by liposomes are in a satisfactory degree monomeric in the tumor cells, and their photooxidative stability is high enough to induce lethal cellular damage. Another positive effect of the examined photosensitizers is the direct early alteration of neoplastic cells under irradiation and a delayed photodamage of the endothelial cells. In contrast Photofrin and other hematoporphyrin derivatives induce direct vascular damages (Gomer, 1989; Karaivanova *et al.*, 1990) which can lead to a lower amount of oxygen in the tumor and then to an reduced photodynamic effect.

All investigated naphthalocyanine photosensitizers exhibit a photodynamic effect, but noticeable differences exist between the different compounds. Because ZnNc6 leads to a strong regrowth delay but only to an average prolongation of AST, the naphthalocyanines with long aliphatic substituents may have some toxic side effects. The localisation on the cellular level probably depends not only on the hydrophilic/lipophilic character of the compound, but also on its size and shape. That could be an explanation that the larger molecules ZnNc7 and ZnNc5 show less activity than ZnNc6 and ZnNc4. Comparing all tested dyes the tetrabenzamido naphthalocyanine ZnNc4 is the most promising compound. This result was confirmed by the comparative PDT-studies with different generations of photosensitizers for the treatment of pigmented melanoma. ZnNc4 is now subject of further investigations.

2.5.4. FUTURE ASPECTS

Exemplarily it was shown that liposome-delivered long wavelength absorbing ZnNc's are good photosensitizers for PDT because of their good tumor localization, fast clearance from skin (<72 h), high phototoxicity at low concentrations (only 0.3 mg kg^{-1} b.w. towards 3–5 mg kg^{-1} b.w. for HpD or Photofrin) and their intracellular localization. An expressed reduction of tumor growth (a significant tumor growth delay), a reliable increase in the survival time and a pronounced delay in the metastasis development were found. In addition it should be pointed out that in contrast to other at shorter wavelength absorbing photosensitizers some tumors like pigmented melanomas could be treated successfully with ZnNc's. Further investigations should evaluate also Cremophor and other oil emulsions as less expensive delivery systems.

In order to enhance the tumor accumulation and to reduce possible side effects, the experiences obtained with other carrier systems (e.g. monoclonal antibodies) or the polyphasic tumor therapy (see Chapter 3.3) should be taken into account. The photodynamic activity of the ligand–metal combination of MNc's has been proven (for example the naphthalocyanine Zn(II) combination). Now suitable structural optimization for the combination with a selective carrier is necessary. Examples are mono- and difunctional naphthalocyanines bearing electrophilic, nucleophilic or ionic substituents. Syntheses of tetra- and octa-substituted MNcs are readily known. Experiences with other less functionalized photosensitizers (see Chapter 3.2) must be used for the synthesis of suitable naphthalocyanine derivatives.

ACKNOWLEDGEMENT

This work was partly supported by the Volkswagen Stiftung (Grant No. I/69407) and Deutsche Forschungsgemeinschaft (Grant No. 436 Bul-133/51/0).

LITERATURE CITED

Berg, K., Bommer, J. C., and Moan, J. (1989): Evaluation of sulfonated aluminum phthalocyanines for use in photochemotherapy. A study on the relative efficiencies of photoinactivation. *Photochem. Photobiol.* **49**, 587–594.

Biolo, R., Jori, G., Soncin, M., Pratesi, R., Vanni, U., Rihter, B., Kenney, M. E., and Rodgers, M. A. J. (1994): Photodynamic therapy of B16 pigmented melanoma with liposome-delivered Si(IV)-Naphthalocyanine. *Photochem. Photobiol.* **59**, 362–365.

Brach, P. J., Grammatica, S. J., Ossanna, O. A., and Weinberger, L. (1970): Improved Synthesis of metal-free Phthalocyanine. *J. Heterocycl. Chem.* **7**, 1403.

Bradbrook, E. F. and Linstead, R. P. (1936): Phthalocyanines. Part VIII. 1,2-Naphthalocyanines. *J. Chem. Soc.* **65**, 1744–1748.

Cook, M. J., Dunn, A. J., Howe, S. D., Thomson, A. J., and Harrison, K. J. (1988): Octa-alkoxy phthalocyanine and naphthalocyanine derivaives: dyes with Q-band absorption in the far red or near infrared. *J. Chem. Soc. Perkin Trans.* **1**, 2453–2458.

Cuomo, V., Jori, G., Rither, B., Kenny, M. E., and Rodgers, M. A. J. (1990): Liposome delivered Si(IV)-Naphthalocyanine as a photodynamic sensitizer for experimental tumors: pharmacokinetic and phototherapeutic studies. *Br. J. Cancer* **62**, 966–970.

Daraio, M. E., Aramendia, P. F., San Roman, E. A., and Braslavsky, S. E. (1991): Carboxylated Zinc-phthalocyanines- II Dimerization and singlet molecular oxygensensitization in hexadecyltrimethylammonium bromide micelles. *Photochem. Photobiol.* **54**, 367–373.

Dougherty, T. J. (1987): Photosensitizers: therapy and detection of malignant tumors. *Photochem. Photobiol.* **45**, 879–889.

Dougherty, T. J. and Potter, W. R. (1991): Of what value is a highly absorbing photosensitizer in PDT? *J. Photochem. Photobiol. B.* **8**, 223–225.

Firey, P. A. and Rodgers, M. A. J. (1987): Photo-properties of a silicon naphthalocyanine: a potential photosensitizer for photodynamic therapy. *Photochem. Photobiol.* **45**, 535–538.

Ford, W. E., Firey, P. A., Sounik, J. R., Rither, B. D., Kenney, M. E., and Rodgers, M. A. J. (1988): Photoproperties of naphthalocyanines. *Proc. SPIE* **997**, 105–106.

Gomer, C. J. (1989): Photodynamic therapy in the treatment of malignancies. *Seminars Hematol.* **26**, 27–34.

Goncharova, G. I., Galpern, M. G., and Lukyanets, E. A. (1982): *J. Gen. Chem. USSR* **52**, 581.

Ho, X., Pandey, R., Sumlin, A., Missert, J., Bellinier, D., and Dougherty, T. (1990): Potential new photosensitizers for photodynamic therapy. *Proc. SPIE, Int. Soc. Opt. Eng.* **1203**, 293–300.

Karaivanova, M., Karanov, St., Shopova, M., Kaicheva, E., Peeva, M., Getov, N., and Prokopanov, H. (1990): Studies of Photodynamic effect of Bulgarian hematoporphyrin derivative. *J. Photochem. Photobiol. B Biol.* **6**, 297–308.

Kitahara, K., Asano, T., Hamano, K., Tokita, S., and Nishi, H. (1990): Synthesis of 2,3, 11,12,20,21,29,30-Octadodecylthio-2,3-naphthalocyanines. *J. Heterocyclic Chem.* **27**, 2219–2220.

Kovshev, E. I. and Lukyanets, E. A. (1972): Phthalocyanines and related compounds XI. Substituted 2,3-naphthalocyanines. *Zh. Obshch. Khim.* **42**, 1593–1597.

Kovshev, E. I. and Lukyanets, E. A. (1972b): Phthalocyanines and related compounds X. Synthesis and electronic absorption spectra of tetra-6-t.butyl-2,3-naphthalocyanines. *J. Gen. Chem. USSR* **42**, 691–693.

Lukyanets, E. A. *et al.* (1989): Electronic spectra of phthalocyanines and derivatives, catalog. Research institute for technical and economical investigations (Tscherkassy, USSR).

Mang, T. S., Dougherty, T. J., Potter, W. R., Boyle, D. G., Somer, S., and Moan, J. (1987): Photobleaching of porphyrins used in photodynamic therapy and implications for therapy. *Photochem. Photobiol.* **45**, 501–506.

Mantareva, V., Kassabov, K., Shopova, M., Müller, S., and Wöhrle, D. (1994): Influence of photodynamic therapie on the delay of metastasis development in Lewis lung carcinoma. *Proc. SPIE* **2325**, 355–360.

Michelsen, U., Kliesch, H., Schurpfeil, G., Sobbi, A. K., and Wöhrle, D. (1996): Unsymmetrically substituted zinc-benzonaphthoporphyrazines: a new class of cationic photosensitizers for the photodynamic therapy of cancer. *Photochem. Photobiol.* **64**, 694–701.

Mikhalenko, S. A. and Lukyanets, E. A. (1969): Phthalocyanines and related Compounds II. Synthesis and certain properties of 2,3-Naphthalocyanines. *J. Gen. Chem. USSR* **39**, 2495–2498.

Müller, S., Mantareva, V., Stoichkova, N., Kliesch, H., Sobbi, A. K., Wöhrle, D., and Shopova, M. (1996): Tetraamido-substituted 2,3-naphthalocyanine Zn(II) complexes as phototherapeutic agents: synthesis, comparative photochemical and photobiological studies. *J. Photochem. Photobiol. B Biol.* **35**, 167–174.

Paquette, B., Ali, H., Langlois, R., and van Lier, J. E. (1990): Biological activities of phthalocyanines. XI. Biological activities of sulfonated aluminium naphthalocyanines towards V-79 Chinese hamster cells. *Photochem. Photobiol.* **51**, 313–318.

Reddi, E., Zhou, C., Biolo, R., Menegaldo, E., and Jori, G. (1990): Liposome- or LDL-administeted Zn(II)-phthalocyanine as a photodynamic agent for tumors. I. Pharmacokinetic properties and phototherapeutic efficiency. *Br. J. Cancer* **61**, 407–411.

Röder, B. and Nähter, D. (1991): Characterization of photophysical properties of sensitizers used in photodynamic therapy. *SPIE* **1525**, 377–384.

Schnurpfeil, G., Sobbi, A. K., Kliesch, H., Müller, S., Eichhorn, H., and Wöhrle, D. (1997): Photochemical Stability and the Correlation with Semiempirical MO-Calculations of Various Porphyrins in Solution. *J. Porphyrins phthalocyamines* **1**, 159–167.

Shopova, M., Wöhrle, D., Stoichkova, N., Milev, A., Mantareva, V., Müller, S., Kacsabov, K., and Georgiev, K. (1994): Hydrophobic Zn-naphthalocyanines as photodynamic therapie agents for Lewis lung carcinoma, *J. Photochem. Photobiol. B* **23**, 35–42.

Shopova, M., Reeva, M., Mantareva, V., Michailov, N., Stoichkova, N., Jori, G., Ricchelli, F., Wöhrle, D., and Müller, S. (1996): Comparative photodynamic therapy of B16 pigmented melanoma with different generations of sensitizers. Manuscript in preparation.

Sounik, J., Schechtman, L., Rither, B., Ford, W., Rodgers, M. A. J., and Kenney, M. E. (1990): Synthesis and characterisation of naphthalocyanines and phthalocyanines of use in sensitizer studies. *Proc. SPIE, Int. Soc. Opt. Eng.* **1203**, 224–232.

Svaasand, L. O., Martinelli, E., Gomer, C. J., and Profio, A. E. (1990): Optical characteristics of intraocular tumours in the visible and near-infrared. In Photodynamic Therapy: Mechanisms II. Vol. 1203 (Edited by T. J. Dougherty and A. Katzir), *SPIE, Bellingham* WA, 2–21.

Vogeler, A. and Kunkely, H. (1980): Template synthesis and optical spectra of zinc-2,3-naphthalocyanines. *Inorg. Chem. Acta* **44**, 209–210.

Wheeler, B. L., Nagasubramanian, G., Bard, A. J., Schechtman, L. A., Dininny, D. R., and Kenny, M. E. (1984): A silicon phthalocyanine and a silicon naphthalocyanine: Synthesis, electrochemistry and electrogenerated chemiluminescence. *JACS* **106**, 7404–7410.

Wöhrle, D., Schnurpfeil, G., and Knothe, G. (1992): Efficient synthesis of phthalocyanines and related compounds in the presence of organic bases. *Dyes and Pigments* **18**, 91–102.

Wöhrle, D., Wendt, A., Weitemeyer, A., Stark, J., Spiller, W., Schneider, G., Müller, S., Michelsen, U., Kliesch, H., and Ardeschirpur, A. (1994): Metal Chelates of Porphyrin Derivatives as Sensitizers in Photooxidation Processes of Sulfur Compounds and in the Photodynamic Therapy of Cancer. *Russ. Chem. Bull., Izvi. Akad. Nauk. Ser. Khim.*, 2071–2082.

Wöhrle, D., Shopova, M., Müller, S., Milev, A. D., Mantareva, V. N., and Krastev, K. K. (1993): Liposome-deliverd Zn(II)-2,3-naphthalocyanines as potential sensitizers for PDT: synthesis, photochemical, pharmacokinetic and phototherapeutic studies. *J. Photochem. Photobiol. B Biol.* **21**, 155–165.

Yates, N. C., Moan, J., and Western, A. (1990): Watersluble metal naphthalocyanines – near-IR photosensitizers: cellular uptake, toxicity and photosensitizing properties NHIK 3025 human cancer cells. *J. Photochem. Photobilol. B: Biol.* **4**, 379–390.

Zhou, C. (1989): Mechanism of tumor necrosis induced by photodynamic therapy. *J. Photochem. Photobilol. B Biol.* **3** (1989), 299–318.

Zuk, M. M., Rither, B. D., Kenney, M. E., Rodgers, M. A. J., and Kreimer-Birnbaum, M. (1994): Pharmakokinetic and tissue distribution studies of the photosensitizer bis(di-isobutyl octadecylsiloxy)silicon-2,3-naphthalocyanine (isoBOSINC) in normal and tumor-bearing rats. *Photochem. Photobiol.* **59**, 66–72.

2.6. UNSYMMETRICALLY SUBSTITUTED PORPHYRAZINES

ANDREA WEITEMEYER, H. KLIESCH, ULRIKE MICHELSEN, ANDREAS HIRTH and DIETER WÖHRLE

2.6.1. FUNDAMENTAL ASPECTS

In recent years unsubstituted and symmetrically substituted phthalocyanines, tetrabenzoporphyrazines, naphthalocyanines and tetranaphtoporphyrazines have been intensively investigated as second generation photosensitizers for PDT. (Spikes, 1986; Rosenthal, 1991; see Chapters 2.4 and 2.5). In addition to their longer wavelength absorptions (Pc's 660–730 nm and Nc's 750–840 nm) their absorption coefficients ($>10^5\,l\,mol^{-1}\,cm^{-1}$) are higher than those of the first generation sensitizers like HpD. The longer wavelength absorption leads to a therapeutic penetration depth of light into tissue which is ten till hundred times higher than in the case of HpD (Wan *et al.*, 1981; Jori, 1992). Mainly the macrocylic metal complexes with aluminum and zinc as central metal ion are interesting for PDT because they show high values for the product of triplet quantum yield times triplet lifetime. Therefore these compounds exhibit the best singlet oxygen quantum yields (Röder *et al.*, 1991). This is very important because singlet oxygen is the main cytotoxic agent in PDT (Weishaupt *et al.*, 1976). A number of examinations showed that aluminum and zinc porphyrazines are excellent sensitizers for PDT but they have the disadvantage of limited selectivity for accumulation in tumor tissue which is the general disadvantage for all the other classes of dyes investigated until now (Rosenthal, 1991; Fingar *et al.*, 1993).

Photosensitizers specially designed to target tumor cells can be called the "third generation" of sensitizers. A variety of strategies is reported to achieve this aim. One possibility is the incorporation of the dyes into liposomes or Cremophor emulsions (see Chapter 2.5). This application method is likely to lead to a higher affinity of the sensitizer to low density proteins (LDL) which is believed to be the main transport system of dyes to tumor cells in human serum (Reddi *et al.*, 1990). It should be mentioned that direct coupling of the sensitizers to LDL also enhances tumor selectivity (Jori *et al.*, 1993). But not only tumor cells bear LDL receptors, and therefore a LDL mediated transport always results in a limited accumulation. A potential alternative is the coupling of dyes to more selective carrier systems like monoclonal antibodies. Several investigations with antibody linked sensitizers were carried out in the past (Dawson *et al.*, 1991; Schultes *et al.*, 1992; Morgan *et al.*, 1994; Oseroff *et al.*, 1986). *In vivo* experiments with sulfonated aluminum phthalocyanines covalently bound to antibodies showed a 1000 : 1 accumulation in tumor tissue over normal tissue (Dawson *et al.*, 1991). Problems of the use of monoclonal antibodies are the high costs, inactivation of antibodies during modification and the limited number of dye molecules that can be linked to one antibody without destroying the biological activity (Klyashchitsky *et al.*, 1994). In order to increase the number of sensitizer molecules transported by one antibody other concepts than the direct coupling are necessary. A polymer loaded with photosensitizers linked to the antibody is a promising alternative (Jiang *et al.*, 1991). Such polymer–sensitizer conjugates can be obtained more easily by using monofunctional photosensitizers instead of tetrafunctional derivatives due to the impossibility of crosslinking reactions. The same crosslinking problem can occur by direct coupling of polyfunctional dyes to antibodies. Another opportunity to multiply the number of sensitizers per antibody is the polyphasic avidine/biotine/cyclodextrin delivery system which is described in more detail in the following section (see Chapter 3.3). This concept requires photosensitizers like porphyrazines with a high affinity to cyclodextrines. Hydrophobic tert.-butyl substituents at the photosensitizers fulfill good requirements for the incorporation into the hydrophobic pocket of cyclodextrines.

The combination of hydrophobic and hydrophilic substituents in one sensitizer molecule results in an intramolecular polarity axis. By this way a better accumulation in subcellular compartments occurs which is a prerequisite for an effective PDT (Brasseur *et al.*, 1988; Berg *et al.*, 1989; Lengoed *et al.*, 1993). After *in vitro* and *in vivo* studies with sulfonated macrocyclic chelates of phthalocyanine type structure, partially sulfonated benzonaphthoporphyrazines showed the best cell uptake (Margaron *et al.*, 1992). Figure 1 summarizes one demand for the configuration of a photosensitizer.

In addition, other necessary characteristics are summarized as follows (and compared with other photosensitizers in Fig. 2):

- absorption at 680–800 nm with high absorption coefficients for deeper penetration of light;
- limited stability, for better therapeutical depth of light (see Section 2.6.3.1) and clearance in peritumoral tissues.

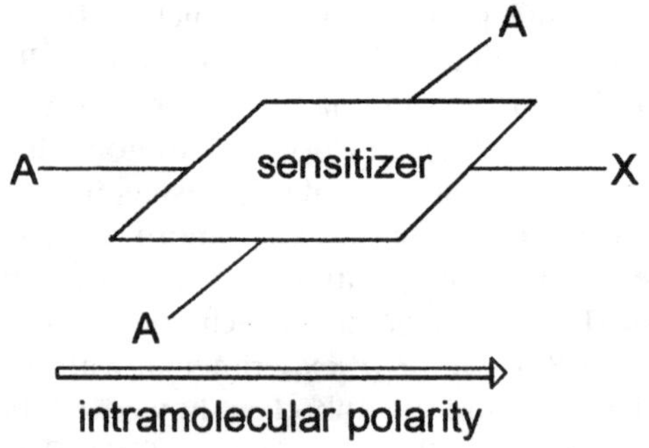

Figure 1 Configuration of an optimized photosensitizer with intramolecular polarity axis: hydrophilic, reactive substituent X for covalent binding to delivery systems; hydrophobic substituents A for better solubility, incorporation into cyclodextrines or delivery systems (LDL, liposomes, Cremophor emulsions).

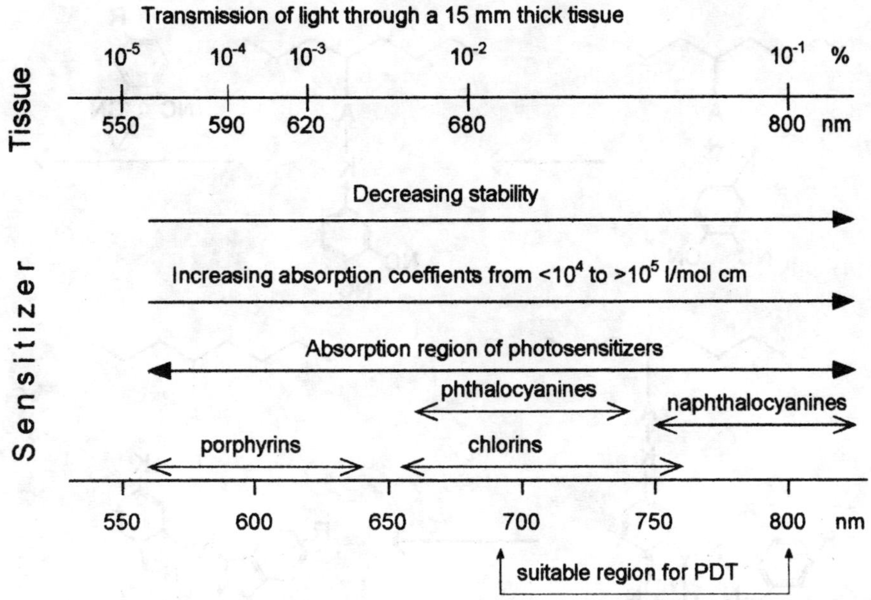

Figure 2 Optical properties of photosensitizers and transmission of light in tissues.

In the following, synthesis and properties of unsymmetrically substituted photosensitizers of porphyrazine-type structure which fulfill the requirements mentioned above are discussed.

Synthetical Pathways

Several possibilities exist to synthesize unsymmetrically substituted porphyrazines: polymer-supported route, ring enlargement of subphthalocyanine, statistical synthesis.

a. Polymer-Supported Route

This method uses the construction of a functionalized porphyrazine at insoluble organic or inorganic carrier (Wöhrle *et al.*, 1986; Leznoff *et al.*, 1991, 1992; Hirth, 1995) (Fig. 3). At first a dinitrile coupled to a functionalized carrier is cyclotetramerized with another dinitrile yielding polymer bound monofunctionalized phthalocyanines. The next step is the cleavage of the bound between the carrier and the phthalocyanine following isolation of the macrocyclic compound.

Differently substituted porphyrazines were obtained by this way. But some disadvantages are related to this procedure. Due to the limited capacity of the carrier only small amounts of porphyrazines can be obtained. Moreover, coupling and cleavage reactions are complicated and the yields are not always satisfactory. Therefore this route may not be a suitable method for production of monofunctionalized porphyrazines in a larger scale.

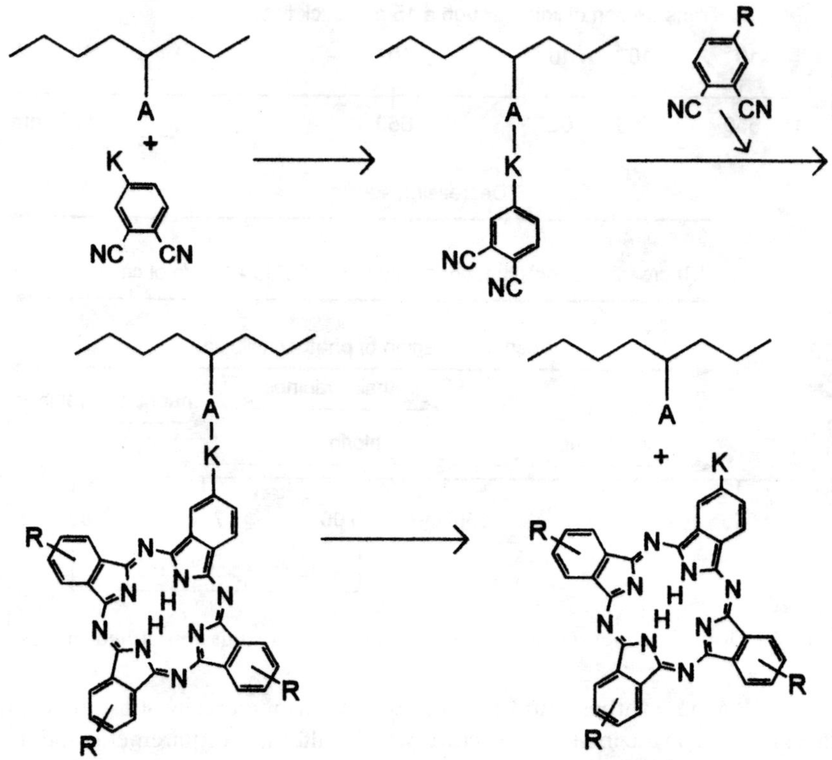

Figure 3 Synthesis of monofunctional phthalocyanines by the polymer supported route.

b. Ring Enlargement of Subphthalocyanine

In 1990 the ring enlargement reaction with subphthalocyanine was described (Kobayashi *et al.*, 1990). This route seemed to be a very promising method for the selective synthesis of unsymmetrically substituted porphyrazines. One substituted 1,3-diiminoisoindolenine is inserted into a subphthalocyanine leading to ring enlargement. After the reports in the literature several unsymmetrical porphyrazines were obtained by this method (Musluoglu *et al.*, 1992; Kasuga *et al.*, 1992; Dabak *et al.*, 1994; Kobayashi *et al.*, 1991). But it was shown by more detailed investigations that the ring enlargement of subphthalocyanines can result in a mixture of differently substituted porphyrazines instead of the one expected compound (Weitemeyer *et al.*, 1995; Sastre *et al.*, 1995). Furthermore the yields are often in the unsatisfactory range of only 4–6% and the metal free dyes must be metaled (e.g. into the zinc(II) chelates) which are photodynamically more active.

The ring enlargement of the unsubstituted subphthalocyanine was improved by the employment of a dinitrile instead of diiminoisoindolenine in a one step procedure with zinc(II) acetate as template (see Fig. 4) (Weitemeyer *et al.*, 1995). The obtained mixtures were separated by HPLC.

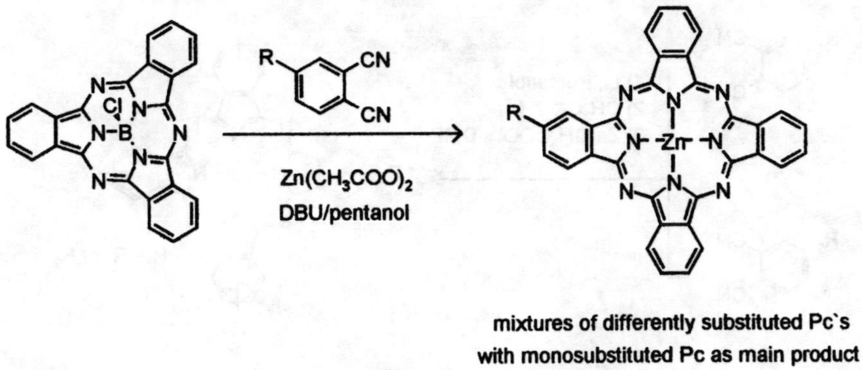

Figure 4 Modified ring enlargement reaction.

Monosubstituted zinc(II) phthalocyanines were received now in yields of 10–20%. Also substituted subphthalocyanines can be employed but they are obtained only in low yields (Rauschnabel *et al.*, 1995). The main disadvantages of the ring enlargement pathway are the multi-step synthesis and low yields. In addition, it is necessary to separate the product mixtures.

c. *Statistical Synthesis*

The classical and most used routes are the statistical modification of unsubstituted phthalocyanines and the statistical synthesis of unsymmetrically substituted porphyrazines.

Mono and disulfonated phthalocyanines, frequently used in PDT, are often synthesized by sulfonation of unsubstituted phthalocyanine by sulfuric acid (Chatlani *et al.*, 1991; Rosenthal, 1991; see Chapter 2.4). The substitution reactions lead to complex mixtures of differently sulfonated phthalocyanines which are difficult to separate by common chromatographic methods.

The most potent method for the preparation of unsymmetrically substituted porphyrazines bearing different kind of substituents is the statistical cyclotetramerisation of two different dinitriles (Cook *et al.*, 1988; Kliesch *et al.*, 1995), diiminoisoindolenines (Wada *et al.*, 1994) or dicarboxylic acids (Margaron *et al.*, 1992). Employing two different dicarbonitriles, six different substituted porphyrazines – in addition constitutional isomers – can be formed. After cyclotetramerisation the reaction mixture must be separated by chromatographic methods. Different reaction conditions for the cyclisation were applied, e.g. the cyclisation in DBU/$C_nH_{(2n+1)}$ (Linßen *et al.*, 1994), in DMAE (Wada *et al.*, 1994), or in substance without any solvent (Kudrevich *et al.*, 1994). These reactions can be carried out in the presence of a metal salt yielding directly the desired metal chelate. Some dinitriles do not react sufficiently under these conditions. In these cases the lithium alkoxyde-catalyzed statistical condensation method is more successful (see Fig. 5) (Cook *et al.*, 1988; Kliesch *et al.*, 1995). The unstable

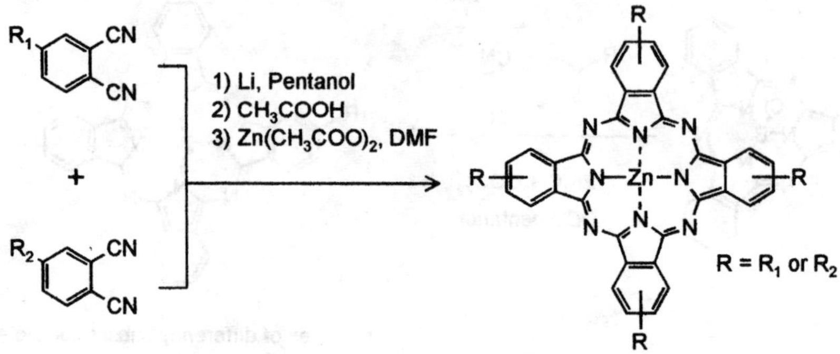

Figure 5 General procedure for the statistical synthesis.

dilithium compounds obtained were transformed into the metal free porphyrazines by acid. These were then treated with a zinc(II) salt to yield the corresponding zinc(II) chelates.

The main advantage of the statistical cyclotetramerisation is the one step procedure which is completed within few minutes in often high yields (40–80°C). More deficient is the separation of the reaction mixtures because of the tendency of porphyrazines to form aggregates. The formation of aggregates of differently substituted porphyrazines can lead to insufficient separation on the columns. In order to overcome this problem one interesting way is the use of silicagels modified with covalently bound phthalocyanines (Leznoff *et al.*, 1993). But also chromatographic separations on common stationary phases with different solvent mixtures were successfully carried out (Linßen *et al.*, 1994; Wada *et al.*, 1994; Kliesch *et al.*, 1995).

2.6.2. EXAMPLES FOR FUNCTIONALIZED PHOTOSENSITIZERS

In our research group a number of functionalized unsymmetrical porphyrazines bearing sulfonic acid, carboxylic acid, phenolic, alcoholic, amino and pyridyl-oxy group were synthesized (see Fig. 6) (Kliesch *et al.*, 1995; Wöhrle *et al.*, 1995; Michelsen *et al.*, 1996). The lithium alkoxydecatalyzed reaction was the most suitable tetramerisation method. Separation of the reaction mixtures was carried out on silica with an ether/DMF gradient. After chromatographic purification the compounds were obtained in overall yields up to 20%. Compounds **3a–f** were obtained after methylation of the analogous pyridyloxy substituted porphyrazines. All zinc(II) chelates possess the intramolecular polarity axis mentioned above. Most of the compounds are substituted with tert.-butyl groups bound to aromatic systems for incorporation into cyclodextrines. All compounds absorb in the deep red region from 680–750 nm ($\varepsilon > 10^5\,\mathrm{l\,mol^{-1}\,cm^{-1}}$). The introduction of naphthalene units results in a red shift of > 700 nm (see Fig. 7). Furthermore it should be mentioned that monosulfonated phthalocyanines were obtained

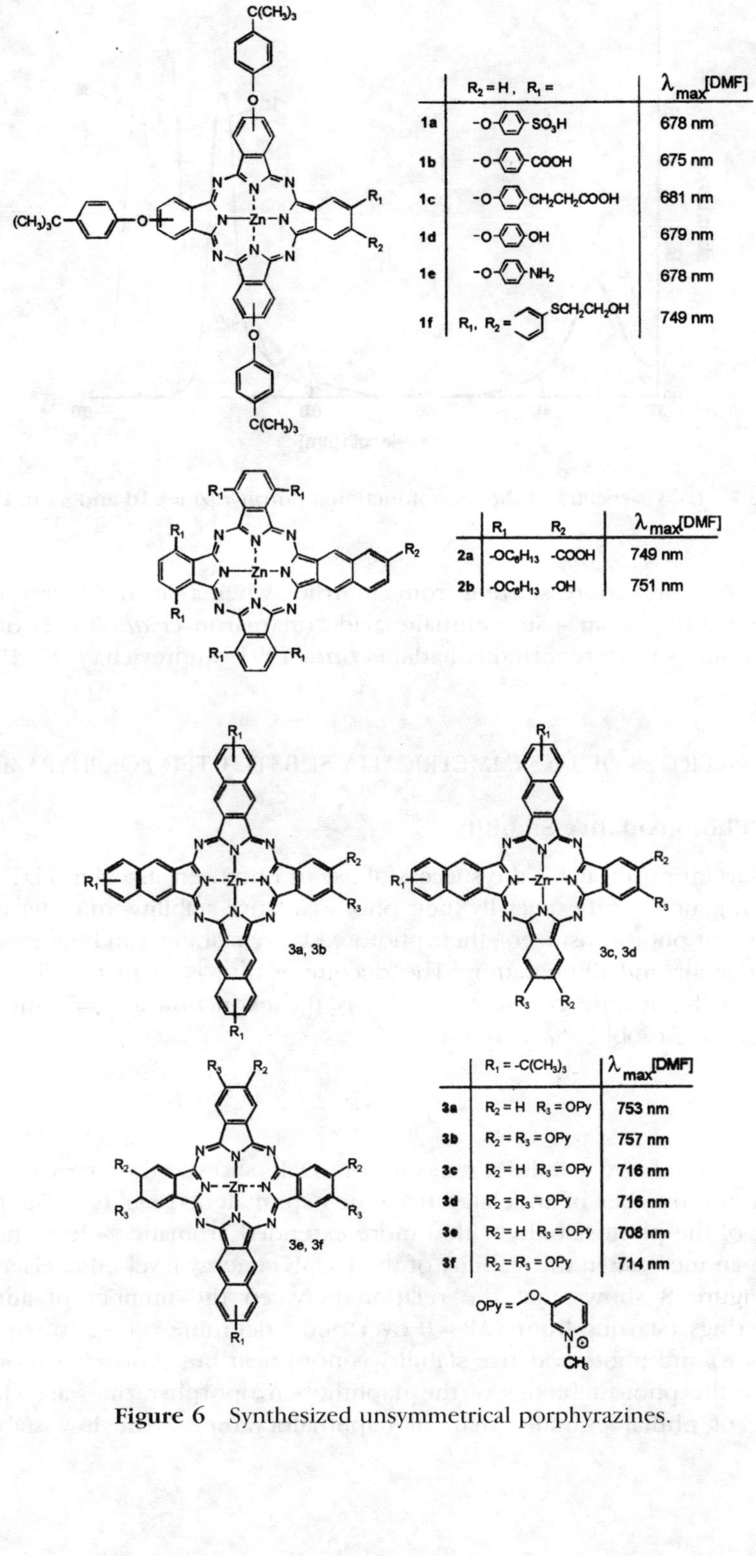

Figure 6 Synthesized unsymmetrical porphyrazines.

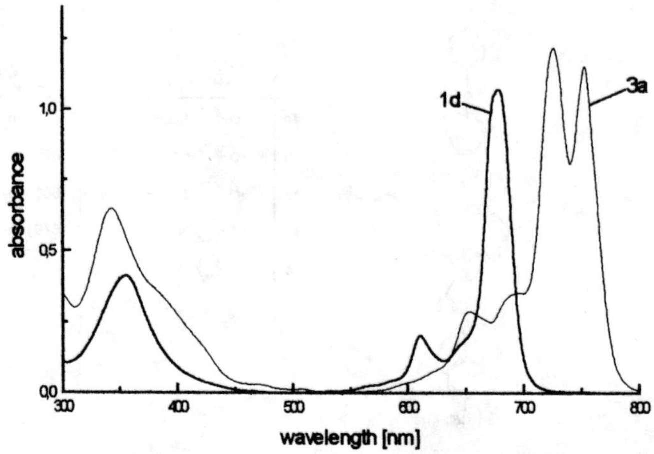

Figure 7 UV/Vis-spectra of the monofunctional porphyrazines 1d and 3a in DMF.

by a one step procedure starting from dinitriles whereas in the literature only syntheses starting from 4-sulfophthalic acids (Margaron *et al*., 1992) or other phthalocyanines were reported (Chatlani *et al*., 1991; Kudrevich *et al*., 1994).

2.6.3. PROPERTIES OF UNSYMMETRICALLY SUBSTITUTED PORPHYRAZINES

2.6.3.1. Photooxidative Stability

One important property for the successful use of photosensitizers in PDT is their stability in general and especially their photooxidative stability. In order to compare different photosensitizers, their photooxidative stability can be measured in DMF under air and illumination. The decomposition is of first order kinetics (Eq. (1)) with the rate constant k_1 ($E_{R,0}$ is the extinction at $t=0$ and $E_{R,t}$ at different times) (Sobbi *et al*., 1993).

$$\ln \frac{E_{R,0}}{E_{R,t}} = k_1 \cdot t. \qquad (1)$$

The photooxidative stabilities measured in DMF showed the expected dependence on the number of annelated benzene/naphthalene rings (see Fig. 8). The decrease of the photostability with a more extended aromatic π-electron system is due to an increase in the stability of the HOMO-energy level (Michelsen *et al*., 1996). Figure 8 shows that the relation between the number of annelated benzene rings (starting from TAP = 0 over phthalocyanine = 4 up to naphthalocyanine = 8) and photooxidative stability is not linear but probably exponential. Therefore the photostabilities of the naphthobenzoporphyrazines are closer to that one of phthalocyanines than of naphthalocyanines. The low stability of

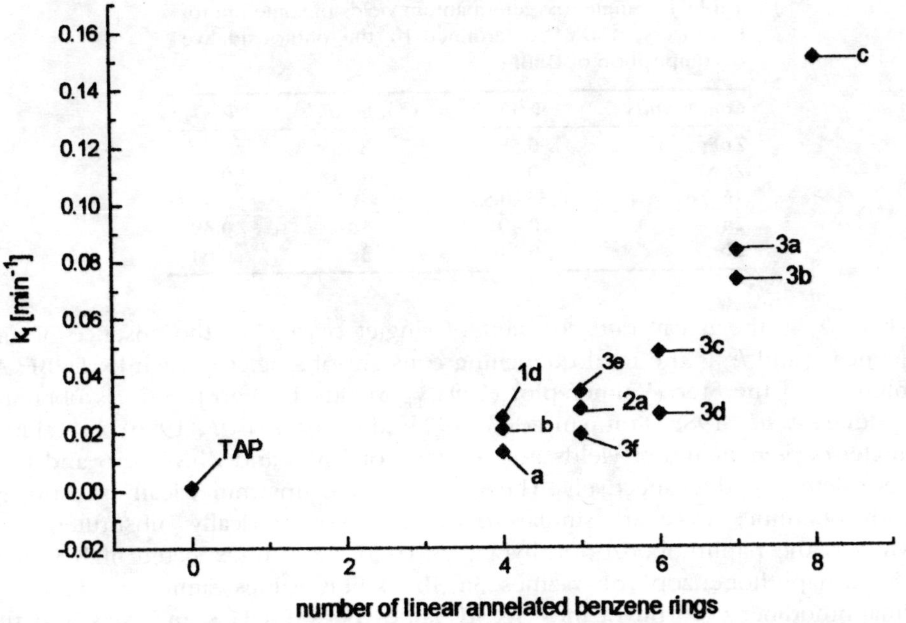

Figure 8 Rate constant k_1 for the photooxidative stability versus the number of linearly anellated benzene rings (TAP = 0; Pc = 4; Nc = 8). TAP = octathiomethyltetraazaporphyrinzinc; a = methylated octapyridyloxy ZnPc; b = ZnPc; c = tetratert.-butyl Nc.

naphthalocyanines is a problem during their preparation and especially their purification. Due to their low stability also *in-vivo* (see Chapter 2.4) only a limited time for photodynamic treatment exists (Paquette *et al.*, 1990). The limited photostability of the naphthobenzoporphyrazines **1f**, **2a**, **b**, **3a–3f** compared with phthalocyanines may increase the therapeutical depth of the laser light because sensitizers in the upper cellular layers photobleach faster than those in deeper layers (Dougherty *et al.*, 1991).

2.6.3.2. Singlet Oxygen Quantum Yields

A high singlet oxygen quantum yield is important for the potential use of photosensitizers in PDT. Besides photophysical measurements the photooxidative decomposition of 1,3-diphenylisobenzofuran (DPBF) in polar solvents like DMF is a suitable chemical method for the determination of the quantum yield of $^1O_2$ formation. According to the Eq. (2) the singlet oxygen quantum yields Φ_Δ were calculated from the quantum yields of the photoreaction with respect to the starting concentration:

$$\frac{1}{\Phi_{[\mathrm{DPBF}]}} = \frac{1}{\Phi_\Delta} + \frac{1}{\Phi_\Delta} \cdot \frac{k_\mathrm{d}}{k_\mathrm{a}} \cdot \frac{1}{[\mathrm{DPBF}]}, \tag{2}$$

Table 1 Singlet oxygen quantum yields of some photosensitizers in DMF determined by the photooxidative decomposition of DPBF

Compounds	$\Phi\,^1O_2$	*Compounds*	$\Phi\,^1O_2$
ZnPc	0.55	**3a**	0.49
ZnNc	0.45	**3b, 3f**	0.44
1a–1e	0.55–0.51	**3c**	0.43
2a	0.49	**3d**	0.39
2b	0.11	**3e**	0.64

where k_d is the decay rate constant of singlet oxygen in the absence of any quencher and k_a is the total quenching constant of singlet oxygen by DPBF. As intercept of the Stern-Volmer plot ($1/\Phi_{[DPBF]}$ versus 1/[DPBF]) $1/\Phi_\Delta$ is obtained (Valduga *et al.*, 1988; Roitman *et al.*, 1994; Michelsen *et al.*, 1996). In Table 1 singlet oxygen quantum yields are shown. For ZnPc and ZnNc 0.56 and 0.45 were determined, respectively. The values for the unsymmetrically substituted phthalocyanines **1a–e** are similar to those of symmetrically substituted Pc's, whereas the naphthobenzoporphyrazines **1f–3f** show unexpected high values. The trinaphthobenzoporphyrazines **3a, 3b** exhibit values similar to Pc's, the dinaphthodibenzoporphyrazines **3c, 3d** values between Pc's and Nc's and the tribenzonaphthoporphyrazines **1f, 2a, 2b, 3e, 3f** values which are even higher than those of Pc's (Michelsen *et al.*, 1996). The singlet oxygen quantum yield depends on two contrary effects which are the symmetry of the macrocycles and the number of annelated benzene rings. Decreasing symmetry leads to a higher quantum yield, whereas increasing number of anellated benzene rings results in a lower quantum yield. Therefore a decrease of the singlet oxygen quantum yield of substances of the same symmetry (for example Pc's > Nc's or **3a** > **3b** > **3e** > **3f**) with the number of annelated benzene rings was observed. An exception are the unsymmetrically substituted phthalocyanines **1a–1e**. They have the same low symmetry as compounds **1f, 2a, 2b, 3a, 3b, 3e, 3f** but the substituent (causing the lower symmetry) do not affect the central core, and therefore no influence on the singlet oxygen quantum yield is observed.

2.6.4. CONCLUSION

It was shown that unsymmetrically substituted porphyrazines are readily available by the statistical synthesis. These compounds are characterized by long wavelength absorption with high absorption, excellent singlet oxygen quantum yields and suitable limited photooxidative stability. Monofunctional derivatives are qualified for coupling to delivery systems for selective tumor targeting. The orientation of hydrophobic and hydrophilic substituents results in an intramolecular polarity necessary for good cell penetration. *In vitro* and *in vivo* investigations are now in progress (for some first advanced results see Chapter 3.3). Positive results are expected for the compounds described in Chapter 2.6.2. Partially sulfonated Al(III)- and Zn(II)-benzonaphthoporphyrazines exhibit after *in vitro* and *in vivo* experiments good photodynamic effects at low concentrations. Tumor response 72 h after PDT at EMT-6 mouse mammary tumor implanted in BALB/c mice was up to 83% after i.v. of only 0.8 mg/kg b.w. partially sulfonated Al(III)-benzonaphthoporphyrazines compared to only 33% with 5 mg/kg b.w. Photofrin II (Margaron *et al.*, 1992). No dark toxicity of the partially sulfonated compounds was found.

ACKNOWLEDGMENT

This work was partly supported by the German BMFT (grant No. 13N6290).

LITERATURE CITED

Berg, K., Bommer, J. C., and Moan, J. (1989): Evaluation of sulfonated aluminum phthalocyanines for use in photochemotherapy. A study on the relative efficiencies of photoinactivation. *Photochem. Photobiol.* **49**, 587–594.

Brasseur, N., Ali, H., Langlois, R., and van Lier, J. E. (1988): Biological activities of phthalocyanines-IX. Photosensitization of V-79 Chinese hamster cells and EMT-6 mouse mammary tumor by selectively sulfonated zinc phthalocyanines. *Photochem. Photobiol.* **47**, 705–711.

Chatlani, P. T., Bedwell, J., MacRobert, A. J., Barr, H., Boulos, P. B., Krasner, N., Phillips, D., and Bown, S. G. (1991): Comparison of distribution and photodynamic effects of di- and tetrasulfonated aluminum phthalocyanines in normal rat colon. *Photochem. Photobiol.* **53**, 745–751.

Cook, M. J., Dunn, A. J., Howe, S. D., Thomson, A. J., and Harrison, K. J. (1988): Octa-alkoxy phthalocyanine and naphthalocyanine derivatives: dyes with Q-band absorption in the far red or near infrared. *J. Chem. Soc. Perkin Trans.* **1**, 2453–2458.

Dabak, S., Gül, A., and Bekaroglu, O. (1994): Hexaalkylthia-substituted unsymmetrical phthalocyanines. *Chem. Ber.* **127**, 2009–2018.

Dawson, J. W., Morgan, J., Barr, H., Davidson, B. R., MacRobert, A. J., Savage, F., Dean, C., and Boulos, P. B. (1991): Targeted photosensitisation of colorectal and ovarian cancers; enhanced tumour selectivity and cytotoxicity of a new antibody-photosensitiser conjugate. *Photochem. Photobiol.* **53**, 25S.

Dougherty, T. J. and Potter, W. R. (1991): Of what value is a highly absorbing photosensitizer in PDT? *J. Photochem. Photobiol. B* **8**, 223–225.

Fingar, V. H., Wieman, T. J., Karavolos, P. S., Doak, K. W., Quellet, R., and van Lier, J. E. (1993): The effects of photodynamic therapy using differently substituted zinc phthalocyanines on vessel constriction, vessel leakage and tumor response. *Photochem. Photobiol.* **58**, 251–258.

Hirth, A. (1995): Synthese monofunktionalisierter Phthalocyanine durch Aufbau und Abspaltung an Silicagel. Diplomarbeit Universität Bremen.

Jiang, F. N., Liu, D. J., Neyndorff, H., Chester, M., Jiang, S., and Levy, J. G. (1991): Photodynamic killing of human squamous cell carcinoma cells using a monoclonal antibody-photosensitizer conjugate. *J. Natl. Cancer Inst.* **83**, 1218–1225.

Jori, G. (1992): Far red-absorbing photosensitizers: their use in the photodynamic therapy of tumors. *J. Photochem. Photobiol. A: Chem.* **62**, 371–378.

Jori, G. and Reddi, E. (1993): The role of lipoproteins in the delivery of tumour-targeting photosensitizers. *Int. J. Biochem.* **25**, 1369–1375.

Kasuga, K., Idehara, T., Handa, M., and Isa, K. (1992): Preparation of unsymmetrical phthalocyanine by means of a ring expansion of subphthalocyanine. *Inorg. Chim. Acta* **196**, 127–129.

Kliesch, H., Weitemeyer, A., Müller, S., and Wöhrle, D. (1995): Synthesis of phthalocyanines with one sulfonic acid, carboxylic acid or amino group. *Liebigs Ann.* 1269–1273.

Klyashchitsky, B. A., Nechaeva, I. S., and Ponomarov, G. V. (1994): Approaches to targeted photodynamic tumor therapy. *J. Cont. Release* **29**, 1–16.

Kobayashi, N., Kondo, R., Nakajima, S., and Osa, T. (1990): New route to unsymmetrical phthalocyanine analogues by the use of structurally distorted subphthalocyanines. *J. Am. Chem. Soc.* **112**, 9640–9641.

Kobayashi, N., Kondo, R., Ashida, T., Nakajima, S., and Osa, T. (1991): Synthesis and spectroscopic properties of phthalocyanine analogues with lower symmetry. *J. Chem. Soc., Chem. Commun.*, 120–121.

Kudrevich, S. V., Ali, H., and van Lier, J. E. (1994): Syntheses of monosulfonated phthalocyanines, benzonaphtoporphyrazines and porphyrines via the Meerwein reaction. *J. Chem. Soc. Perkin Trans.* **1**, 2767–2774.

Lengoed, H. L. L. M. van, van der Veen, N., Versteeg, A. A. C., Ouellet, R., van Lier, J. E., and Star, W. M. (1993): *In vivo* photodynamic effects of phthalocyanines in a skin-fold observation chamber model: role of central metal ion and degree of sulfonation. *Photochem. Photobiol.* **58**, 575–580.

Leznoff, C. C., Svirskaya, P. I., Khouw, B., Cerny, R. L., Seymour, P., and Lever, A. B. P. (1991): Syntheses of monometalated and unsymmetrically substituted binuclear phthalocyanines and a pentanuclear phthalocyanine by solution and polymer support methods. *J. Org. Chem.* **56**, 82–90.

Leznoff, C. C., Mc Arthur, C. R., and Quin, Y. (1993): Phthalocyanine modified silica gels and their application in the purification of unsymmetrical phthalocyanines. *J. Chem.* **73**, 1319–1326.

Leznoff, C. C. and Hall, T. W. (1982): The synthesis of soluble, unsymmetrical phthalocyanine on a polymer support. *Tetrahedron Lett.* **23**, 3023–3026.

Linßen, T. G. and Hanack, M. (1994): Synthesis, separation and characterisation of unsymmetrically substituted phthalocyanines. *Chem. Ber.* **127**, 2051–2057.

Margaron, P., Langlois, R., van Lier, J. E., and Gaspard, S. (1992): Photodynamic properties of naphtosulfobenzoporphyrazines, novel asymmetric, amphiphilic phthalocyanine derivatives. *J. Photochem. Photobiol. B: Biol.* **14**, 187–199.

Michelsen, U., Kliesch, H., Schnurpfeil, G., Sobbi, A. K., and Wöhrle, D: Unsymmetrically substituted zinc-benzonaphthoporphyrazines: a new class of cationic photosensitizers for the photodynamic therapy of cancer. *J. Photochem. Photobiol.*, submitted.

Morgan, J., Lottman, H., Abbou, C. C., and Chopin, D. K. (1994): A comparison of direct and liposomal antibody conjugation of sulfonated aluminum phthalocyanines for selective photoimmunotherapy of human bladder carcinoma. *Photochem. Photobiol.* **60**, 486–496.

Musluoglu, E., Gürek, A., Ahsen, V., Gül, A., and Bekaroglu, O. (1992): Unsymmetrical phthalocyanines with a single macrocyclic substituent. *Chem. Ber.* **125**, 2337–2339.

Oseroff, A. R., Ohuoha, D., Hasan, T., Bommer, J. C., and Yarmush, M. L. (1986): Antibody-targeted photolysis: Selective photodestruction of human T-cell leukemia cells using monoclonal antibody-chlorin e_6 conjugates. *Proc. Natl. Acad. Sci.* **83**, 8744–8748.

Paquette, B., Ali, H., Langlois, R., and van Lier, J. E. (1990): Biological activities of phthalocyanines. XI. Biological activities of sulfonated aluminium naphthalocyanines towards V-79 Chinese hamster cells. *Photochem. Photobiol.* **51**, 313–318.

Rauschnabel, J. and Hanack, M. (1995): New derivatives and homologues of subphthalocyanine. *Tetrahedron Lett.* **36**,1629–1632.

Reddi, E., Zhou, C., Biolo, R., Menegaldo, E., and Jori, G. (1990): Liposome- or LDL-administered Zn(II)-phthalocyanine as s photodynamic agent for tumours. I. Pharmacokinetic properties and phototherapeutic efficiency. *Br. J. Cancer* **61**, 407–411.

Röder, B. and Nähter, D. (1991): Characterization of photophysical properties of sensitizers used in photodynamic therapy. *SPIE* **1525**, 377–384.

Roitman, L., Ehrenberg, B., and Kobayashi, N. (1994): Spectral properties and absolute determination of singlet oxygen production yield by naphthaloporphyrins. *J. Photochem. Photobiol. A: Chem.* 7723–7728.

Rosenthal, I. (1991): Phthalocyanines as photodynamic sensitizers. *Photochem. Photobiol.* **53**, 859–870.

Sastre, A., Torres, T., and Hanack, M. (1995): Synthesis of novel unsymmetrical monoaminated phthalocyanines. *Tetrahedron Lett.* **36**, 8501–8504.

Schultes, B. C., Spaniol, S., Popat, S., Ertmer, W., and Schmidt, S. (1992): Photodynamic treatment of ovarian cancer by antibody coupled phthalocyanine: an *in vitro* and *in vivo* study, in Photodynamic Therapy and Biomedical Lasers. Eds. P. Spinelli, M. Dal Fante, and R. Marchesini, Elsevier Sci. Publ.

Sobbi, A. K., Wöhrle, D., and Schlettwein, D. (1993): Photochemical stability of various porphyrins in solution and as thin film electrodes. *J. Chem. Soc. Perkin Trans.* **2**, 481–488.

Spikes, J. D. (1986): Yearly Review, Porphyrin photosensitization and phototherapy. *Photochem. Photobiol.* **43**, 681–690.

Valduga, G., Nonell, S., Reddi, E., Jori, G., and Braslavsky, S. E. (1988): The production of singlet molecular oxygen by zinc(II) phthalocyanine in ethanol and in unilamellar vesicles. Chemical quenching and phosphorescence studies. *Photochem. Photobiol.* **48**, 1–5.

Wada, T., Yamada, A., and Sasabe, H. (1994): Synthesis and characterization of a novel unsymmetrical metal-free phthalocyanine with donor–acceptor substituents. *J. Heterocyclic Chem.* **31**, 1017–1020.

Wan, S., Parrish, J. A., Anderson, R. R., and Madden, M. (1981): Transmittance of nonionizing radiation in human tissues. *Photochem. Photobiol.* **34**, 679–681.

Weishaupt, K. R., Gomer, C. J., and Dougherty, T. J. (1976): Identification of singlet oxygen as the cytotoxic agent in photoinactivation of a murine tumor. *Cancer Res.* **36**, 2326.

Weitemeyer, A., Kliesch, H., and Wöhrle, D. (1995): Unsymmetrically substituted phthalocyanine derivatives via a modified ring enlargement reaction of unsubstituted subphthalocyanine. *J. Org. Chem.* **60**, 4900–4904.

Wöhrle, D. and Krawczyk, G. (1986): Porphyrines and their precursors 2. Solid phase synthesis of a monosubstituted phthalocyanine. *Polym. Bull.* **15**, 193–200.

Wöhrle, D., Weitemeyer, A., Sobbi, A., Michelsen, U., and Kliesch, H: Monofunctional phthalocyanines derivatives as potential sensitizers for PDT. *SPIE Conf. Proc.* Vol. 2625 (in press).

2.7. PRECLINICAL PHOTODYNAMIC THERAPY STUDIES WITH ENDOGENOUS AND NEW EXOGENOUS PHOTOSENSITIZERS

GENADY KOSTENICH, ARIE ORENSTEIN, ZVI MALIK and BENJAMIN EHRENBERG

INTRODUCTION

A new generation of photosensitizers with various improvements in their photophysical and biological properties have been synthesized over the last few years (Jori, 1992; Dougherty, 1993; Levy, 1994). Different methodological approaches and biological models which were used to study the agents' efficacy complicate the possibility of correctly evaluating their prospects for further clinical trials. This poses a problem in developing an accepted and united experimental protocol for testing, comparing and determining the agents' prospects.

Experimental and clinical experience shows that the conception of an "ideal photosensitizer" should be focused not only on searching for agents with long wavelength light absorption bands, high extinction and high phototoxicity, but also on low dark toxicity and high selectivity. In fact, lower extinction and/or location of the absorption maximum at the shorter end of the red range may be compensated by increased therapeutic drug and light doses. From this point of view, more important properties of new agents must be their low dark toxicity (allowing administration of higher doses), high rate of clearance from normal tissues and high selectivity of biodistribution and photochemically induced tumor damage. Thus, *in vivo* pharmacokinetic studies and selectivity assessment remain the most important initial stages allowing for real practical evaluation of a drug's prospects for use in PDT.

EXPERIMENTAL APPROACH

The methodological scheme shown in Fig. 1 was used in the present investigation for an *in vivo* comparative study of four agents with different photophysical properties: lutetium texaphyrin (Lu-Tex), chlorin e_6 (Chl), 5-aminolevulinic acid (ALA) and Photofrin® (as a standard classical photosensitizer).

Examination methods and criteria used for assessment are presented in this scheme.

C26 colon carcinoma transplanted subcutaneously into the footpad of mice was used as a tumor model. The foot without the tumor was used as normal tissue control.

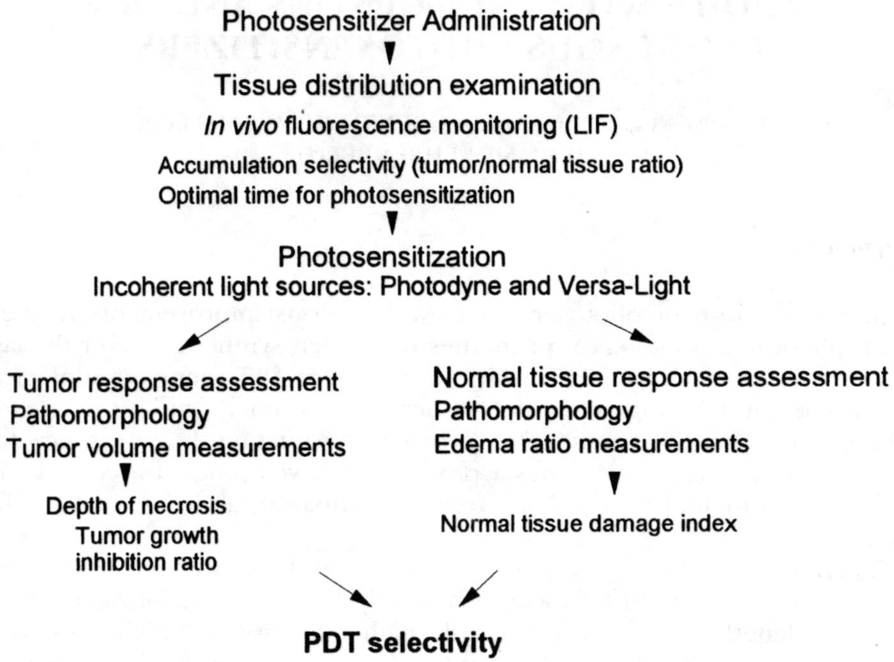

Figure 1 Scheme for *in vivo* experimental study of new photosensitizers.

PHOTOSENSITIZERS

Lutetium texaphyrin (Pharmacyclics Inc., Sunnyvale, CA) is a promising new photosensitizer belonging to a class of porphyrin-like compounds absorbing in the near infrared region about 740 nm (Fig. 2) and generating singlet oxygen efficiently. These molecules contain a system of 22 conjugated π electrons in an expanded aromatic macrocycle, which exhibits the spectroscopic Soret and Q-type transition characteristics. Modification of texaphyrin molecules by complexing with metals leads to fluorescence quenching and enhanced production of singlet oxygen. Earlier studies with metal complexes of texaphyrins showed that the photophysical characteristics of these photosensitizers make them attractive for preclinical investigations (Harriman *et al.*, 1989; Ehrenberg *et al.*, 1992; Lavi *et al.*, 1994; Sessler *et al.*, 1991, 1993; Ehrenberg *et al.*, 1993; Young *et al.*, 1996).

Figure 2 shows the structural formula, absorption and fluorescence spectra of the new sensitizer Lu-Tex in an aqueous solution and when bound to the lipid layer of phosphatidylcholine liposomes. The figure demonstrates the common behavior of solvent effect on the location of absorption bands. The sharp absorption spectra in both water and in a lipid layer indicate that there is no aggregation of the dye in either environment.

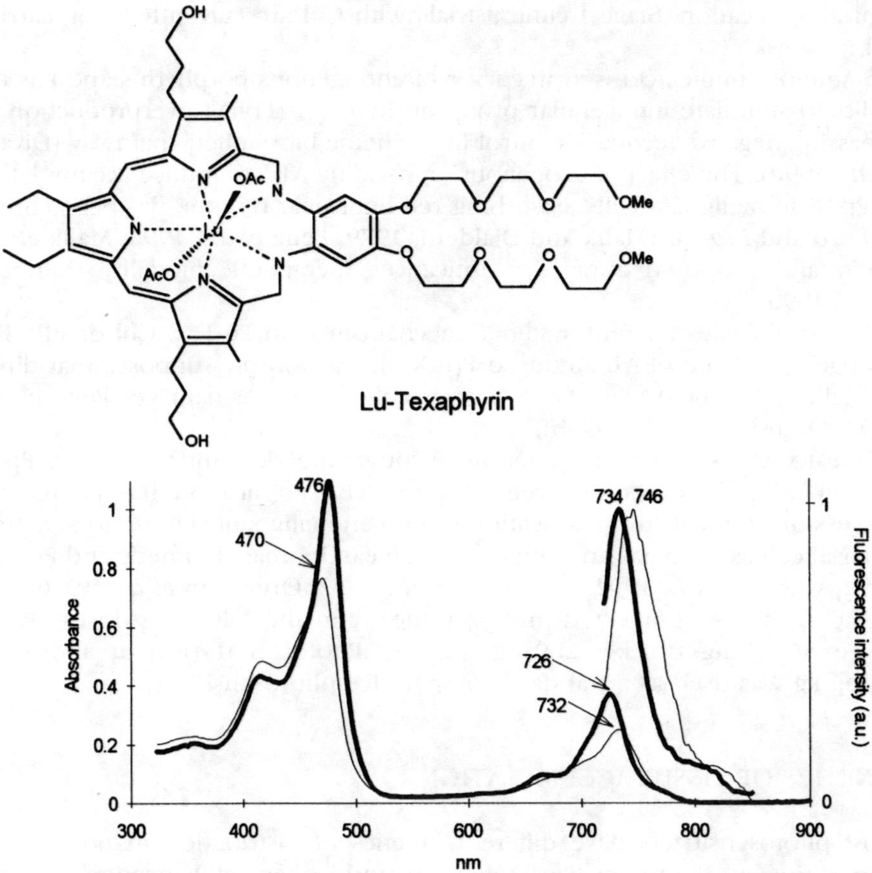

Figure 2 Structural formula, absorption (left scale) and fluorescence (right scale; arbitrarily normalized to 1) spectra of Lu-Tex (10 μM) in water (thin lines) and in a suspension containing 1 mg sonicated phosphatidyl-choline small unilamellar liposomes (thick lines).

Chlorin e_6 is a water soluble chlorophyll A derivative with strong absorption in the red spectrum (near 660 nm), and good photophysical properties (Frolov *et al.*, 1989, 1990; Spikes, 1990). It has been shown with some chlorins that blood circulation disturbances with hemostasis as the dominant factor and direct cytotoxic effect as an additive factor are probably involved in the mechanism of tumor necrosis after PDT (Nelson *et al.*, 1988; Kostenich *et al.*, 1991; McMahon *et al.*, 1994). Detailed preclinical investigations of Chl including studies of toxicity, pharmacokinetics and photodynamic effect on different tumor strains have been performed in the Byelorussian Research Institute of Oncology and Medical Radiology (Kostenich *et al.*, 1991, 1993, 1994). A drug form of this photosensitizer has been developed for clinical application. Stage I clinical trials with Chl are currently being carried out in Minsk.

5-Aminolevulinic acid is a precursor of endogenous porphyrins and has the ability to stimulate intracellular protoporphyrin IX (Pp-IX) overproduction by bypassing negative feedback control in the heme biosynthetic pathway (Divaris *et al*., 1990). The effect of exogenously providing ALA to induce accumulation of Pp-IX in malignant cells, absorbing red light near 632 nm, has been shown *in vitro* and *in vivo* (Malik and Djaldetti, 1979; Peng *et al*., 1992; Malik *et al*., 1995) and proposed as a new anticancer therapeutic modality (Kennedy *et al*., 1990).

ALA-PDT has a different systemic mechanism than Lu-Tex, Chl or PII. The endogenous route of ALA-induced Pp-IX production pre-supposes that direct cell killing may be a main factor responsible for tumor damage (Peng *et al*., 1992; Orenstein *et al*., 1996b).

Due to ALA's ability to penetrate through the skin and to induce Pp-IX accumulation in cancerous cells, topical ALA application has been used successfully for selective eradication of human malignant skin tumors, mainly of basal cell carcinomas and squamous cell carcinomas (Kennedy and Pottier, 1992; Warloe *et al*., 1992; Svanberg *et al*., 1992; Orenstein *et al*., 1996a).

The agents were injected intraperitoneally in the following doses: 10 mg Lu-Tex/kg; 5 mg Chl/kg; 200 mg ALA/kg. Photofrin II (PII) at a dose of 10 mg/kg was used as a standard comparative photosensitizer.

KINETICS OF TISSUE ACCUMULATION

Most photosensitizers have different kinetics of distribution in normal and tumor tissues. Photosensitizer retention and enhanced concentration in a tumor as compared to adjacent normal tissue is the basis of selective photochemically-induced tumor destruction caused by PDT. The exact mechanism of this phenomenon is not known, but it is supposed that peculiarities of blood circulation, enhanced vascular permeability, low rate of lymphatic drainage and distinct drug uptake by the tumor cells may be the factors influencing this process (Jain, 1987; Dvorak *et al*., 1988; Bugelski *et al*., 1981). The individual character of agent/tissue distribution, including blood transport, interstitial distribution, binding with extracellular and intracellular structures (biomolecules), and removal from the tissue, is dependent on the agent's biochemical properties (Maziere *et al*., 1991; Kongshaug, 1992).

It is important for PDT to find optimal time after agent injection when the maximal ratio between tumor and adjacent normal tissues is observed. *In vivo* fluorescence monitoring by the method of laser induced fluorescence (LIF) is very suitable for such investigations (Kennedy *et al*., 1992; Frisoli *et al*., 1993). We applied this method for the determination of tumor/normal tissue ratio (R_{tn}) and the optimal time interval for photosensitization. Three main components were used in our LIF system: an argon-ion laser for fluorescence excitation, a Perkin-Elmer spectrofluorimeter for fluorescence registration, and a bifurcated fibreoptic bundle for connection of the system instruments with the tissue object (Malik *et al.*, 1995).

In the tumor model used, the tumor/normal tissue ratio was expressed as:

$$R_{tn} = (I_t - I_n)/I_n, \qquad (1)$$

where I_t and I_n are the fluorescence intensities in the foot with the tumor and the normal foot, respectively.

Figure 3 demonstrates the fluorescence spectra of Lu-Tex, Chl, ALA induced Pp-IX and PII obtained *in vivo* on Balb/c mice with subcutaneously located C26 colon carcinoma after a spectroscopic fluorescence study using the LIF system. The fluorescence kinetics of the agents in the foot with the tumor and in the normal foot of the mice are shown in Fig. 4.

The results reveal different accumulation patterns of the agents, reflecting their different biochemical properties. The following patterns of fluorescence kinetics in the tumor as compared to normal tissue, were observed in our experimental model: initial lower tumor accumulation with subsequent retention in the tumor (Lu-Tex); higher tumor accumulation followed by

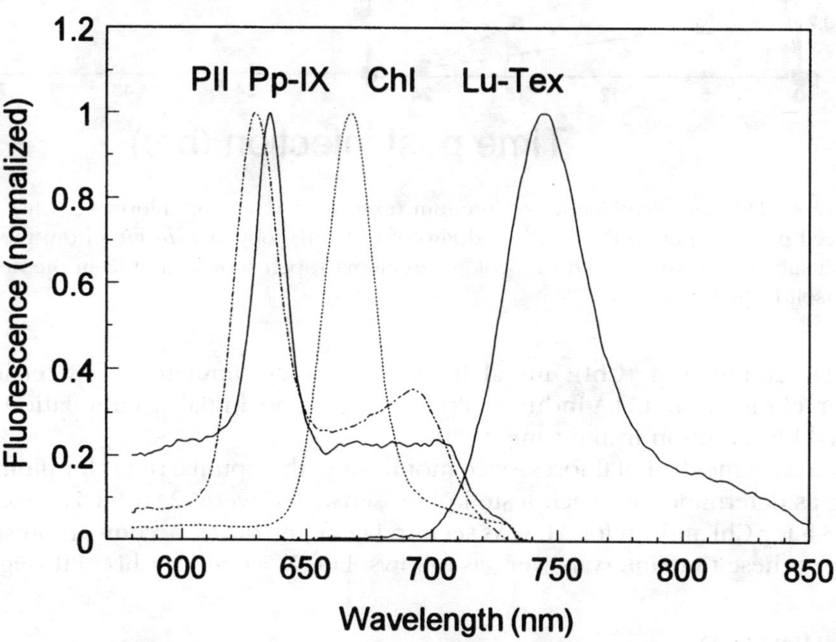

Figure 3 Fluorescence spectra of Photofrin II (PII), ALA-induced protoporphyrin IX (Pp-IX), chlorin e_6 (Chl) and lutetium texaphyrin (Lu-Tex) obtained *in vivo* from subcutaneously located C26 colon carcinoma of mice. Fluorescence was excited by the 502 nm (PII, Pp-IX, Chl) and 488 nm (Lu-Tex) lines of an argon-ion laser.

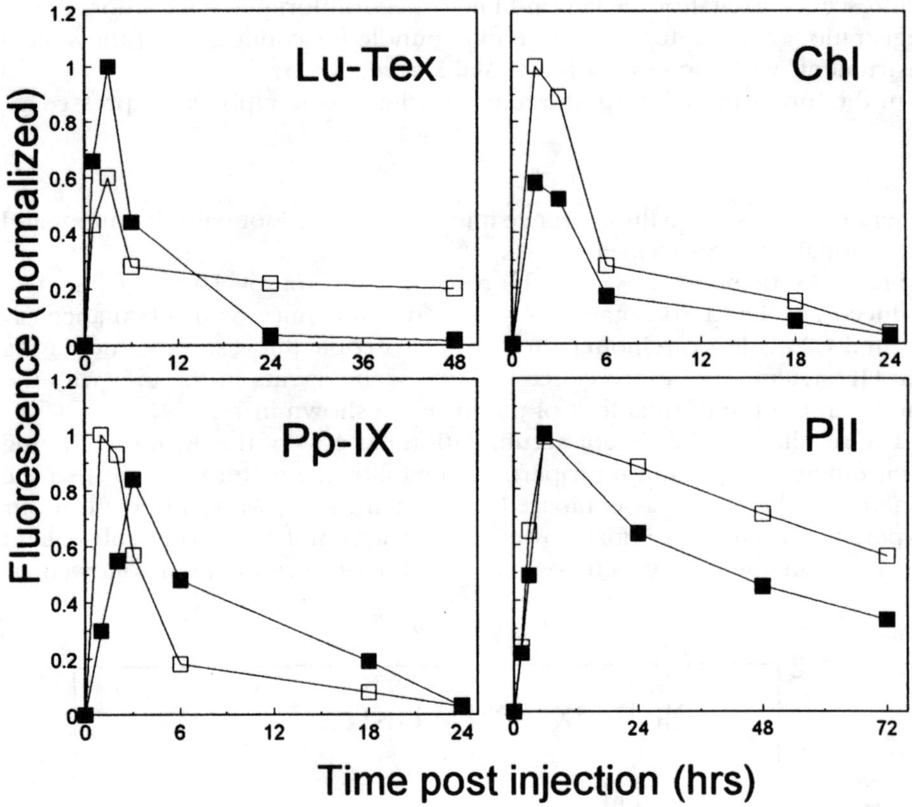

Figure 4 Fluorescence kinetics of lutetium texaphyrin (Lu-Tex), chlorin e_6 (Chl), ALA-induced protoporphyrin IX (Pp-IX) and Photofrin II(PII), obtained *in vivo* from the foot with a subcutaneously located C26 colon carcinoma (open square) and from the normal foot (solid square) of mice.

similar elimination (Chl); initial higher tumor accumulation with ensuing faster elimination (ALA-induced Pp-IX); the same initial accumulation followed by retention in the tumor (PII).

Based on the data of fluorescence monitoring, the optimal times for illumination, as determined for each tested photosensitizer, were: 24 h for Lu-Tex and PII, 3 h for Chl and 1 h for ALA. As seen in Fig. 5, the drugs' accumulation selectivity at these time intervals were as follows: Lu-TX > Pp-IX > Chl > PII (Fig. 5).

ILLUMINATION

Two incoherent illumination systems, which were developed for PDT by ESC Medical Sytems LTD (Haifa, Israel), were used in our PDT study: VersaLight (continuous wave, CW) and Photodyne (high-intensity pulsed light).

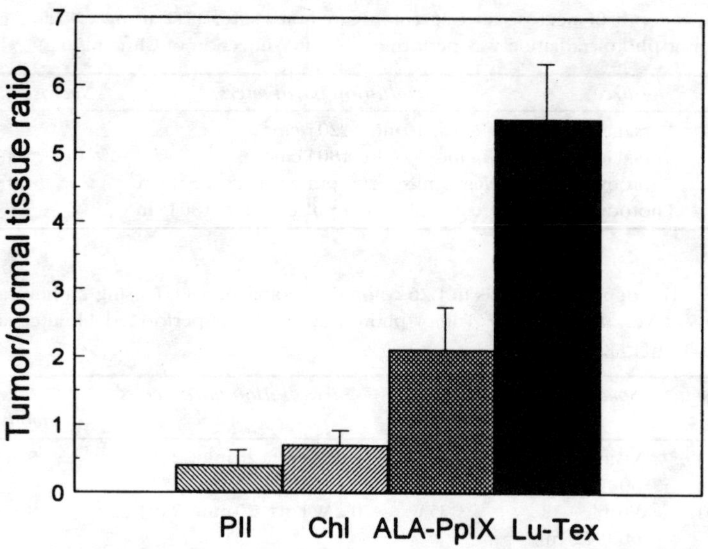

Figure 5 Accumulation selectivity for Photofrin (24 h after injection), chlorin e_6 (3 h after injection), ALA induced Pp-IX (1 h after injection) and lutetium texaphyrin (24 h after injection) determined by the LIF method on a C26 colon carcinoma model.

The spectral characteristics and output parameters of these illumination sources are given in Table 1.

The broad-band photoirradiation provided by these systems allows the testing of photosensitizers with different spectral characteristics. The results of comparison evaluation showed that the same effect can be obtained in a C26 tumor model after Chl injection and application of either CW or pulsed light sources (Table 2). The advantage of pulsed photoirradiation as compared to CW was in the shorter treatment time (3–5 min vs. 10–15 min). Table 3 demonstrates the possibility of using the additive effect of hyperthermia produced by the VersaLight system in ALA-PDT.

For a comparative study of Lu-Tex, Chl, ALA and PII, both feet were illuminated simultaneously by the Photodyne system, using 0.6 J/cm^2 pulses providing total light doses from 90 to 300 J/cm^2.

Table 1 The Spectral Characteristics and Output Parameters of Illumination Sources used for PDT

Source	*Spectral range*	*Maximal output*	*Pulse*		
			Energy	*Duration*	*Frequency*
VersaLight (continuous wave, visible only)	600–720 nm	3 W	–	–	–
Photodyne (pulsed light)	600–800 nm	–	0.1–5 J/cm^2	1–3 ms	1–0.1 Hz

Table 2 The depth of necrosis in C26 colon carcinoma after PDT using CW and pulsed light sources. Tumor photoirradiation was performed 3 h after injection of Chl (5 mg/kg)

Treatment	*Source*	*Irradiation parameters*	*Necrosis depth* (mm)
Chl-PDT	VersaLight	$0.2\,W/cm^2$, 10 min, $120\,J/cm^2$	4.7 ± 0.3
Chl-PDT	VersaLight	$0.2\,W/cm^2$, 15 min, $180\,J/cm^2$	5.8 ± 0.5
Chl-PDT	Photodyne	$0.6\,J/cm^2$/pulse, 200 pulses, 1 Hz, $120\,J/cm^2$	4.9 ± 0.1
Chl-PDT	Photodyne	$0.6\,J/cm^2$/pulse, 300 pulses, 1 Hz, $180\,J/cm^2$	5.5 ± 0.2

Table 3 The depth of necrosis in C26 colon carcinoma after PDT using 2 photoradiation regimens of VersaLight system. Tumor photoirradiation was performed 1 h after injection of ALA (200 mg/kg)

Treatment	*Spectral range*	*Maximal output*	*Irradiation parameters*	*Necrosis depth* (mm)
ALA-PDT	Visible 600–720 nm	3 W	$0.2\,W/cm^2$, 20 min, $240\,J/cm^2$	5.2 ± 0.3
ALA-PDT	Visible + IR 600–720 nm 1200–1700 nm	3.75 W	$0.2\,W/cm^2$, 20 min, $240\,J/cm^2$	8.5 ± 0.2

TUMOR AND NORMAL TISSUE RESPONSES

Tissue reaction to PDT is determined by the expression of damage effect and the potency of reparative processes. The expression of the damage effect is dependent on efficiency and tissue concentration of the photosensitizer and the light dose applied. The morphological character of damage effects after PDT on tumor and normal tissues are very similar, displaying vascular reaction (stasis, edema) followed by necrosis. The expression of edema can be more pronounced in the normal tissue than in the tumor, but it may disappear without necrosis formation, depending on the treatment dose applied.

We used inhibition of tumor growth rate as compared to the untreated control as a criterium of tumor response, and expression of edema in the normal foot as a criterium of normal tissue response to PDT.

Tumor growth inhibition ratio (TGIR) was calculated as:

$$\mathrm{TGIR} = [(k_c - k_e)/k_c] \times 100\%, \tag{2}$$

where k_c and k_e are the constants of the tumor growth rate, which were determined by the least squares method in the control and the experimental groups of animals, respectively.

The value of the edema ratio (ER) in the normal foot was calculated as:

$$\mathrm{ER} = (D_t/D_0) - 1 \tag{3}$$

where D_0 and D_t are the size of the foot before and after the treatment, respectively.

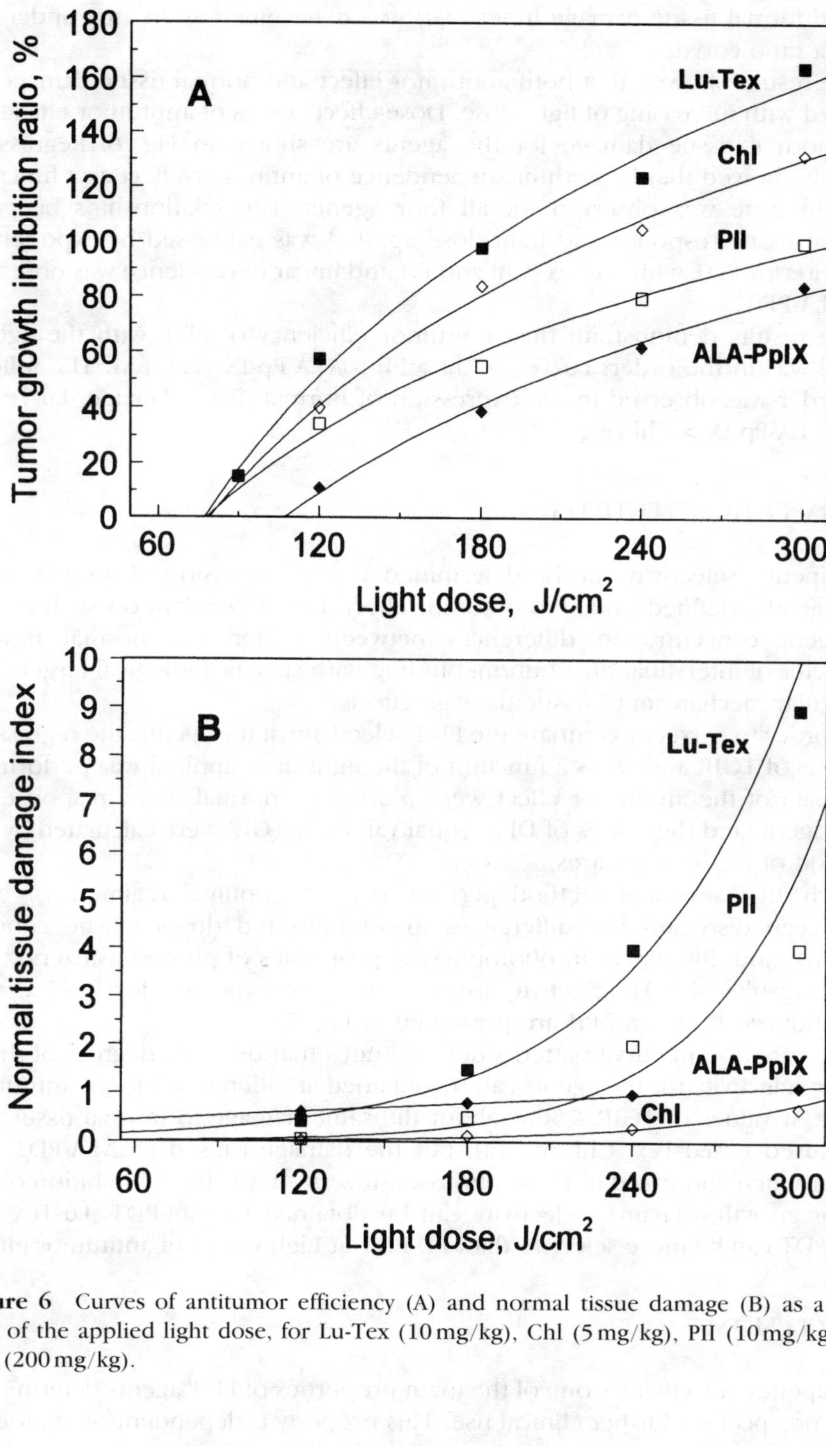

Figure 6 Curves of antitumor efficiency (A) and normal tissue damage (B) as a function of the applied light dose, for Lu-Tex (10 mg/kg), Chl (5 mg/kg), PII (10 mg/kg) and ALA (200 mg/kg).

The normal tissue damage index (DI) was determined as an area under the edema ratio curve.

The results showed that both antitumor effect and normal tissue damage increased with increasing of light dose. Dose-effect curves of antitumor efficiency and normal tissue damage for the agents are shown in Fig. 6. Regression analysis showed that logarithmic dependence of antitumor effect as a function of light dose was observed for all four agents. The relationships between normal tissue response and light dose applied was expressed by exponential behavior for PDT with Lu-Tex, Chl and PII and linear dependence was observed for ALA-PDT.

The results demonstrate that antitumor efficiency of PDT with the agents tested was in the order: Lu-Tex > Chl > PII > ALA-Pp-IX (Fig. 6A). The following order was observed in the expression of normal tissue damage: Lu-Tex > PII > ALA-Pp-IX > Chl (Fig. 6B).

THERAPEUTIC SELECTIVITY

Therapeutic selectivity can be determined as the expression of normal tissue damage at a defined value of antitumor effect. It is dependent on such factors as agent concentration differences between tumor and normal tissues, character of interstitial distribution, binding with specific biological targets and particular mechanism of tissue damage effects.

In order to correctly compare the PDT selectivity of the agents, the regression analysis of TGIR and DI as a function of the light dose applied was performed. The data of the antitumor effect were plotted vs. normal tissue response for each agent, and the values of DI at equal values of TGIR were calculated by the method of the least squares.

Such an assessment method performed at the optimal regimen for each agent can disregard the differences in administered doses (tissue concentrations) and differences in photophysical properties of photosensitizers.

The results of PDT selectivity assessment by this method for Lu-Tex, Chl, ALA-induced Pp-IX and PII are presented in Fig. 7.

The variation in curve patterns demonstrates that different degrees of therapeutic selectivity for the agents can be obtained at different values of antitumor effect. At values of TGIR $\leqslant$ 50%, about the same damage to normal tissue can be caused by Lu-Tex, Chl and PII, but the damage caused by ALA-PDT was higher when compared to these photosensitizers. At 80–100%-inhibition of the tumor growth, maximal selectivity can be obtained for Chl-PDT. Lu-Tex and ALA-PDT can be more selective than PII-PDT at high values of antitumor effect.

CONCLUSIONS

Therapeutic selectivity is one of the main properties of PDT agents determining their prospect for further clinical use. This property is dependent on biological

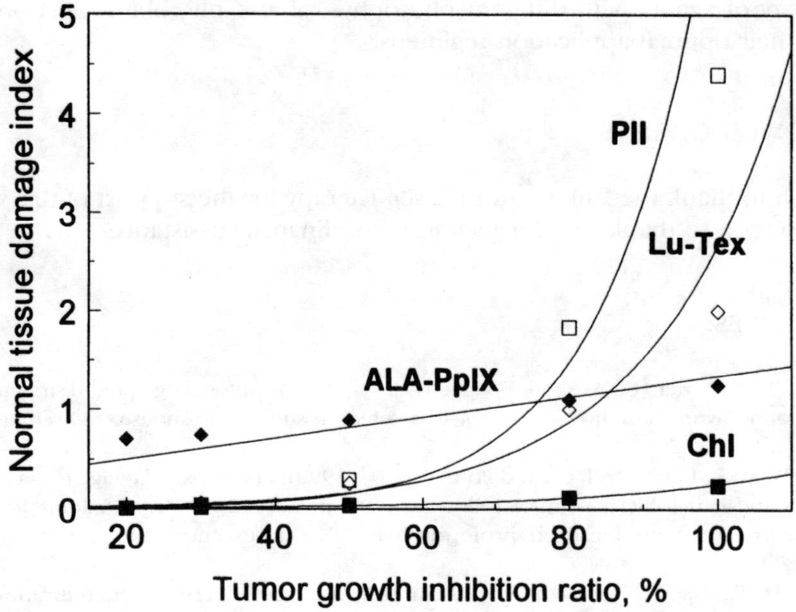

Figure 7 PDT selectivity of Lu-Tex, Chl, ALA and PII (calculated values of normal tissue damage at different values of antitumor effect).

mechanism of specific interstitial distribution (binding sites) and characteristics of tissue-damage effects.

The purpose of the present experimental study was to carry out accumulation kinetics and therapeutic selectivity assessments of the agents with distinct photophysical and biochemical properties.

LIF monitoring revealed different kinetic patterns of accumulation in normal and tumor tissues for the agents tested and allows the determination of the optimal time interval between injection and photoirradiation.

Results of the PDT study showed different antitumor efficiency and expression of the normal tissue damage for all agents at the regimens used. Selectivity assessment tests, based on the regression analysis of normal and tumor tissue responses to PDT as a function of the light dose, revealed that at equal values of antitumor effect Chl, Lu-Tex and ALA-PDT can be more selective than PII-PDT.

The observed differences in kinetics of accumulation and PDT selectivity of the agents reflected distinct biochemical properties and mechanisms of their action. These differences, provoked by individual agent biodistribution, may be confirmed by histopathological and ultrastructural examinations (Nelson *et al.*, 1988; Fingar *et al.*, 1990, 1992; McMahon *et al.*, 1994; Orenstein *et al.*, 1996b).

We suggest that the experimental model and approach used in these experiments allow objective comparison of tissue accumulation and therapeutic selectivity of agents with different photophysical and photobiological properties at their optimal application regimens.

ACKNOWLEDGEMENT

We wish to thank the Falk Chair in Laser Therapy for the support of this work. We also wish to thank ESC for technical and financial assistance.

REFERENCES

Bugelski, P. J., Porter, C. W., and Dougherty, T. J. (1981): Autoradiographic distribution of hematoporphyrin derivative in normal and tumor tissue of the mouse. *Cancer Res.* **41**, 4606–4612.

Divaris, D. X. G., Kennedy, J. C., and Pottier, R. H. (1990): Phototoxic damage to sebaceous glands and hair follicles of mice following systemic administration of 5-aminolevulinic acid correlates with localized protoporphyrin IX fluorescence. *Am. J. Pathol.* **136**, 891–897.

Dvorak, H. F., Nagy, J. A., Dvorak, J. T., and Dvorak, A. M. (1988): Identification and characterization of the blood vessels of solid tumors that are leaky to circulating macromolecules. *Am. J. Pathol.* **133**, 95–109.

Dougherty, T. J. (1993): Photodynamic therapy. *Photochem. Photobiol.* **58**, 895–900.

Ehrenberg, B., Malik, Z., Nitzan, Y., Ladan, H., Johnson, F. M., Hemmi, G., and Sessler, J. L. (1993): The binding and photosensitization effects of tetrabenzoporphyrins and texaphyrin in bacterial cells. *Lasers Med. Sci.* **8**, 197–203.

Fingar, V. H., Wieman, T. J., Wiehle, S. A., and Cerrito, P. B. (1990): The role of thromboxane and prostacyclin release on photodynamic-therapy-induced tumor destruction. *Cancer Res.* **50**, 2599–2603.

Fingar, V. H., Wieman, T. J., Wiehle, S. A., and Cerrito, P. B. (1992): The role of microvascular damage in photodynamic therapy: the effect of treatment on vessel constriction, permeability and leukocyte adhesion. *Cancer Res.* **52**, 4914–4921.

Frisoli, J. K., Tudor, E. J., Flotte, T. J., Hasan, T., Deutsch, T., and Schomacker, K. T. (1993): Pharmacokinetics of a fluorescent drug using laser-induced fluorescence. *Cancer Res.* **53**, 5954–5961.

Frolov, A. A., Kochubeyev, G. A., and Gurinovich, G. P. (1989): Photodynamic effect of chlorin e_6 on biological systems. *Studia Biophysica* **134**, 235–247.

Frolov, A. A., Zenkevich, E. I., Gurinovich, G. P., and Kochubeyev, G. A. (1990): Chlorin e_6–liposome interaction. Investigation by the methods of fluorescence spectroscopy and inductive resonance energy transfer. *J. Photochem. Photobiol. B: Biol.* 7, 43–56.

Jain, R. K. (1987): Transport of molecules in the tumor interstitium: a review. *Cancer Res.* **47**, 3039–3051.

Jori, G. (1992): Far-red-absorbing photosensitizers – their use in the photodynamic therapy of tumours. *J. Photochem. Photobiol. A: Chem.* **62**, 371–378.

Harriman, A., Maiya, B. G., Murai, T., Hemmi, G., Sessler, J. L., and Mallouk, T. E. (1989): Metallotexaphyrins: a new family of photosensitizers for efficient generation of singlet oxygen. *J. Chem. Soc. Chem. Commun.* 314–316.

Kennedy, J. C. and Pottier, R. H. (1992): Endogenous protoporphyrin IX, a clinically useful photosensitizer for photodynamic therapy. *J. Photochem. Photobiol. B: Biol.* **14**, 275–292.

Kennedy, J. C., Nadeau, P., Petryka, Z. J., Pottier, R. H., and Weagle, G. (1992): Clearance times of porphyrin derivatives from mice as measured by *in vivo* fluorescence spectroscopy. *Photochem. Photobiol.* **55**, 569–574.

Kennedy, J. C., Pottier, R. H., and Pross, D. C. (1990): Photodynamic therapy with endogenous protoporphyrin IX: basic principles and present clinical experience. *J. Photochem. Photobiol. B: Biol.* **6**, 143–148.

Kongshaug, M. (1992): Distribution of tetrapyrrole photosensitizers among human plasma proteins. *Int. J. Biochem.* **24**, 1239–1265.

Kostenich, G. A., Zhuravkin, I. N., Furmanchuk, A. V., and Zhavrid, E. A. (1991): Photodynamic therapy with chlorin e_6. A morphologic study of tumour damage efficiency in experiment. *J. Photochem. Photobiol. B: Biol.* **11**, 307–318.

Kostenich, G. A., Zhuravkin, I. N., Furmanchuk, A. V., and Zhavrid, E. A. (1993): Sensitivity of different rat tumour strains to photodynamic treatment with chlorin e_6. *J. Photochem. Photobiol. B: Biol.* **17**, 187–194.

Kostenich, G. A., Zhuravkin, I. N., and Zhavrid, E. A. (1994): Experimental grounds for using chlorin e_6 in the photodynamic therapy of malignant tumours. *J. Photochem. Photobiol. B: Biol.* **22**, 211–217.

Lavi, A., Johnson, F. M., and Ehrenberg, B. (1994): Wavelength dependence of the fluorescence and singlet oxygen quantum yields of new photosensitizers. *Chem. Phys. Lett.* **231**, 144–150.

Levy, J. G. (1994): Photosensitizers in photodynamic therapy. *Semin. Oncol.* **21**, 4–10.

Malik, Z. and Djaldetti, M. (1979): 5-Aminolevulinic acid stimulation of porphyrin and hemoglobin synthesis by uninduced Friend erythroleukemic cells. *Cell Different.* **8**, 223–233.

Malik, Z., Kostenich, G., Roitman, L., Ehrenberg, B., and Orenstein, A. (1995): Topical application of 5-aminolevulinic acid, DMSO and EDTA: protoporphyrin IX accumulation in skin and tumours of mice. *J. Photochem. Photobiol. B: Biol.* **28**, 213–218.

Maziere, J. C., Morliere, P., and Santus, R. (1991): The role of the low density lipoprotein receptor pathway in the delivery of lipophilic photosensitizers in the photodynamic therapy of tumors. *J. Photochem. Photobiol. B: Biol.* **8**, 351–360.

McMahon, K. S., Wieman, T. J., Moore, P. H., and Fingar, V. H. (1994): Effects of photodynamic therapy using mono-L-aspartyl chlorin e_6 on vessel constriction, vessel leakage, and tumor response. *Cancer Res.* **54**, 5374–5379.

Nelson, J. S., Liaw, L. H., Orenstein, A., Roberts, W. G., and Berns, M. W. (1988): Mechanism of tumor destruction following photodynamic therapy with hematoporphyrin derivative, chlorin, and phthalocyanine. *J. Natl. Cancer Inst.* **80**, 1599–1605.

Orenstein, A., Kostenich, G., Roitman, L., Tsur, H., Katanick, D., Kopolovic, J., Ehrenberg, B., and Malik, Z. (1996a): Photodynamic therapy of malignant lesions of the skin mediated by topical application of 5-aminolevulinic acid in combination with DMSO and EDTA. *Lasers Life Sci.* **7**, 1–9.

Orenstein, A., Kostenich, G., Roitman, L., Shechtman, Y., Kopolovic, J., Ehrenberg, B., and Malik, Z. (1996b): A comparative study of tissue distribution and PDT selectivity of chlorin e_6, Photofrin II and ALA-induced protoporphyrin IX in a colon carcinoma model. *Br. J. Cancer* **73**, 937–944.

Peng, Q., Moan, J., Warloe, T., Nesland, M., and Rimington, C. (1992): Distribution and photosensitizing efficiency of porphyrins induced by application of exogenous 5-aminolevulinic acid in mice bearing mammary carcinoma. *Int. J. Cancer* **52**, 433–443.

Sessler, J. L., Hemmi, G., Mody, T. D., and Lynch, V. (1993): Synthesis and structural characterization of lanthanide (III) texaphyrins. *Inorg. Chem*. **32**, 3175–3187.

Sessler, J. L., Hemmi, G., Maiya, B. G., Harriman, A., Judy, M. L., Boriak, B., Matthews, J. L., Ehrenberg, B., Malik, Z., Nitzan, Y., and Ruck, A. (1991): Tripyrroledimethine-derived (Texaphyrin type) macrocycles: potential photosensitizers which absorb in the far red spectral region. *SPIE* **1426**, 318–329.

Spikes, J. D. (1990): Chlorins as photosensitizers in biology and medicine. *J. Photochem. Photobiol. B: Biol*. **6**, 259–274.

Svanberg, K., Anderson, T., and Killander, D. (1992): Photodynamic therapy of human skin malignancies and laser-induced fluorescence diagnostics utilizing photofrin and 5-Aminolevulinic acid. In: Spinelli, P., Dal Fante, M., Marchesini, R. (eds.), *Photodynamic Therapy and Biomedical Lasers*, Elsevier Science Publishers, Amsterdam, 436–440.

Warloe, T., Peng, Q., Moan, J., Qvist, H. L., and Giercksky, K. E. (1992): Photochemotherapy of multiple basal cell carcinoma with endogenous porphyrins induced by topical application of 5-aminolevulinic acid. In: Spinelli, P., Dal Fante, M., Marchesini, R. (eds.), *Photodynamic Therapy and Biomedical Lasers*, Elsevier Science Publishers, Amsterdam, 449–453.

Young, S. W., Woodburn, K. W., Wright, M., Mody, T. D., Fan, Q., Sessler, J. L., Dow, W. C., and Miller, R. A. (1996): Lutetium texaphyrin (PCI-0123): A near-infrared water soluble photosensitizer. *Photochem. Photobiol*. **63**, 892–897.

3. STATE OF THE ART AND FUTURE PROSPECTS

3.1. CHLOROPHYLL AND BACTERIOCHLOROPHYLL DERIVATIVES AS PHOTODYNAMIC AGENTS

VARDA ROSENBACH-BELKIN, LOUISA CHEN, LESZEK FIEDOR, YORAM SALOMON and AVIGDOR SCHERZ

Chlorophyll and bacteriochlorophyll were modified at the propionyl residue by hydrolysis or transesterification using the enzyme chlorophyllase in order to make them water soluble. The new derivatives retain their spectral properties of strong absorption in the near infra red (NIR) and show strong photocytotoxicity in M2R melanoma cell cultures.

INTRODUCTION

Among the novel classes of photosensitizers and treatment protocols that were developed in order to overcome the shortcomings of the presently applied photodynamic therapy (PDT) agents, are the photosynthetic pigments chlorophylls (Chl) and bacteriochlorophylls (Bchl). This natural pigments have high optical extinction coefficient in the ~660 nm and ~780 nm bands, respectively. In the second wavelength domain, light penetration depth is approximately three times that attained at 630 nm, the wavelength currently used in clinics for photosensitization of Photofrin (Amato, 1993; Doiron, 1984; Svaasand, 1984; Wilson *et al.*, 1985). Chlorophyll and Bchl have good yields of excited triplet state with life times similar to those observed for hematoporphyrin derivative (HpD) [30–70% (Leupold, personal communication; Amato, 1993; Fiedor *et al.*, 1993; Krasnovskii, *et al.*, 1985)]. Unfortunately they are water insoluble and were previously administered by others in detergent micelles or liposome vehicles in order to deliver antitumor activity *in vivo* (Henderson *et al.*, 1991).

Since the spectral characteristics of Chl and Bchl are determined by their macrocycle, it was realized that modifications of peripheral groups that are not conjugated to the macrocycle, may further enhance their hydrophilicity while retaining their photodynamic activity as in the cases of chlorins, pheophorbides or purpurins (Bellnier *et al.*, 1993; Hoober *et al.*, 1988; Kessel *et al.*, 1989; Lee *et al.*, 1993; Moser, 1993; Pandey *et al.*, 1992, 1994, 1996; Röder, 1990; Spike, 1990). Indeed, hydrolysis of the phytol chain of Chl a and Bchl a enhanced their solubility in aqueous media by several orders of magnitude. Further increase was observed upon esterification of the propionic side chain with polar amino acid residues such as serine and tyrosine (Scherz *et al.*, 1994), while the optical properties of the Bchl conjugates were found similar to those of native Chl/Bchl molecules (Fiedor *et al.*, 1993). The quantum yield for triplet state formation of the new Bchl complex is much lower than that of native Bchl (unpublished data). Yet, the new compounds showed much higher photocytotoxicity as compared to HpD when tested in M2R melanoma cell cultures (Tregub *et al.*, 1992; Rosenbach-Belkin *et al.*, 1996) and *in vivo* (Scherz *et al.*, 1994; Zilberstein *et al.*,

1994, 1995, 1997), and cleared from mouse tissues within a few hours to days (Rosenbach-Belkin *et al.*, 1996). The shorter retention of these pigment derivatives in the circulation is expected to minimize the serious side effect of cutaneous phototoxicity, presently a major drawback of photofrin based PDT.

Following this strategy, the new Chl/Bchl conjugates can be further conjugated with peptides, hormones or antibodies for targeting purposes (Scherz *et al.*, 1994 Fiedor *et al.*, 1996). This conjugation renders site specificity to the new PDT reagents.

MATERIALS AND METHODS

Photosensitizers

Chlorophyll and Bchl derivatives are prepared from the natural pigments Chl a and Bchl a, respectively, using *Melia Azedarach L., China* tree chlorophyllase (Chlase) (Amir-Shapira *et al.*, 1987).

Bchl a is extracted from lyophilized cells of *Rhodospirillum rubrum* (Scherz *et al.*, 1984). Chl a is similarly extracted from *Spirulina geitleri*.

Enzymatic Synthesis of Bacteriochlorophylide/Chlorophylides (Bchlide/Chlide) (Scherz *et al.*, 1994)

Acetone powder of Chlase (400 mg) is homogenized in 45 ml of 0.2 M sodium phosphate buffer at pH = 7.8, containing 0.8% Triton X-100 (v/v), using a Polytron homogenizer. The suspension is stirred vigorously for 3 h at room temperature and then centrifuged for 15 min at 15,000 × *g*. The supernatant containing solubilized Chlase is collected and stored at − 20°C up to several months. To 10 ml of the Chlase extract, 25 mg sodium ascorbate are added. The enzyme solution is then added to a portion of 10–15 mg solid Bchl a/Chl a and sonicated to suspend the pigment. The reaction mixture is saturated with argon, sealed and stirred for 5–6 h at 37°C in the dark.

Purification of Bchlide/Chlide (Scherz *et al.*, 1994)

The reaction mixture is saturated with NaCl and extracted a few times with 30–40 ml of diethyl ether. The ether extract is dried over solid NaCl, filtered and the solvent is evaporated under vacuum. The blue/green residue of the pigment is dried by lyophilization, dissolved in acetone and loaded on a CM-Sepharose column (1 × 8 cm) equilibrated in acetone. Less polar unreacted pheophytins and Chls are eluted in acetone and 5% MeOH in acetone (v/v). Pheophorbide is eluted with 7% MeOH in acetone and, finally, the product Bchlide/Chlide is collected from the column using 25% MeOH in acetone. The solvent is evaporated and the solid pigment is stored under argon at − 20°C in the dark.

CM-Sepharose Preparation

CM-Sepharose (Pharmacia Fine Chemicals CL-6B) is first washed with water and then 3 times with acetone before packing a column and equilibrating in acetone. The chromatographic material can be reused after thorough rinsing with 2 M NaCl aqueous solution until colorless, washing with water and resuspending in acetone.

Enzymatic Synthesis of Bchl/Chl-Serine (Bchl/Chl-Ser) (Scherz *et al.*, 1994)

400 mg of 1-methyl ester serine hydrochloride (Sigma) and 70 mg ascorbic acid (Merck) are dissolved in 9 ml of water. Using 10 M KOH aqueous solution, the pH of the serine solution is adjusted to 7.7 and 1 ml of 0.5 M sodium phosphate buffer (pH 7.7) is added to maintain the pH during the reaction. Approximately 80 µl of Triton X-100 are added to achieve a final detergent concentration of 0.8% (v/v). In 6 ml of this solution, 200 mg of Chlase acetone powder is homogenized using a Polytron homogenizer. The remaining solution is used to wash the instrument and is then combined with the homogenate. The enzyme suspension is sonicated with 20 mg of solid Bchl a/Chl a, saturated with argon and incubated in the dark for 7 h at 37°C while stirring.

Purification of Bchl/Chl-Ser (Scherz *et al.*, 1994)

The reaction mixture is filtered in a Buchner funnel under vacuum and the residual pigments are washed from the filter paper with acetone. The combined filtrates are saturated with NaCl and the pigments are extracted with diethyl ether. After drying over NaCl, the solvents are evaporated under vacuum. If there is still water left, the blue-green residue is dried in a lyophilizer overnight. Then the residue is dissolved in acetone and subjected to CM-Sepharose column equilibrated in acetone. The column is washed with acetone to elute unreacted material and then with 5% and 7% methanol (v/v) in acetone to elute Bchlide/Chlide, Bpheophorbide/Pheophorbide. The product is then eluted with 25% methanol in acetone. The solvent is evaporated and the solid pigment is stored under argon at −20°C in the dark.

The hematoporphyrin derivative was the commercially available Photosan-3, supplied at a concentration of 3.3 mg/ml in isotonic NaCl by Seehof Laboratory GmbH D-25764 Wesselburenerkoog, Germany, kindly given to us by Dr. J. Moser.

Cell Culture

M2R mouse melanoma cells were cultured as monolayers in Dulbecco's modified Eagle's medium (DMEM)/F12 containing 25 mM HEPES pH 7.4, 10% Fetal Bovine Serum (FBS), glutamine 2 mM, penicillin 0.06 mg/ml and streptomycin 0.1 mg/ml at 37°C in a humidified atmosphere of 8% CO_2 as previously described (Gerst *et al.*, 1986).

Light Source

The light source for irradiation was a homebuilt 250 W halogen lamp focused through a 10 cm water filter on a glass support and fitted with a cut-off filter that blocked light under 550 nm in the case of photosan as a photosensitizer or under 610 nm for cells treated with Chl-Ser and Bchl-Ser. The light dose was adjusted to 45 mW/cm^2 in all cases.

Cell Photocytotoxicity Studies

M2R mouse melanoma cells (1×10^5/well) were cultured in 24 well microplates and grown for 24 h to about 2×10^5 cells/well, approximately 70–80% confluency. Chl-Ser or Bchl-Ser were dissolved in culture medium and dispersed by sonication.

Photosan was diluted to its final concentration in culture medium. The medium was replaced with serum-free medium and cells were incubated in dark with the desired concentration of photosensitizers. Following 2 h of incubation the cells were irradiated at room temperature for 5 min from the bottom of the plate. The medium was replaced by serum containing medium and the culture plates were placed back in the incubator for 24 h. Cytotoxic efficiency in the cell culture was determined by (i) microscopic examination of cell morphology (ii) fluorescence microscopy of cells following treatment with vital stain, [propidium Iodide (PID) 2,7-diamino-9-phenyl-10-(diethylaminopropyl)-phenathridinium iodide methiodide] which selectively accumulates in nuclei of damaged cells (Yeh *et al.*, 1981) and (iii) [^{3}H] thymidine incorporation as further described below. Control experiments included (1) untreated cells kept in the dark, (2) untreated cells illuminated and (3) cells treated with the drug but kept in the dark.

[^{3}H] Thymidine Incorporation

Twenty-four hours after PDT, cell cultures were pulsed with 1 μCi/ml [^{3}H] thymidine for 2 h at 37°C. Cultures were then washed twice with phosphate buffered saline (PBS), treated with 7.5% cold trichloroacetic acid (TCA) for 30 min at 4°C and washed twice with ethanol. Sodium hydroxide 1 N (300 μl/well) was added and the plates were kept for 10 min at 37°C. Samples of 100 μl were transferred to scintillation vials, neutralized with 100 μl 1 N HCl and radioactivity was counted by liquid scintillation counting in 4 ml (20 : 8 (v/v)) xylene scintillator lumax mixture according to Chen *et al.* (1988).

Light Microscopy

Cell monolayers were examined by phase and fluorescence (rhodamine optics) microscopy using a Zeiss Axiovert 35 inverted microscope.

RESULTS AND DISCUSSION

Optical Absorption of Bchl/Chl Derivatives

The optical absorption spectra of Bchl-Ser and Chl-Ser in acetone is shown in Fig. 1 and are the same as that of Bchlide/Chlide and of the natural photosynthetic pigments Bchl/Chl in acetone. Figure 1 also shows the optical absorption of HPD at the same concentration as the Bchl/Chl-Ser. One can see that the strong absorption of the chlorophyllous pigments in the red and near infrared regions render their superiority for PDT.

The extinction coefficients of the derivatives were calculated by monitoring the atomic absorption of the central Magnesium atom in methanol (Rosenbach-Belkin, 1988). For calibration we used curves that describe the absorption of different concentrations of Chl in Methanol. The extinction coefficients were found to be the same as those of the natural (B)Chl (unpublished data).

Photocytotoxicity of Bchl/Chl Derivatives

All new derivatives showed photodynamic activity both *in vitro* (Tregub *et al.*, 1992; Rosenbach-Belkin *et al.*, 1996) and *in vivo* (Scherz *et al.*, 1994; Zilberstein

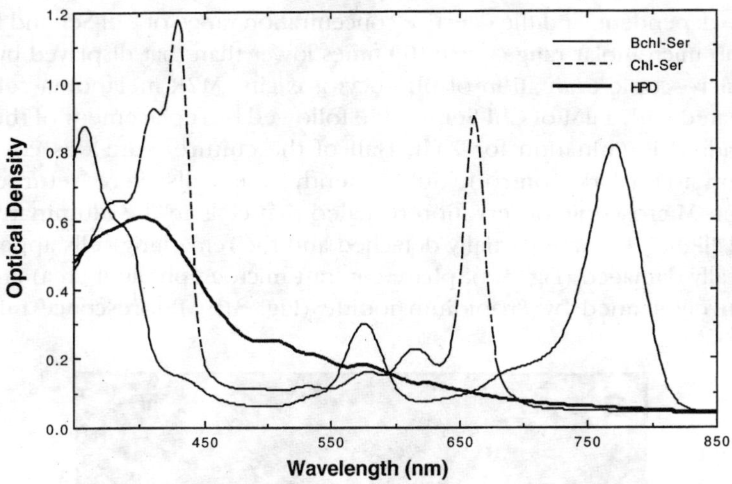

Figure 1 Absorption spectra of Bchl-Ser, Chl-Ser and HPD. All pigment (Bchl-Ser, Chl-Ser, HPD (Photosan)) are at the same concentration of 1.1×10^{-5} M in acetone.

et al., 1994, 1995). Their photocytotoxicity in melanoma cell cultures was compared to that of the commercial hematoporphyrin derivative (HPD, Photosan) by following [^{3}H] thymidine incorporation after incubation of cell cultures with increasing concentrations of Chl-Ser, Bchl-Ser or photosan in the dark (control) or under illumination (Fig. 2). It can be seen that cytotoxicity of all pigment derivatives is light

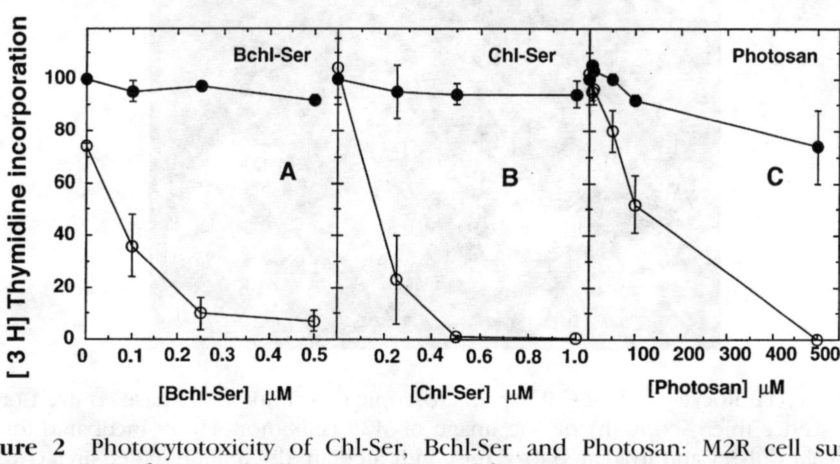

Figure 2 Photocytotoxicity of Chl-Ser, Bchl-Ser and Photosan: M2R cell survival determined by [^{3}H] thymidine incorporation. [^{3}H] thymidine incorporation in M2R cells following treatment with the indicated photosensitizer concentrations (Bchl-Ser, Chl-Ser and Photosan) in the dark or after illumination (5 min) is shown. Cell survival is given as [^{3}H] thymidine incorporation (2 h pulse) performed 24 h after PD treatment relative to untreated controls. Values are the mean ± SD of 8, 2 and 7 experiments respectively performed by duplicate determinations each. Reproduced with permission by *Photocem. Photobiol.*

and dose dependent, and the effective concentration range of Chl-Ser and Bchl-Ser is in the sub micromolar range, over 100 times lower than that displayed by HpD.

For microscopic evaluation of photocytotoxicity, M2R melanoma cell cultures were treated with 1 μM of Chl-Ser for 1 h, followed by replacement of the medium and standard illumination for 24 h. Half of the culture plate was covered with aluminum foil (dark control). Subsequently, the cells were returned to the incubator. Microscopic observation revealed that cells in the illuminated regions (marked "light") became partially detached and the remaining cells appeared morphologically damaged (Fig. 3(a), phase contrast micrograph, light area) and became all positively stained by Propidium iodide (Fig. 3(b) fluorescence micrograph,

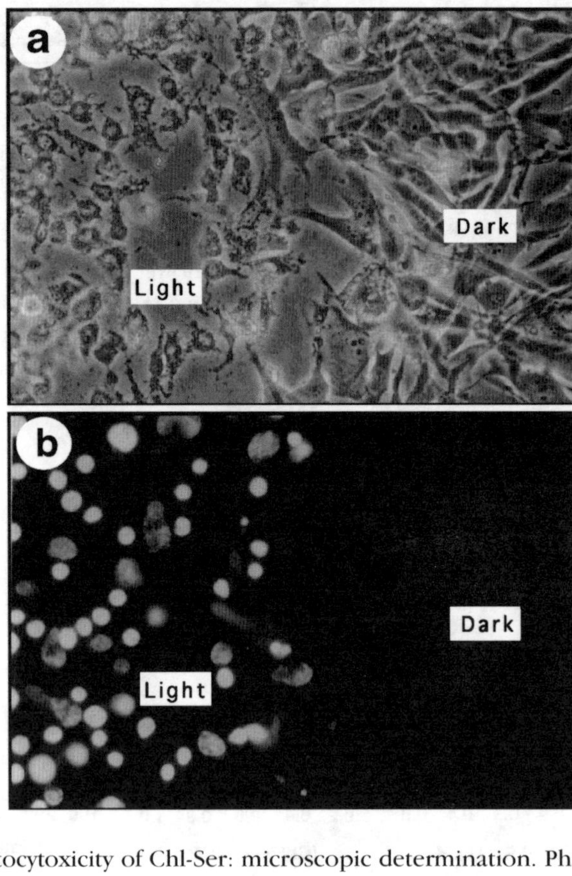

Figure 3 Photocytoxicity of Chl-Ser: microscopic determination. Phase contrast (a) or fluorescence microscopy (b) of one image of M2R cells monolayers incubated for 1 h with 1 μM Chl-Ser and irradiated for 5 min. Indicated are the unilluminated area covered with aluminium foil (dark) and the illuminated area (light). Magnification × 900. Cells in the dark area have a normal shape (a) and exclude the vital stain propidium iodide (b). Cells in the illuminated area (Light) appear damaged (a) and their nuclei become stained with propidium iodide (b). Reproduced with permission by *Photochem. Photobiol*.

light area). In contrast, cells in the aluminum covered area (served as "dark" controls) appeared normal (Fig. 3(a), dark area) and excluded the dye (Fig. 3(b) dark area). Cells in illuminated untreated controls, appeared identical to untreated or dark treated control cultures.

The superior spectral properties and the hydrophilic nature of (B)Chl derivatives seem to make them good potential photodynamic agent as is shown by their significant photodynamic activity *in vivo* and *in vitro*.

ACKNOWLEDGMENTS

Y.S. is the incumbent of the Charles and Tillie Lubin Chair of Biochemical Endocrinology. This study was supported in part by grants from: The Lynne and William Frankel Fund for the Diagnosis and Treatment of Ovarian and Breast Cancer, The Jaffe Family Foundation and Yeda Research and Development Co. Ltd., Israel, and the Ministry of Science and Technology, Israel, the Commission of the European Communities. The authors are in debt to S. Zuckerman for her generous support of this research. The authors wish to thank R. Benjamin and M. Kopelowitz for their excellent secretarial assistance.

REFERENCES

Amato, I. (1993): Hope for a magic bullet that moves at the speed of light. *Science* **262**, 32–33.

Amir-Shapira, D., Goldschmidt, E. E., and Altman, A. (1987): Chlorophyll catabolism in senescing plant tissues: *in vitro* breakdown intermediates suggest different degradative pathways for citrus fruit and parsley leaves. *Proc. Natl. Acad. Sci. USA* **84**, 1901–1905.

Bellnier, D. A., Henderson, B. W., Pandey, R. K., Potter, W. R., and Dougherty, T. J: Sensitizer. 2-[1-hexyloxyethyl]-2-devinyl pyropheophorbide-a. *J. Photochem. Photobiol. B: Biol.* **20**, 55–61.

Chen, L., Mory, Y., Zilberstein, A., and Revel, M. (1988): Growth inhibition of human breast carcinoma, and leukemia/lymphoma cell lines by recombinant interferon. *Proc. Natl. Acad. Sci. USA* **85**, 8037–8041.

Doiron, D. R. (1984): Photophysics and instrumentation for porphyrin detection and activation. In Porphyrin Localization and Treatment of Tumors (Edited by D. R. Doiron and C. J. Gomer), pp. 41–73. Liss, New York.

Fiedor, L., Gorman, A. A., Hamblett, I., Rosenbach-Belkin, V., Salomon, Y., Scherz, A., and Tregub, I. (1993): A pulsed laser and pulse radiolysis study of amphiphilic chlorophyll derivatives with PDT activity toward malignant melanoma. *Photochem. Photobiol.* **58**, 506–511.

Fiedor, L., Rosenbach-Belkin, V., Sai, M., and Scherz. A. (1996) Preparation of tetrapyrrole–amino acid covalent complexes. *Plant Physiol. Biochem.* **34**, 393–398.

Gerst, J. E., Sole, J., Mather, J. P., and Salomon, Y. (1986): Regulation of adenylate cyclase by β-melanotropin in the M2R melanoma cell line. *Mol. Cell. Endocrinol.* **46**, 137–147.

Henderson, B. W., Sumlin, A. B., Owczarczak, B. L., and Dougherty, T. J. (1991): Bacteriochlorophyll-a as photosensitizer for photodynamic treatment of transplantable murine tumors. *J. Photochem. Photobiol. B: Biol.* **10**, 303–313.

Hoober, J. K., Sery, T. W., and Yamamoto, N. (1988): Photodynamic sensitizers from chlorophyll: purpurin-18 and chlorin p6. *Photochem. Photobiol.* **48**, 579–582.

Kessel, D. and Smith, K. (1989): Photosensitization with derivatives of chlorophyll. *Photochem. Photobiol.* **49**, 157–160.

Krasnovskii, A. A., Jr., Vichegzhanina, I. V., Drozdova, N. N., and Krasnovskii, A. A. (1985): Generation and quenching of singlet molecular oxygen by bacteriochlorophyll and bacteriopheophytin a and b. *Dokl. Akad. Nauk SSSR* **283**, 474–477.

Lee, S.-J. H., Jagerovic, N., and Smith, K. M. (1993): Use of the chlorophyll derivative, purpurin-18, for syntheses of sensitizers for use in photodynamic therapy. *J. Chem. Soc. Perkin Trans.* **I**, 2369–2377.

Moser, J. G. (1993): Attempts to treat malignant melanoma by photodynamic therapy using bacteriopheophorbide ester as a sensitizer. *SPIE Conf. Proc.* **1881**, 116–125.

Pandey, R. K., Shiau, F.-Y., Sumlin, A. B., Dougherty, T. J., and Smith, K. M. (1992): Structure/activity relationships among photosensitizers related to pheophorbides and bacteriopheophorbides. *Bioorg. Med. Chem. Lett.* **2**, 491–496.

Pandey, R. K., Shiau, F.-Y., Sumlin, A. B., Dougherty, T. J., and Smith, K. M. (1994): Syntheses of new bacteriochlorins and their antitumor activity. *Bioorg. Med. Chem. Lett.* **4**, 1263–1267.

Pandey, R. K., Constantine, S., Goff, D. A., Kozyrev, A. N., Dougherty, T. J., and Smith, K. M. (1996): Chlorophyll-a derivatives in photodynamic therapy: effect of position of heptyl ether side-chains on *in vivo* photosensitizing activity. *Bioorg. Med. Chem. Lett.* **6**, 105–110.

Röder, B. (1990): Photosensitizing properties of phorbides. *J. Photochem. Photobiol. B: Biol.* **5**, 519–521.

Rosenbach-Belkin, V. (1988): The primary reactants in bacterial photosynthesis modeling by *in vitro* preparation. Ph.D. thesis, The Weizmann Institute of Science, Rehovot, Israel.

Rosenbach-Belkin, V., Chen, L., Fiedor, L., Tregub, I., Pavlotsky, F., Brumfeld, V., Salomon, Y., and Scherz, A. (1996): Serine conjugates of chlorophyll and bacterio-chlorophyll: photocytotoxicity *in vitro* and tissue distribution in mice bearing melanoma tumors. *Photochem. Photobiol.* **64**, 174–181.

Scherz, A. and Parson, W. W. (1984): Oligomers of bacteriochlorophyll and bacterio-pheophytin with spectroscopic properties resembling those found in photosynthetic bacteria. *Biochim. Biophyis. Acta* **766**, 653–665.

Scherz, A., Salomon, Y., and Fiedor, L. (1994): Chlorophyll and bacteriochlorophyll derivatives, preparation and pharmaceutical compositions comprising them as photo-sensitizers for photodynamic therapy. *Chem. Abs.* **120**, 386.

Spikes, J. D. (1990): Chlorins as photosensitizers in biology and medicine. *J. Photochem. Photobiol. B: Biol.* **6**, 259–274.

Svaasand, L. O. (1984): Optical dosimetry for direct and interstitial photoradiation therapy of malignant tumors. In Porphyrin Localization and Treatment of Tumors (Edited by D. R. Doiron and C. J. Gomer), pp. 91–114. Liss, New York.

Tregub, I., Schmidt-Sole, J., DeJordy, J., Rosenbach-Belkin, V., Brumfeld, V., Fiedor, L., Salomon, Y., and Scherz, A. (1992): Application of chlorophyll and bacteriochlorophyll derivatives to PDT of malignant melanoma. In Proceedings of the Second International Congress on Interaction of Light with Biological Systems (Edited by M. Holick and A. Kligman), pp. 354–361. W. de Gruyter, New York.

Wilson, B. C., Jeeves, W. P., and Lowe, D. M. (1985): *In vivo* and post mortem measurements of the attenuation spectra of light in mammalian tissue. *Photochem. Photobiol.* **42**, 153–162.

Yeh, C. -J. G., Hsi, B. -L., and Faulk, W. P. (1981): Propidium iodide as a nuclear marker in immunofluorescence. II. Use with cellular identification and viability studies. *J. Immunol. Methods* **43**, 269–275.

Zilberstein, J., Scherz, A., Bromberg, A., Bendel, P., Neeman, M., and Salomon, Y. (1994): Chlorophyll based PDT of melanoma: follow up by MRI and by tissue inserted oxygen sensor. In abstract book of the conference: The Tumor Microenvironment: Its Characterization, Modification and Clinical Implication. Faculty of Medicine, University of Granada, Granada, Spain.

Zilberstein, J., Scherz, A., Bromberg, A., Bendel, P., Neeman, M., and Salomon, Y. (1995): Mechanisms involved in chlorophyll based photoinduced cell damage: photodynamic therapy of melanoma. In *Proc. Soc. Magn. Reson.* **3**, 1681.

Zilberstein, J., Bromberg, A., Franz, A., Rosenbach-Belkin, V., Kritzmann, A., Pfeferman, R., Salomon, Y., and Scherz, A. (1997): Light dependent oxygen consumption in bacteriochlorophyll-serine treated melanoma tumors: on line determination using a tissue inserted oxygen microsensor. *Photochem. Photobiol.* **65**, 1012–1020.

Zilberstein, J., Bloemers, M. C. W. M., Neeman, M., Scherz, A., and Salomon, Y. (1997): Therapy of solid melanoma tumors by vascular infraction and perfusion arrest in bacteriocholorphyll-serine based photochemotherapy, *Cancer Res.* Submitted.

3.2. CARRIER AND DELIVERY SYSTEMS

JOERG G. MOSER

The dream of the "*magic bullet*" carrying a photochemotherapeutic drug to its target, especially tumors, has not yet been fulfilled (Fazio and Paganelli, 1993). Several photodynamic drugs show an enrichment at tumor sites by a factor of 2–7, in some reported cases of brain tumors just by a factor of 30. But this means only that the surrounding tissue doesn't store the respective sensitizer to any measurable extent. For muscle as the surrounding tissue this has been discussed at the 5th IPA Meeting (1994) by Bonnet. Nonspecific storage is the basis of the severe side effects in PDT and has to be avoided in future.

The several trials to overcome nonspecific storage and to deliver the sensitizer to its target can be systematically summarized into 4 items:

(1) Delivery vehicles using lipophilic properties of the sensitizers
(2) High molecular weight non-specific carriers
(3) Monophasic Immunotargeting: Immunotoxins
(4) Polyphasic Tumor Targeting (PTT)

These items can be described in short together with a choice of the respective recent literature.

3.2.1. DELIVERY VEHICLES BASED ON LIPOPHILIC PROPERTIES OF THE SENSITIZER

Photophysics of different sensitizers included into liposomes and detergent micelles have been described by Gensch *et al*. (1995). These investigations showed that the sensitizer molecules at not too high concentrations are inserted into the lipophilic surroundings in monomeric form displaying similar photophysical properties (e.g. fluorescence lifetimes) as in monomeric organic solutions. Such sensitizers are easily taken up into the lipoproteins of serum, especially LDL, and transported this way to lipoprotein receptors of living cells which keep them up together with the lipoproteins to the cells interior (Jori and Reddi, 1993). Detergent micelles are not useful because they damage the lipoprotein layers of the cells. For lipoproteins a skillful technology has been developed at Ciba-Geigy (Isele *et al*., 1993) to integrate phthalocyanine photosensitizers into liposomes for use in PDT. Another drug frequently used to solubilize and to deliver phthalocyanines is Cremophor™, a polyethylene glycol derivative. Reddi (1996) has recently pointed out a considerable tumor-specific enrichment of several apolar photosensitizing drugs by injecting it into the bloodstream as Cremophor adducts. Bacteriopheophorbides are complexed so closely into Cremophor micelles that transfer to cultured tumor cells is completely inhibited (unpublished observations). Methods of inclusion into different solubilizers seem to influence subcellular distribution of a sensitizer as demonstrated for tin etiopurpurin by Kessel *et al.* (1991) (cf. the chapter on purpurins of this book by Garbo). Surfaces of liposomes have been decorated with tumor-specific antibodies to enhance specificity to tumors without any reasonable success (e.g. Lesermann *et al.*, 1980).

3.2.2. HIGH MOLECULAR WEIGHT NONSPECIFIC CARRIERS

Grashew *et al.* (1990) have first published the idea and some results using the voracity of tumors for building materials to incorporate sensitizers as conjugates to high molecular weight drag carriers like albumin or polyethylene glycols. This elicited an upsetting chemistry to develop such conjugates (Ardeschirpur *et al.*, 1991) and to apply this methodology in human patients (Hünerbein *et al.*, 1991). Several drugs of this kind were patented by Sinn (1992). Since several years it has become astonishingly quiet with this excitement possibly just because of the high burden of several healthy organs which could not be prevented by this method.

The waste technology of this approach has raised two different discoveries: the reduction of immunostimulating effects of protein molecules by coupling to polyethylene glycols, and the synthesis of carriers containing more than one sensitizer molecule to enhance photodynamic effects of immunotoxins.

3.2.3. MONOPHASIC IMMUNO-THERAPY: IMMUNOTOXINS

The immunotoxin concept originated from coupling of diphtheria toxin to polyclonal antibodies damaging just erythrocytes by the toxicity of the coupled drug. The next step was coupling ricin a to polyclonal and monoclonal antibodies showing much more specificity because of the intracellular site (polysomes) of intended damage. This was followed finally by coupling of monoclonal antibodies with gelonin using different kind of spacers which could or could not deliver the drug to intracellular targets (SPDP vs. adipinic acid as the spacer, respectively). These techniques are followed up to today with more drawbacks than dubious success (e.g. Lambert *et al.*, 1985, and the literature cited therein).

This can be best exemplified on a photodynamic drug developed by a group to Boston, MA (Oseroff *et al.*, 1986), showing excellent phototoxicity in *in vitro* experiments on lymphoid cancer cell lines, namely 30 molecules of chlorin e6 coupled to a dextran carrier of 30 kDa molecular weight. This carrier molecule was connected to a monoclonal antibody and showed excellent phototoxicity *in vitro* with nearly unchanged absorption spectrum as compared with the original sensitizer. This drug as given in a mouse model failed totally from curing the tumor bearing animal *in vivo* (personal communication by Oseroff). The basis of this failure became clear from investigating the reticulo-endothelial cells of the liver which contained all the sensitizer without any delivery to the tumor.

Every antibody modified in such an extreme way will have the same fate: *it will be recognized by the reticuloendothelial system as a foreign molecule and will be caught and destroyed*. Sometimes such drugs or their degradation products are transported secondarily to tumors by macrophages (Korbelik and Krosl, 1994). Exactly this happens with all the immunotoxins synthesized yet despite the extremely expensive international congresses held every year on these topics. The same is true for direct conjugates of photosensitizers to monoclonal antibodies which are published every year for new. What we need is a reduction in size and minimum deviation from natural structure of humanized antibodies or antibody fragments to overcome recognition by the reticulo-endothelial system and, by the same time, the intratumoral pressure gradient counteracting to tumor localization of photodynamic drugs (Jain, 1991).

3.2.4. POLYPHASIC TUMOR TARGETING (PTT)

To illustrate the present situation in chemotherapy and photochemotherapy a simple table should be helpful showing the side effects of frequently applied drugs (Table 1).

This table shows clearly the needs to reduce the side effects of general chemotherapy as well as of photochemotherapy. What is the reason of these severe side effects including longterm neurotoxicity and genotoxicity? The reason is non-specific uptake in all organs of the patient combined with permanent storage of biologically inert, i.e. nondegradable, substances. How to prevent this?

Experiments with polysulfonated phthalocyanines and *meso*-tetraphenyl porphins have clearly shown that these drugs are repelled from the cell surface due to its negative charge and are never taken up by a living cell. The same is the case with hydrophilic drugs like tetrahydroxylated porphins. On the other hand the semipolar drugs, e.g. pheophorbide a or $TPPS_{2a}$ (Moan *et al.*, 1989), show the most effective uptake in cells due to its intramolecular polarity, as expressed by its dipole momentum, promoting rearrangement in between the lipoprotein double layer of the cell membrane structure. Model experiments using liposomes and detergent micelles have described clearly this process in physical terms (Gensch *et al.*, 1995).

These results allow us the decisive statement that drugs to be targeted to a tumor should be structured to provide a high dipole momentum on one hand, but on the other hand should be strongly hydrophilic or electronegative during transport through the whole body.

The next question is: how can such a drug find a tumor selectively? Such questions are answered in the mean time by methodologies developed on the field of immunoscintigraphy (Fazio and Paganelli, 1993; Fazio *et al.*, 1994). The cited literature has shown a selective targeting just of liver metastases in a normally highly burdened surrounding using tumor marker specific antibodies coupled with only minimum deviation substituents alike biotin or ethylene triamine pentaacetic acid as a binder for 111-In or 99m-Tc. These slightly

Table 1 Side Effects of Commonly Applied Chemotherapeutics and Phototherapeutics (According to Vervoorts, 1997)

	BENDAMUSTIN	BUSULFAN	CARMUSTIN	CHLORAMBUCIL	CYCLOPHOSPHAMID	IFOSAMID	LOMUSTIN	MELPHALAN	NIMUSTIN, TROFOSAMID	THIOTEPA	CYTARABIN	FLUOROURACIL	MERCAPTOPURIN	METHOTHREXAT	TIOGUANIN	VINBLASTIN	VINCRISTIN	VINDESIN, VINORELBIN	ACLARUBICIN	BLEOMYCIN	DACTINOMYCIN	DAUNORUBICIN, DOXORUBICIN	IDARUBICIN, EPIRUBICIN	MITOMYCIN	CARBOPLATIN, CISPLATIN	HYDROXYPHEOPHORBIDE, LIGHT	PHOTOPHRIN II
Fever, Allergies	•			•	•						•	•	•	•		•	•		•	•	•	•	•	•	•	•	•
Nausea, Diarrhoe, Vomitation	•	•	•	•	•	•	•	•	•	•	•	•	•	•	•	•	•	•	•	•	•	•	•	•	•		
Stomatitis, Oesophagitis			•		•	•	•	•	•		•	•	•	•	•	•	•	•	•	•	•	•	•	•	•		
Skin alterations, Alopecia	•	•	•	•	•	•	•	•	•	•			•			•	•	•	•	•	•	•	•	•	•	•	•
Cardiotoxicity		•			•	•						•							•	•	•	•	•	•			
Lung fibrosis, Pneumonitis		•	•	•	•		•	•												•							
Hepatotoxicity	•	•	•	•	•	•	•		•				•	•	•	•	•	•						•	•		
Nephrotoxicity	•		•		•	•	•		•	•						•	•	•			•			•	•		
Hämorrhagic cystitis		•			•	•	•				•																
Blood clotting alterations	•		•	•	•	•	•	•				•		•			•								•		
Neuropathy			•	•	•	•	•		•			•		•		•	•	•							•		
Genetic alterarions				•	•							•						•	•		•	•	•		•		•
Ulcer of mucous membranes	•	•	•		•	•	•		•	•		•	•	•	•	•	•	•	•		•	•	•				
Infertility		•	•	•	•	•	•	•	•	•			•			•	•	•	•		•	•	•		•		
Secondary neoplasia		•	•										•								•	•					
Immunosuppression			•		•	•	•		•			•	•	•	•	•	•	•	•		•	•	•		•		
Shock																										•	
Retina destruction																										•	•

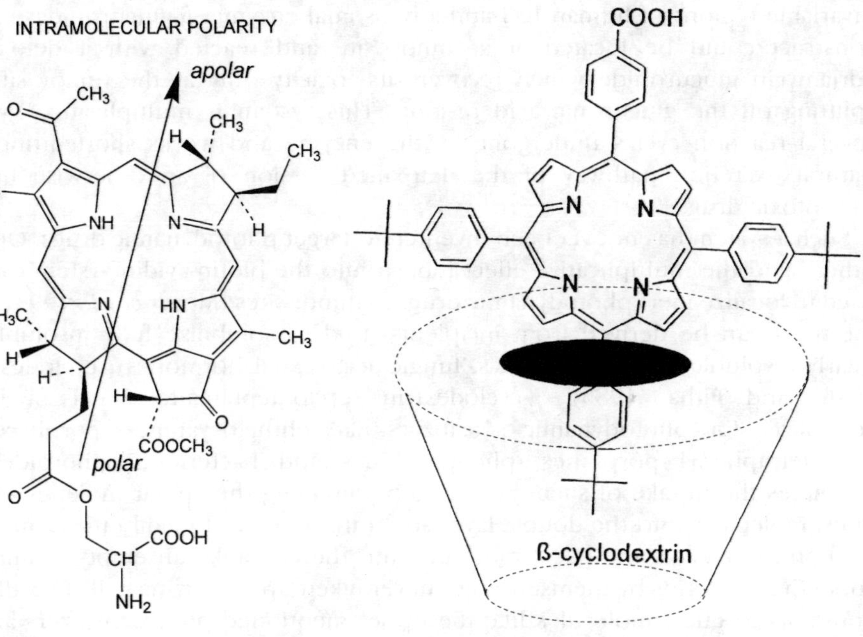

Figure 1 Polarity of photosensitizer molecules and acquired polarity using cyclodextrin inclusion complexes.

modified antibodies or antibody fragments, ($F(Ab)_2$), are not recognized as foreign elements by the reticuloendothelial system. After clearing the system from a surmount of biotinylated antibodies with avidin biotinylated antibodies can be labelled with sufficient amounts of a 111-In complexing biotinylated drug to visualize metastases of melanoma and other carcinomas. The maximum amount of isotope labelling with a triphasic procedure of this kind can be calculated in the order of 1.5×10^4 radiating atoms per tumor cell.

All results obtained *in vitro* on efficient tumor labelling with photodynamic drugs have shown that the minimum amount of loading a cell with photosensitizers is in the order of 10^6–10^7 molecules per cell for effective photodynamic therapy (see the foregoing chapters of this book). Some work done with monophasic tumor labelling of ovarian carcinoma (Schultes *et al.*, 1993) allowed to calculate this minimum amount to the order of 10^6 molecules per cell. This is much higher as the amount necessary to visualize tumors and tumor metastases. This means that we need a multiplicative system to overcome this barrier. One of the most attractive systems showing the necessary multiplicative effects is the Antibody Directed Enzyme Prodrug Therapy (ADEPT) as invented by Bosslet *et al.* (1988, 1992) according to first suggestions by Bagshawe. In its final version an ingenious construct containing the active centre of a monoclonal mouse antibody directed against carcinoembryonic antigen (CEA; 20,000–50,000 binding sites at the surface of an adenocarcinoma cell) was combined with the invariable regions of human IgG and a lysosomal enzyme, β-glucuronidase. This construct could be located at a tumor site and reacted with a detoxified adriamycin glucuronide which recovers its toxicity only at the tumor site by splitting off the glucuronic acid residue. This system is multiplicative by the several reaction cycles undergone by the enzyme and works shortcutting the natural excretion pathway of the detoxified version of an otherwise highly cardiotoxic drug.

Such a system has not yet been invented to target photodynamic drugs. On the other hand the multiplicative effect inborn into the biotin-avidin system can be used to localize inert photodynamic drugs at tumor sites (Moser *et al.*, 1994). The inertness can be derived from incipients used to solubilize fully insoluble or nearly insoluble drugs (virostatics, fungicides, sexual hormones): cyclodextrins (Pitha and Pitha, 1985). β-cyclodextrin (cyclo-heptamaltoside) is a good solubilizer for photodynamic sensitizers like phthalocyanines, porphycenes, *meso*-tetraphenyl porphines, pheophorbides and bacteriopheophorbides. It promotes the uptake of such molecules by directing the apolar moieties of the guest molecules into the double layer structure of the cell membrane swimming off upon uptake of the guest molecule into the cell alike an empty swimming rope. Cyclodextrins by themselves are never taken up by a living cell. The affinity constants to guest molecules like the upper mentioned photosensitizers are in the order of 10^3–10^4 l/mole. These can be enhanced by dimerization of the cyclodextrins over a spacer molecule. Considerable chemistry has been done during the last 2 years to optimize these constructs and to functionalize these inert shells with biotin (Ruebner *et al.*, 1997) (Table 2 and Fig. 2).

Complexation of porphyrinoids in these chlathrates is strong enough to prevent transfer of the drugs to the serum lipoprotein system as shown by gel permeation chromatography and by UV/Vis spectra (Moser *et al.*, 1995). Cell membranes with its higher affinity to semipolar drugs are not as inert as LDL. Tailoring of the spacers as well as of the guest molecules itself may be helpful to form stable complexes. The future affinity constants should be of the order of 10^8 to 10^{10} l/mole. Very simple models showing affinity constants of the postulated order were investigated by Breslow and his group (Breslow and

Table 2 Binding constants of different β-cyclodextrin dimersto defined chemically synthesized porphyrinoid derivatives. From Ruebner *et al.* (1997)

Cyclodextrin dimer	*Porphyrinoid*		
	*Tri(tbutyl)carboxy m*TPP	*Tri(tbutylphenoxy) sulfophenoxy Pc*	*Tri(tbutyl)methyl-pyridyloxy ZnPc*
Di-β-CD($2NA_3C_2A_3$)	$4.5 \pm 1.3 \times 10^5$	$3.3 \pm 0.5 \times 10^5$	$2.1 \pm 0.5 \times 10^5$
Di-β-CD($2NA_3C_4A_3$)	$3.1 \pm 0.8 \times 10^5$	$1.3 \pm 0.3 \times 10^5$	$6.3 \pm 1.9 \times 10^5$
Di-β-CD($2NA_4C_3A_4$)	$1.3 \pm 0.5 \times 10^5$	*$1.5 \pm 0.3 \times 10^7$*	$8.4 \pm 1.8 \times 10^5$
Di-β-CD($2NA_4C_4A_4$)	$1.4 \pm 0.3 \times 10^5$	$4.1 \pm 0.9 \times 10^6$	$8.7 \pm 0.4 \times 10^5$
Di-β-CD($6NA_2C_3A_2$)	$5.8 \pm 1.7 \times 10^4$	$4.0 \pm 0.7 \times 10^6$	$5.0 \pm 0.5 \times 10^5$
Di-β-CD($6NA_2C_4A_2$)	n.d.	$1.4 \pm 0.4 \times 10^6$	$2.4 \pm 0.4 \times 10^5$
Me-β-CD	n.d.	$6.8 \pm 1.3 \times 10^4$	n.d.

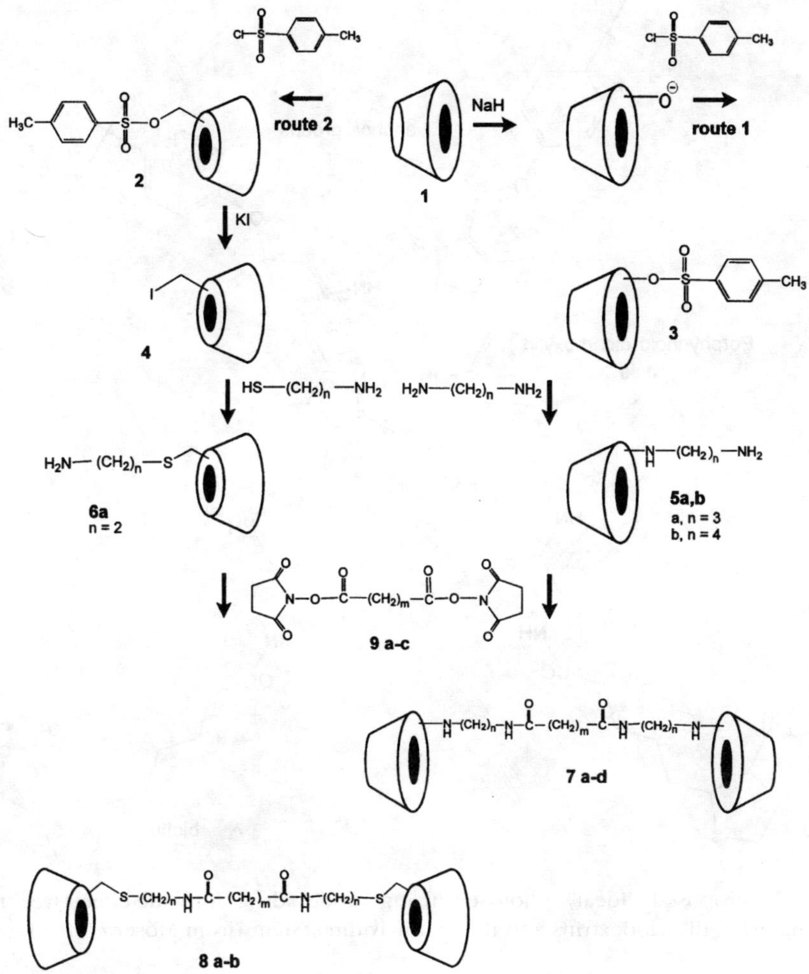

Figure 2 Chemistry leading to cyclodextrin dimers for formation of porphyrinoid inclusion complexes. Modified from Ruebner *et al.* (1997).

Chung, 1990). The substituent forming the highest affinities was tert. butyl phenol as ether or ester. This group seems to interfere with the π-electron ring current of the porphyrinoids giving rise to energy losses into the cyclodextrin cavity.

So an isolator should have better chances to conserve the energy contents of the ring system. Proposed are cyclohexyl derivatives of the sensitizers or chinoid structures like isonicotinic acid derivatives. The established chemistry has to be extended to natural photosensitizers like bacteriochlorins or bacteriopheophorbides to get the most effective but degradable drug for targeting tumors in

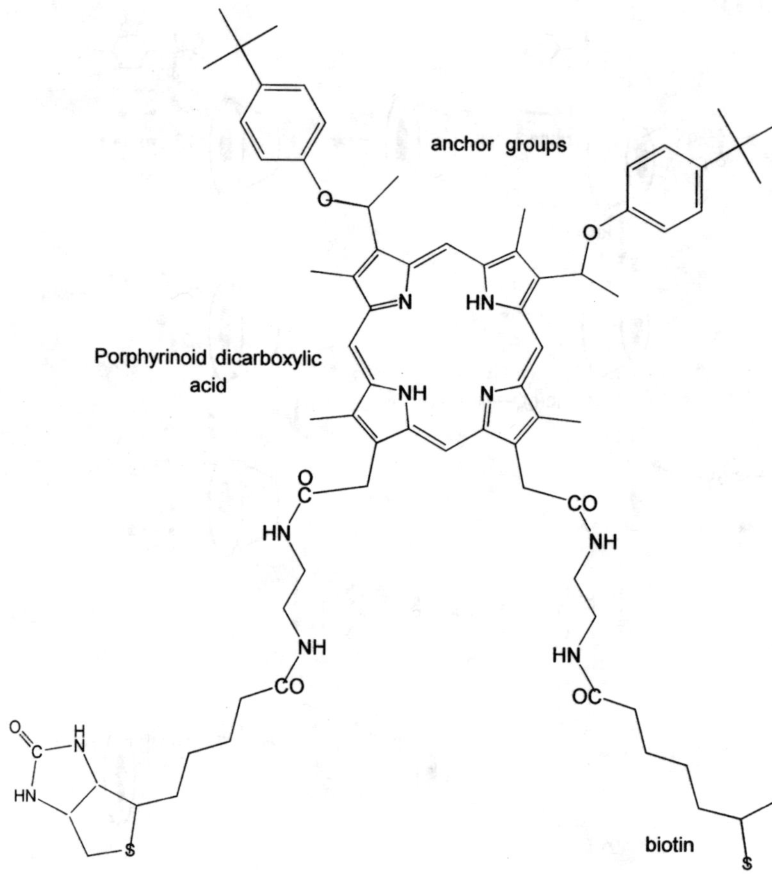

Figure 3 Proposed "ideal" photosensitizing model drug for side-effect free tumor targeting using dicyclodextrins and the biotin-avidin system (from Moser *et al.*, 1996).

future (Fig. 3). Model substances of this kind are now synthesized in our laboratory (Moser *et al.*, 1996) in order to improve selectivity of photodynamic substances to tumors. This selectivity is and will be in future the key problem in photodynamic tumor therapy at all.

Returning to Table 1, we emphasize to take into account possible consequences of this research into a modification of general chemotherapy.

As in photodynamic therapy, the side effects of chemotherapeutic drugs might be reduced in future by forming inert inclusion complexes for a transport of these drugs through the blood stream. This should be reduce or just extinguish the severe side effects of these drugs to the patient. With some natural anti-cancer drugs, like taxol, work is underway to form transport inclusion complexes with the drug.

LITERATURE CITED

Ardeschirpur, A., Heuermann, A., Müller, S., Wöhrle, D., Rinneberg, H., and Graschew, G. (1991): Fluorescence properties and biodistribution of new sensitizers with potential use in PDT. Int. Conf. PDT & Laser Medicine, Peking (China): **10**, 14.

Bonnet, R. (1995): Remarks during a panel discussion at the 5th IPA Meeting (Amelia Island FL, USA).

Bosslet, K., Steinstraesser, A., Schwarz, A., Harthus, H. P., Lueben, G., Kuhlmann, L., and Sedlacek, H. H. (1988): Quantitative considerations supporting the irrelevance of circulating serum CEA for the immunoscintigraphic visualization of CEA expressing carcinomas. *Eur. J. Nucl. Med.* **14**, 523–528.

Bosslet, K., Czech, J., Lorenz, P., Sedlacek, H. H., Schuermann, M., and Seemann, G. (1992): Molecular and functional characterization of a fusion protein suited for tumour specific prodrug activation. *Br. J. Cancer* **65**, 234–238.

Breslow, R. and Chung, S. (1990): Strong binding of ditopic substrates by a double-linked occlusive C_1 "clamshell" as distinguished from an aversive C_2 "loveseat" cyclodextrin. *J. Am. Chem. Soc.* **112**, 9659–9660.

Fazio, F. and Paganelli, G. (1993): Antibody-guided scintigraphy: targeting of the "magic bullet". *Eur. J. Nucl. Med.* **20**, 138–1140.

Fazio, F., Paganelli, G., Magnani, P., Zito, F., and Lucignani, G. (1994): Pretargeted immunodetection in glioma patients: tumour localization and single photon emission tomography imaging of ^{99m}Tc-pnAO-biotin. *Eur. J. Nucl. Med.* **21**, 314–321.

Graschew, G., Müller, W., Sinn, H., Aderhold, S., Wöhrle, D., Friedrich, E., Stern, J., and Schlag, P. (1990): A new porphyrine derivative (P4P-mD) for tumor diagnosis and PDT. 3rd Int. Congr. PDT (IPA) Buffalo NY, USA.

Gensch, T., Roeder, B., Pfeifer, L., and Moser, J. G. (1995): Photophysical properties of 13^2-hydroxy bacteriopheophorbide a methyl ester in ethanol and micellar solutions (*J. Photochem. Photobiol.* delivered).

Hünerbein, M., Stern, J., Friedrich, E., Sinn, H., Graschew, G., Maier-Borst, W., and Schlag, P. (1991): The preferential accumulation of macromolecular bound photosensitizers in tumors. *Antibodies, Immunoconjugates, and Radiopharmaceuticals* **4**, 483–491.

Isele, U., van Hoogevest, P., Leuenberger, H., Capraro, H. G., and Schieweck, K. (1993): Pharmaceutical development of CGP 55847, a liposomal Zn-phthalocyanine formulation using a controlled organic solvent dilution method. *SPIE Biomed. Optics* **2078**, 397–403.

Jain, R. K. (1991): Therapeutic implications of tumor physiology. *Curr. Opinions Oncol.* **1991**, 1105–1108.

Jori, G. and Reddi, E. (1993): The role of lipoproteins in the delivery of tumour targeting photosensitizers. *Int. J. Biochem.* **25**, 1369–1375.

Kessel, D., Morgan, A., and Garbo, G. M. (1991): Sites and efficiency of photodamage by tin etiopurpurin *in vitro* using different delivery systems. *Photochem. Photobiol.* **54**, 193–196.

Korbelik, M. and Krosl, G. (1994): Tumor associated macrophages (not tumor cells) are the determinants of photosensitizer localization. *SPIE Biomed. Optics* **2371**, 344–346.

Lambert, J. M., Senter, P. D., Yau-Yong, A., Blattler, W. A., and Goldmacher, V. S. (1985): Purified immunotoxin that are reactive with human lymphoid cells. *J. Biol. Chem.* **260**, 12035–12041.

Lesermann, L., Barbet, J., and Kouritzky, F. (1980): Targeting to cells of fluorescent liposomes covalently coupled with monoclonal antibody or protein A. *Nature* **188**, 602–604.

Moan, J., Peng, Q., Evensen, J. F., Berg, K., Western, A., and Rimington, C. (1987): Photosensitizing efficiencies, tumour- and cellular uptake of different photosensitizing drugs relevant for photodynamic therapy of cancer. *Photochem. Photobiol.* **46**, 713–721.

Moser, J. G., Heuermann, A., Oehr, P., Scheer, H., Vervoorts, A., and Andrees, S. (1994): Carrier systems in PDT: On the way to novel anti-tumor drugs. *SPIE Biomed. Optics* **2325**, 92–99.

Moser, J. G., Ruebner-Heuermann, A., Weitemeyer, A., Michelsen, U., Woehrle, D., Rueck, A., Strauss, W. S. L., Kirsch, D., Andrees, S., and Schroers, C. (1995): Independent pathway for inclusion complexes of porphyrinoid drugs to tumors: The separation from the lipoprotein pathway in plasma. *SPIE Biomed. Optics* **2625**, 138–145.

Moser, J. G., Ruebner, A., Vervoorts, A., and Wagner, B. (1996): Cyclodextrin dimers used to prevent side effects of photochemotherapy and general tumor chemotherapy. Publ. 8th Cyclodextrin Symp. Budapest, pp. 71–76.

Oseroff, A., Ohuoha, D., Hasan, T., Bommer, J. C., and Yarmush, M. L. (1986): Antibody-targeted photolysis: Selective photodestruction of human T-cell leukemia cells using monoclonal antibody-chlorin e_6 conjugates. *Proc. Natl. Acad. Sci. USA* **83**, 8744–8748.

Pitha. J. and Pitha, J. (1985): Amorphous water-soluble derivatives of cyclodextrins: non-toxic enhancing excipients. *J. Phamaceut. Sci.* **74**, 987–990.

Reddi, E. (1996): *SPIE Biomed. Optics* **2924** (unpublished).

Ruebner, A., Kirsch, D., Andrees, S., Decker, W., Roeder, B., Spengler, B., Kaufmann, R., and Moser, J. G. (1997): Dimeric cyclodextrin carriers with high binding affinity to porphyrinoid photosensitizers. *J. Inclusion Phenomena* **27**, 69–84.

Schultes, B., Spaniol, H. J., Ertmer, S., Schmidt, S., Biersack, H. J., and Krebs, D. (1993): Photodynamic laser therapy with antibody-coupled phthalocyanine. *SPIE Biomed. Optics* **2078**, 148–160.

Sinn, H. J., Schrenk, H. H., Friedrich, E. A., Schilling, U., and Maier-Borst, W. (1990): Design of compounds having enhanced tumor uptake using serum albumin as a carrier. Part A: *Nucl. Med. Biol.* **17**, 819–827; Part B: Schilling, U. *et al.* (1992): *Nucl. Med. Biol.* **19**, 685–696.

Sinn, H., Schrenk, H. H., Friedrich, F. A., Maier-Borst, W., and Graschew, G. *et al.* (1990): Konjugate zur Tumorlokalisation oder Therapie: Verfahren zu ihrer Herstellung sowie diese enthaltende Diagnostica und/oder Therapeutica. Patent DE 3912792 A1.

Vervoorts, A. (1997): Laser-Doppler-Spektroskopie an den extraembryonalen Membranen von Hühnerembryonen. Ph.D Thesis. Duesseldorf, 1997.

3.3. IRRADIATION MODALITIES AND IRRADIATION CONTROL

RUDOLF W. STEINER, IVAN S. MELNIK and MARKUS KLOTZ

Dosimetry of laser irradiated tissue is rather complex. Many variant applicators are described to homogeneously irradiate the surface of tissue either in the bladder, the esophagus, the stomach or only the skin surface. Scattering spheres, or reflecting cones are used as fiber tips to radially distribute the light in hollow organs. Another approach is to use fiber tips with notches over a length of several cm, gradually outcoupling the light to form a cylindrical or sectoral irradiation profile.

The crucial question however is, how deep laser light penetrates into the tissue and how the fluence rate in the tissue can be measured *in vivo*. A practical approach is described in this chapter, elements which are commercially available now.

3.3.1. PRINCIPAL DEFINITIONS

Definition of the Fluence Rate

The fluence rate $\psi(r)$ at a given point r in the tissue is a total radiant power that passes through the surface of an infinitesimal small sphere divided by the cross sectional area of that sphere [1]. Fluence rate is expressed in power per area, W/cm^2. The local fluence rate follows from the radiance at that point by integrating over all possible directions in space:

$$\Psi(r) = \int L(r, \alpha)\, \mathrm{d}\omega, \qquad (1)$$

where $\mathrm{d}\omega$ denotes an infinitesimal solid angle pointing in the direction α. The fluence rate has more practical significance than the radiance because absorption of photons at location r inside the tissue does not depend on the direction of photon propagation.

According to this definition a suitable probe for measurement of $\Psi(r)$ must have an isotropic response and spherical form with minimum diameter. The best isotropic response, reported in previous studies, was $\Delta S = \pm 10\%$ within an angular range $\theta = \pm 150°$ [2–5] and diameters of probes were in the range of 0.35–3.2 mm [2–8]. There is an inverse ratio between the diameter of probe and isotropy response: a smaller diameter of the probe corresponds to higher anisotropy response [5]. This effect occurs because of insufficient light scattering in the small volume of scattering material.

Determination of the Anisotropy Response

As a rule, anisotropy response is determined as the angular light distribution measured at inverse conditions for light source and photodetector, namely, the light source is coupled into the bare end of the fiber and the photodetector is mounted in front of the diffusely scattering tip at the other end of the fiber. It is necessary to take that into account. Because of the finite size of the probe there is a difference between light distribution in near field and far field. However, due to the light scattering in the tissue and in the probe, this difference can be neglected and fluence rate can be expressed as

$$\Psi(r) = \int L(r,\alpha)\, S(\alpha)\, \mathrm{d}\omega, \tag{2}$$

where $S(\alpha)$ expresses the sensitivity of the probe to the irradiance L in direction α or the anisotropy response of the probe. Consider two cases:

(1) Irradiance $L(r,\alpha)$ does practically not change with direction in a given point r. This case corresponds to measurement of fluence rate in a homogeneous tissue by a very small probe. In this case one can write from (2):

$$\Psi(r) = L(r) \int S(\alpha)\, \mathrm{d}\omega. \tag{3}$$

It is evident that anisotropy response does not influence the accuracy of measurement of fluence rate if the probe was previously calibrated.

(2) Irradiance $L(r,\alpha)$ is changed with direction α. Such a condition might occur in multilayer tissues or near the tissue surface (skin) or if diameter of the probe is larger than penetration depth of light. In this case correlation function of elementary fluence rate $\mathrm{d}\Psi(r)$ equals

$$K_{\mathrm{d}\Psi}(\alpha') = K_L(\alpha') \times K_S(\alpha'). \tag{4}$$

Therefore, standard deviation during the measurement of fluence rate is related with deviation of $L(\alpha)$ and $S(\alpha)$ as $\sigma_{\mathrm{d}\Psi} = \sigma_L \sigma_S$.

This means, the accuracy of a fluence rate measurement using isotropic detector is proportional to the standard deviation of the anisotropy response but not to the maximum anisotropy ΔS as it was used early. Assuming normal distribution of $S(\alpha)$ one can connect the relationship between $\Delta S_{\max}$ and σ_S as [9]

$$\sigma_S = \Delta S_{\max} / \sqrt{3}. \tag{5}$$

For $\Delta S = \pm 10\%$ or $\Delta S_{\max} = 20\%$ we have the admissible standard deviation $\sigma_S = 20/\sqrt{3} = 11.5\%$.

Relation of Diameter of the Probe to Diameter of the Fiber and Angular Range of Isotropy Response

As already mentioned, the diameter of scattering sphere attached to a fiber tip should be as small as possible. Reducing of sphere size leads to a decrease of isotropy response and in addition to a decrease of the angular range of isotropy θ (Fig. 1).

Angular range of isotropy is related to the ratio R_f/R_s

$$\theta = 180^\circ - \arcsin(R_f/R_s). \tag{6}$$

For $R_f = 110\,\mu m$ and $R_s = 400\,\mu m$ the angular range is $\theta = \pm 164^\circ$. In practice, this range might be changed in both directions because of light leakage and refraction in the small contact zone between fiber and scattering sphere.

Total Transmission of Isotropic Detector

For an absolute measurement of the fluence rate it is necessary to know the ratio between photodetector signal and real fluence rate in tissue. This relation reflects the efficiency of transformation of fluence rate given in mW/cm^2 into electrical signal of photodetector (mV). Coefficient of transformation η can be represented as a product

$$\eta = T_i S_p, \tag{7}$$

where T_i is a total transmission coefficient and S_p is real sensitivity of photodetector to light irradiation of given spectral range of wavelengths λ. Coefficient T_i is determined as ratio of spatial irradiance Φ_p of photodetector sensitive area to total spatial irradiance of the probe Φ_0. It defines light losses in isotropic sphere due to light backscattering, Fresnel reflection, absorption, light leakage in contact zone and light losses in the fiber. Furthermore, in fluorescent probes [10–12], this coefficient includes light losses caused by low efficiency of fluorescence transformation. As maximum quantum efficiency of fluorescence is of about percents and light absorption by fluorescent material is high, the coefficient T_i in fluorescent probes is more than a factor 100 smaller than that in light scattering probes. Total transmission coefficient could be calculated by ray tracing or be measured during a calibration procedure. The maximum value of the total transmission coefficient T_i is of about $T_i = 0.5$ in light scattering probes.

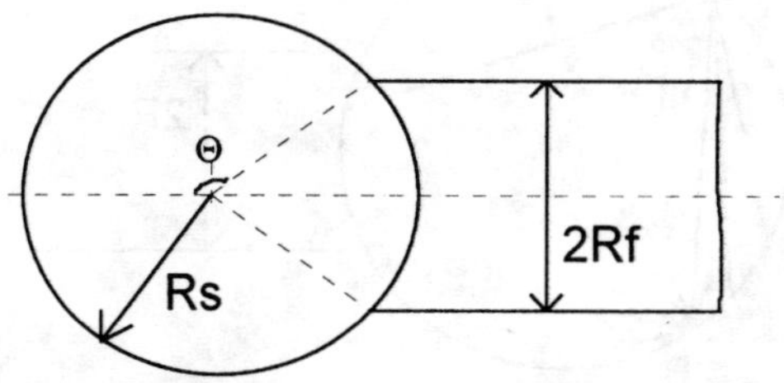

Figure 1 Limitation of angular range θ.

3.3.2. MANUFACTURING THE ISOTROPIC PROBE

One could think of three alternatives to fabricate isotropic probes:

- the sphere is fabricated by melting the fiber tip and then coating it with a layer of scattering material;
- the sphere is fabricated from solid scattering material;
- the sphere is fabricated from fluorescent material or coated by fluorescent layer.

The last approach has a significantly lower total transmission coefficient T_i which is estimated as $T_i = 0.005$. Assuming that the irradiance of tissue surface is about $100\,\mathrm{mW/cm^2}$ and total attenuation coefficient of the tissue is $\tau = 1\,\mathrm{mm}^{-1}$ one can calculate the spatial irradiance on photodetector of about $4 \cdot 10^{-9}\,\mathrm{W}$ at the depth h of 5 mm. It is difficult to registrate this small signal even if noise equivalent power of modern Si-photodiodes is $10^{-12}\,\mathrm{W}$ [13]. Therefore, the method of probe fabrication using fluorescence leads to limitations at larger tissue depths.

Initial successful results in producing small isotropic probes by melting of fiber tip [5, 14] have stimulated further investigations of this technology. However, fabrication of the spheres from solid scattering material (opaque glass) leads to mechanically and optically the best probes.

Calculation of Isotropic Response by Ray-Tracing

Calculation of isotropic response was performed by ray-tracing in a similar way as reported earlier for modified fiber tips [15]. A scheme in Fig. 2 shows a general idea of ray-tracing program.

Uniform light distribution along the fiber end was assumed and Gaussian spatial irradiance was given in each point using a factor $\exp(-2i^2/\beta^2)$; half divergence angle β can vary from 5° to 90°.

Each beam reaching the sphere surface is refracted or/and reflected depending on different conditions:

(a) sphere coated by semi-transparent layer with coefficient of reflection named as "reflectance";

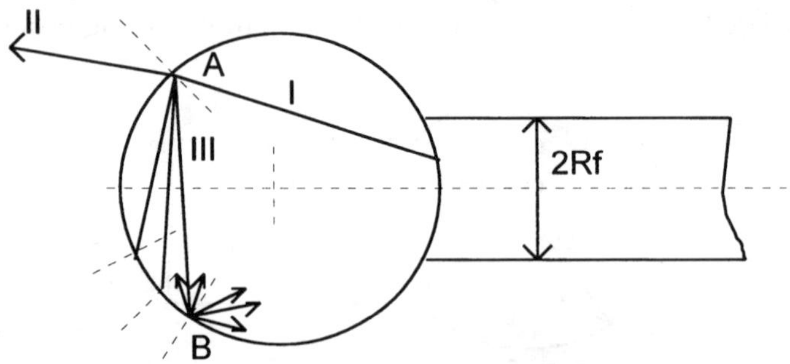

Figure 2 Illustration to the ray-tracing.

(b) sphere coated by diffuse scattering layer with light scattering inside and outside of the sphere.

In case (a), beam I is refracted in point (A). Intensity of refracted beam II is reduced by factor $(1-\rho_0)\tau$, where ρ_0 is a reflection coefficient of the semi-transparent layer and τ is a transmission coefficient calculated by Fresnel-equations. Reflected beam III is directed to the next point (B), where it is divided in two beams in the same way. The calculation procedure is continued until threshold flux level is achieved. Absorption of light in the sphere τ_a is taken into account by Beer's law $\tau_a = \exp(-ax)$. The resulting isotropic response is calculated as a sum of refracted beam intensities at the distance R_{view} from the sphere center in the discrete angle defined as "step flux". Standard deviation σ_S is calculated from isotropic response and related to the mean value.

Case (b) differs from above mentioned condition by modelling of light scattering in the thin layer. In this case, besides reflection, light beams are scattered in every point of sphere surface. This process is represented by an indicatrix of diffusion given by function

$$y = \cos^m(\varphi), \tag{8}$$

where power $m = 1$ corresponds to Lambert diffusion. Angle $\varphi = 0°$ corresponds to direction specular reflection.

For case (a) total transmission is higher in water than that in air by a factor 1.23. It occurs due to reduction of total reflection in sphere-medium interface. It is necessary to note, that this value is smaller than calibration factor of 1.52 given for scattering bulb [3].

A strong forward scattering is a reason of high anisotropy in probe with light scattering layers; typical isotropic response is shown in Fig. 3.

To avoid this large anisotropy, a volume scattering glass material was chosen for producing the probe.

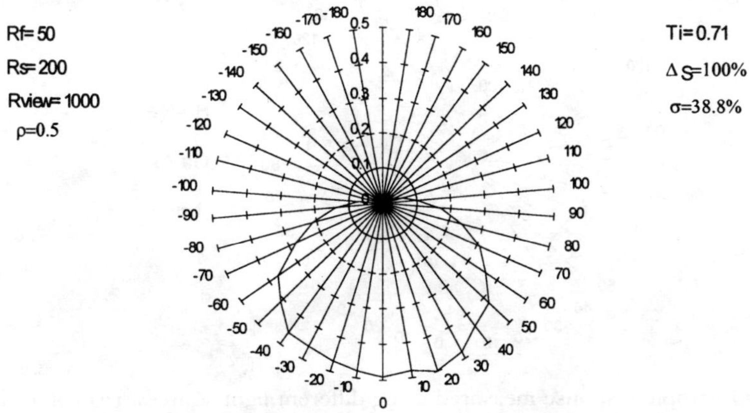

Figure 3 Typical isotropic response of the probe coated by a light scattering layer.

Coherence of the Light Influences Isotropic Response

Speckle structure in light distribution caused by coherent light was detected in all experiments with He–Ne and Ga–As lasers. This phenomenon has effected the isotropy response of probes. It causes an additional anisotropy and sensitivity of experimental setup to small displacements and vibrations of fiber. An additional anisotropy was not observed with incoherent illumination. Figure 4 represents the isotropy response for a 404 μm sphere with 1 layer scattering coating of 100% concentration measured using three different light sources.

Melting and coating of fiber tip allows to manufacture very small probes with high mechanical strength which is limited by mechanical properties of the fiber. However, melting way of probe production gives very high anisotropy. Insufficient light scattering in thin layers provides mostly forward light distribution in the probe. It is necessary to cover the sphere by 4 or 5 layers to reduce the anisotropy less than 10%. Increase of isotropic response by multiple covering is achieved at the expense of inadmissible decrease of total transmission. Results with melting technology could be better if the materials with higher scattering and small absorption are used.

Significant disadvantage of melting technology is a low reproduction and repetition of isotropic response. It is difficult to control the painting process on the miniature sphere and, as a result, to predict the resulting parameter of the probe.

It is necessary to use a noncoherent light source during manufacturing and testing of probes since light coherence leads to additional anisotropy of light distribution. Influence of light coherence will be less *in vivo* measurements because of light coherence decrease in the scattering medium.

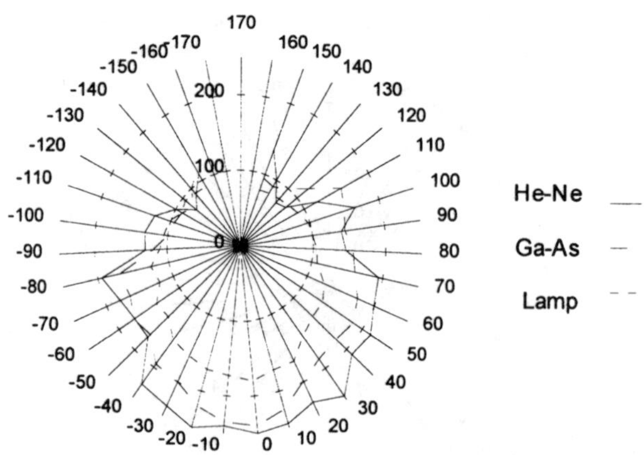

Figure 4 Isotropic response measured using different light sources. Diameter of sphere is 404 μm. Sphere coated with one layer of scattering material of 100% concentration. Note variation of light distribution given by coherent and incoherent light.

Technique Using Light Scattering Balls

A solid sphere attached to the fiber tip has been used as a more promising way of probe manufacturing. This method includes two main procedures: manufacturing of scattering balls and their connection with fiber.

The diameters of balls should be very small: 2 times smaller than that described previously [3]. Besides this, the balls should be identical with spherical shape. Balls were manufactured using a grinding of optical milk glass. Three types of the optical milk glass, namely MC19, MC20 and MC23 (Lytkarino, Russia) were used in our experiments. They have better scattering properties and low light absorbance (Table 1) [16]. Balls were performed at the Arsenal Corp., Kiev. The diameters of balls ranged from 410 to 420 μm.

Anisotropy of scattering g could be calculated from the light distribution $p(\theta)$ [17] as an integral

$$g = \langle \cos(\theta) \rangle = \int p(\theta)\cos(\theta) 2\pi \sin(\theta)\, d\theta, \tag{9}$$

where function $p(\theta)$ is expressed as $p(\theta) = P_0 p^\circ(\theta)$ and maximum value P_0 is calculated taking into account the conserved energy:

$$P_0 = \frac{1}{\int p^\circ(\theta)\, 2\pi \sin(\theta)\, d\theta}. \tag{10}$$

Calculated by this way anisotropy of scattering was performed for glasses MC19, MC20 and MC23 with the values 0.78, 0.43 and 0.62, respectively. Absorption coefficients α_a were calculated from Table 1 using Beer's law. They were equal 0.03, 0.10 and 0.12 mm^{-1} for glasses MC19, MC20 and MC23, respectively. Scattering coefficients, α_s were obtained through the reduced scattering coefficient

$$\alpha_s' = (1 - g)\,\alpha_s. \tag{11}$$

Coefficient α_s' was measured at the Optoelectronic Laboratory, KPI using a 5 cm integrating sphere. They were equal to 0.26, 2.25 and 1.26 mm^{-1} for glasses MC19, MC20 and MC23, respectively. Scattering coefficients, α_s were calculated from (11) and equal 1.20, 3.95 and 2.63 mm^{-1}. Optical parameters of milk glasses used in our experiments are listed in Table 2.

The balls were connected with optical fibers using an optical glue. To improve the mechanical contact the probe was coated by a protection layer.

Two probes were measured for anisotropy showing the characteristics of Fig. 5.

Table 1 Integral Transmittance of Optical Milk Glasses

Type of glass	*Refractive index*	*Thickness* mm	*Transmittance*
MC19	1.472	2	0.91
MC20	1.520	2	0.53
MC23	1.520	2	0.61

Table 2 Optical Parameters of Milk Glasses

Type of glass	*Absorption coefficient* α_a mm^{-1}	*Scattering coefficient* α_s mm^{-1}	*Anisotropy of scattering, g*
MC19	0.03	1.20	0.78
MC20	0.10	3.95	0.43
MC23	0.12	2.63	0.62

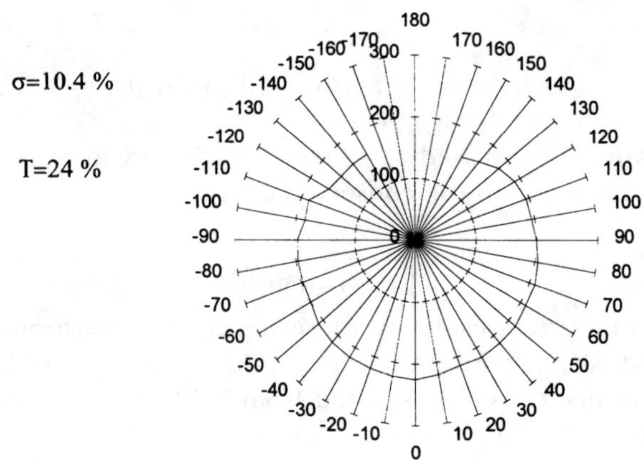

a)

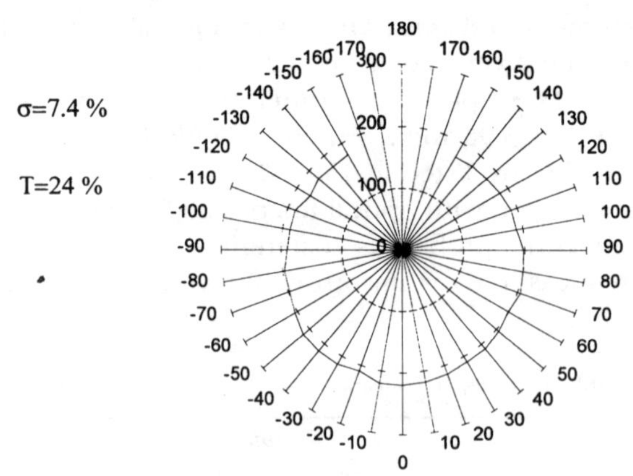

b)

Figure 5 Isotropic response of the probes manufactured of glass: MC20 (a, b).

Presented data allow to conclude: the glass MC20 is the best in respect of isotropic response. The total transmission of the probe, $T_i = 24\%$ is still sufficient. Influence of fiber positioning with small displacements of the center of the ball to the fiber axis has no dramatic effect.

Influence of Light Coherence on Measurements of Isotropic Response

As coherence of light leads to variations of isotropic response, we have also studied the influence on anisotropy of solid probes. Two light sources: He–Ne laser and 200 W lamp were coupled consecutively with the same probe. Light distribution was measured as mentioned above. Five probes were tested. Small (15–25%) increase of anisotropy was registrated in case of coherent illumination. Data are represented in Fig. 6 for one probe.

Correction of Anisotropy During Manufacturing of Probes

Because of its own light absorption and scattering, the protective celluloid layer can change the isotropic response of the probe. We have investigated this effect to decrease the forward light distribution which is a general source of anisotropy in solid probes. For this purpose, different numbers of protective layers surrounded the distal tip of the probe (Fig. 7).

Measured light distributions are represented in Fig. 8. Isotropic response of probes fabricated of solid scattering balls is better than that provided by melting technology. It occurs due to higher light scattering in milk glass than in thin scattering layers.

Glued probes have sufficient mechanical strength to be used for *in vivo* measurements of fluence rate. The tensile strength of glued probes is more than 70% of fiber tensile strength. However, it is necessary to cover the whole scattering ball by a protective layer to achieve high mechanical strength. This

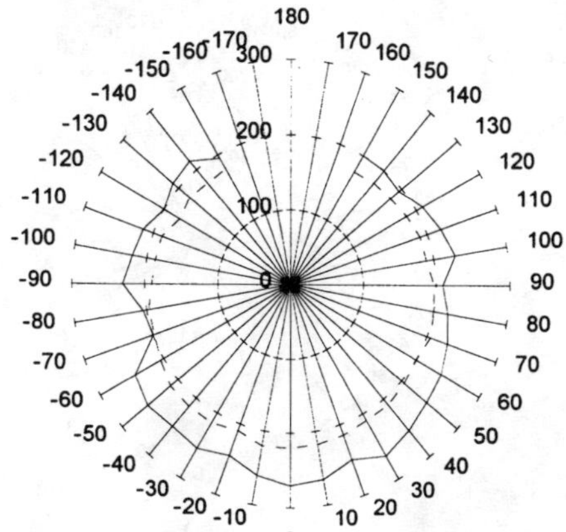

Figure 6 Isotropic response measured using He–Ne laser (solid line) and lamp (dotted line). Anisotropy is 10.0% and 7.8%, respectively.

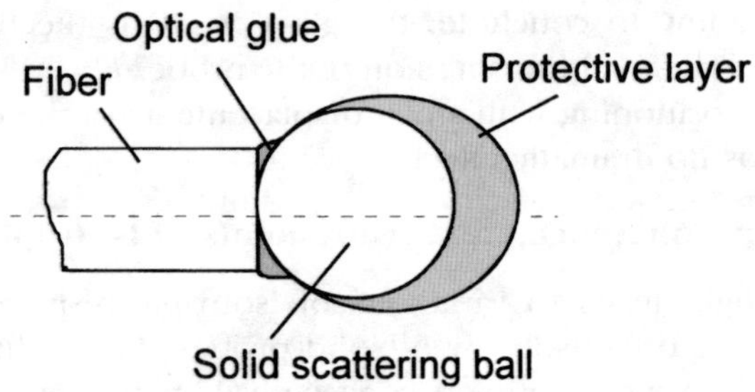

Figure 7 Compensation of forward light distribution by multi-layer protective covering.

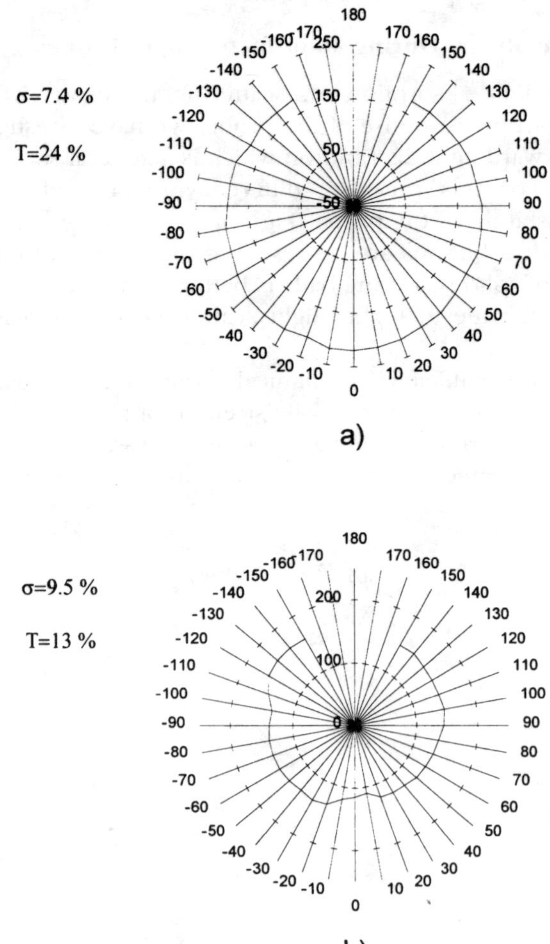

Figure 8 Changes of light distribution in solid probe with number of protective layers: 1 layer (a); 4 layers (b).

additional covering increases the diameter of probes. In contrary, multi-layer protective covering allows to compensate the forward light distribution.

Influence of light coherence on isotropic response was less in glued probes than in melted ones. If noncoherent light source was replaced by He–Ne laser anisotropy increased only by a factor 1.2. In addition, glued technology is more convenient in respect of probe reproduction.

As disadvantages of glued probes one can say difficulties with performing of very small glass balls using conventional polishing technique and necessity of precise control during manufacturing of probes.

3.3.3. *IN VIVO* MEASUREMENTS

Fibers with the isotropic probe were mounted into an applicator with the needle of a syringe. The scattering sphere is protected by sliding into the needle. The probe can be sterilized and be introduced in a sterile needle. For *in vivo* measurements the applicator with the needle is injected into the tissue at an angle of about 45° to the surface of the tissue, withdrawn for 2 mm and the fiber with the sphere pushed out of the needle for 2–3 mm. This procedure is demonstrated in Figs. 9 and 10.

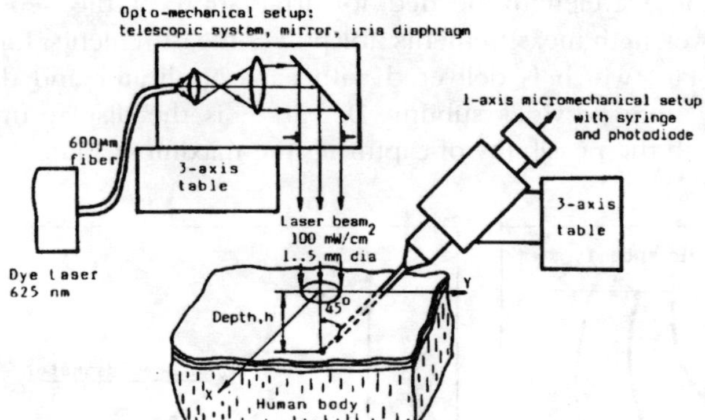

Figure 9 Experimental scheme for the *in vivo* measurements of light distribution in the tissue.

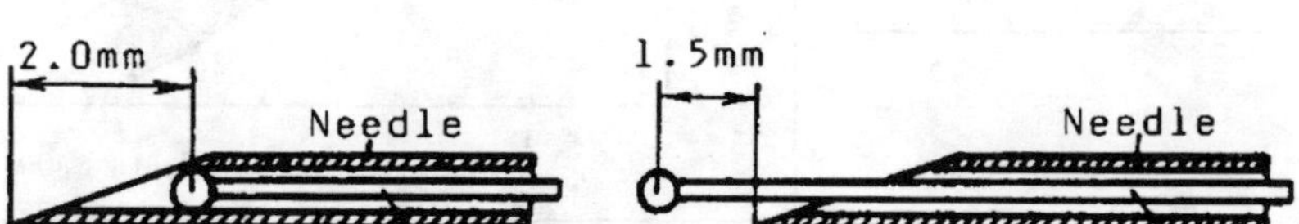

Figure 10 Protection of the isotropic sphere, $d = 420\,\mu m$, during injection of the needle and measuring conditions.

Depth dependent light intensity can be measured by slowly pulling back the applicator. An example of light distribution measured in the muscle of the leg is shown in Fig. 11.

From the graph in Fig. 11b two essential features can be derived. The intensity in the tissue just below the surface is higher due to the scattering of the laser light than the irradiance of the laser beam. From this value, a factor of about 2.2, the optical constants of the tissue can approximately be calculated. The other significant point is that the penetration depth of the laser light, here for $\lambda = 630$ nm, varies with the spot size at the surface. With a beam diameter of 1 mm, the penetration depth for a decrease of light intensity to 10% of the superficial irradiance is about 2.5 mm. For a spot size of 5 mm this depth increases to 5 mm. Also this phenomenon can be explained due to the scattering of the light in the tissue when the scattering length is much smaller than the absorption length.

The electronic registration unit (Fig. 12) contains several functions which are necessary to display an absolute value for the fluence rate in the tissue. These functions are marked with letters from A to E in Fig. 12. The subunit A has an exit for a calibration laser diode of 1 mW power. Segment B is the amplifier of the input signal. The applicator is connected to this subunit by a standard SMA-plug. In section C is a special wavelength dependent detector which measures the wavelength of the laser light. This wavelength meter is important for dye lasers to select exactly the wavelength needed for irradiation of the sensitizer. Mode selection for wavelength measurements, for power measurements, for input of the calibration constant which is delivered with each applicator and display of the absolute fluence rate provides subunit D. Part E is the display unit with zero calibration or with the possibility of capturing the maximum value.

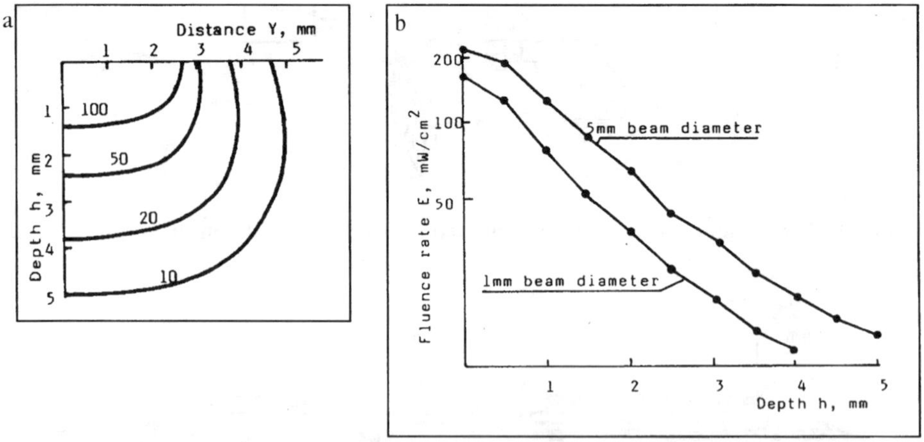

Figure 11 (a) Light distribution in muscle of a human leg with lines of equal fluence rates. (b) Axial light intensity in the tissue with depth at 1 mm laser spot and 5 mm laser spot of equal irradiance.

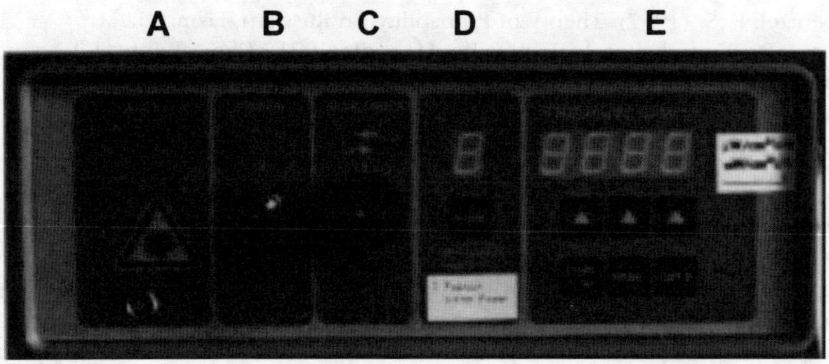

Figure 12 Electronic registration unit. A, power supply for calibrating laser diode, B, SMA-plug for input signal of the applicator, C, wavelength selective detector for measurement of the irradiation laser wavelength, D, mode switch, E, display unit.

The input power meter automatically changes the sensitivity according to the signal level. Illuminated diodes show the actual measuring range and the units, either related to fluence rate or the total power. Electronic device and the applicator with the micro probe are one calibrated unit to objectively determine the laser light distribution in tissue *in vivo*.

REFERENCES

[1] Van Gemert, M. J. C. and Welch, A. J. (1991): Optical and thermal modeling of tissues: dosimetry. In: Optronic Techniques in Diagnostic and Therapeutic Medicine. Ed: R. Pratesi. Plenum Press, NY, pp. 45–57.

[2] Marijnissen, J. P. A., Versteeg, A. A. C., and Star, W. V. (1989): *In vivo* light dosimetry for interstitial photodynamic therapy: results of clinical importance. *SPIE* **1065**, 109–114.

[3] Marijnissen, J. P. A. and Star, W. V. (1987): Quantitative light dosimetry *in vitro* and *in vivo*. *Lasers Med. Sci.* **2**, 235–242.

[4] Stroka, R., Baumgartner, R., Beyer, W. *et al.* (1990): Light monitoring by isotropic and by integrated fiber detectors. *SPIE* **1201**, 320–326.

[5] Melnik, I. and Steiner, R. (1992): *In vivo* measurements of laser irradiation in human tissue by small isotropic detector. *Lasermedizin* **8**, 73–77.

[6] McKenzie, A. L. (1985): Can diffusion be assumed in correcting for oblique incidence in laser photodynamic therapy? *Phys. Med. Biolog.* **31**, 285–234.

[7] Driver, J. J., Feather, J. W., King, P. R., and Dawson, J. B. (1989): Coagulation of blood at the tip of optical fibres used for light delivery in photodynamic therapy. *Lasers Med. Sci.* **4**, 125–1129.

[8] Marijnissen, J. P. A., Jansen, H., and Star, W. M. (1989): Treatment system for whole bladder wall photodynamic therapy with *in vivo* monitoring and control of light dose rate and dose. *Journal of Urology* **22**, 1351–1355.

[9] Ventzel, E. S. (1967): Theory of Probability (in Russian), Fizmatgiz.
[10] Bays, R., Winterhalter, L., Funakubo, H. *et al.* (1991): Clinical optical dose measurement for PDT: invasive and non-invasive techniques. *SPIE* **1525**, 397–408.
[11] Linge, L., Flotte, J., and Wilson, B. C. (1990): A fluorescent-tip optical fiber probe for quantitative light dosimetry in light scattering media and in tissue. *SPIE* **1203**, 106–117.
[12] Linge, L., Haw, T., and Wilson, B. C. (1993): Miniature isotropic optical fibre probes for quantitative light dosimetry in tissue. *Phys. Med. Biol.* **37**.
[13] Ishanin, M. B. (1989): Light Sources and Photodetectors. L, Mashinostroenie.
[14] Melnik, I., Kravchenko, I., and Rozumenko, V. (1993): Light penetration in human and rabbit brain: measurements using isotropic detector. *SPIE* **2077**, 238–242.
[15] Melnik, I., Hibst, R., Fischer, M., and Flemming, G. (1993): New modified optical fiber tips for medical applications. *Opt. Eng.* **32**, 227–232.
[16] Panov, V. A., Kruger, M. Y., Kulagin, V. V. *et al.* (1980): Reference Book for Designer of Opto-Mechanical Devices. Ed: Panov, V. A., Leningrad, Mashinostroenie.
[17] Jacques, S. L., Alter, C. A., and Prahl, S. A. (1987): Angular dependence of HeNe laser light scattering by human dermis. *Lasers Life Sci.* **1**(4), 309–333.

3.4. OPTIMIZATION OF WAVELENGTH IN PHOTODYNAMIC THERAPY

KRISTIAN BERG and JOHAN MOAN

The first law of photochemistry states that "only light absorbed by a molecule can produce photochemical change in that molecule" (Grotthus, 1815; Draper, 1841). The basis for the use of porphyrins and other photosensitizers in photodynamic therapy (PDT) is that they can absorb light at clinically relevant wavelengths. The spectral properties of photosensitizing molecules vary with their surroundings. The light sources used in PDT are usually lasers emitting light within a narrow wavelength range. It is therefore of outermost importance that optimal wavelengths are chosen as recently discussed by Star (1995). Methods related to the wavelength dependency of photosensitization, *in vitro* and *in vivo*, will be reviewed.

3.4.1. ABSORPTION SPECTRA

When light encounters a molecule, it can either be scattered or absorbed. A molecule which has absorbed a quantum of light is said to be *excited* and molecules which can be excited by absorption of visible light are named *chromophores*. In photobiology a chromophore is usually thought of as a molecule starting a photochemical reaction. Excitation energy can either be released as heat, emitted as fluorescence of a wavelength equal to or longer than that of the excitation light or undergoing intersystem crossing (for more details, see Bensasson *et al.*, 1993). The absorption spectrum of a molecule reflects its probability of transition between the ground state and any of the vibrational levels of its first and higher excited states. The absorption spectrum, characterized by the molar extinction coefficient at a particular wavelength, is described by Beer–Lambert's law:

$$I = I_0 \, 10^{-\varepsilon dc} \quad \text{or} \quad \log_{10}\left(\frac{I_0}{I}\right) = \varepsilon dc = \mathrm{OD} = A, \tag{1}$$

where ε is the molar extinction coefficient, I_0 is the fluence rate of the incoming light, I is the fluence rate of the transmitted light, d is the thickness of the sample, c is the molar concentration and OD is the optical density. Absorption can be reported either as % *transmittance* ($100 \times I/I_0$) or as absorbance ($\log_{10}(I/I_0)$). The wavelength of the peak of absorbance (λ_{max}), ε and the spectral shape are dependent on the local concentration of absorbing molecules, pH, polarity of the solvent, binding to other molecules, aggregation and temperature.

When an absorption spectrum is to be used for evaluation of photochemical effects, it should be measured under conditions as similar to the conditions of photochemical treatment as possible. Cell suspensions should be washed, i.e. the surrounding solution replaced with solutions without the dye, at least 3 times and resuspended in a non-absorbing solution such as phosphate-buffered saline (PBS) or 0.9% NaCl. If the absorption spectrum cannot be measured immediately, the suspension should be kept icecold to reduce the metabolic activity of the cells and the diffusion of the chromophore out of the cells. Monolayer cells can be scraped off the substratum with a rubber policeman. The rubber should be soft to reduce the damage to the cells. Absorption measurements on cell suspensions should never be performed later than 1 h after isolation of the cells.

Cells do not only absorb light but they also scatter light (van de Hulst, 1981). Scattering will give rise to artificially high absorbances. The scattering is usually wavelength dependent. Corrections of absorption spectra may be performed by extrapolation of the scattering spectrum from a wavelength region where the chromophore does not absorb light. Absorption and scattering in the cells themselves may be corrected for by using a suspension of untreated cells in the reference cuvette. However, small differences between similar cell suspensions may reduce the accuracy of the measurements of samples with low absorbances. Light scattering from cells in suspension may also introduce an instrumental problem since the artificial absorption can be quite high and the scattering reduces the fluence rate of the light beam so that the noise increases. For example, the apparent optical density of a suspension of 1×10^6 BHK cells/ml is approximately 0.75 at 400 nm (1 cm light path) and about 0.4 at 800 nm in a conventional spectrophotometer. Thus, the use of a spectrophotometer with an integrating sphere, which can detect more of the scattered light, is recommended. The integrating sphere is located close to the cuvette and together with a cuvette with $\leqslant 0.5$ cm pathlength approximately 50% of the scattered light will be captured by the light detector of the spectrophotometer.

3.4.2. QUANTUM YIELD OF PHOTOINACTIVATION

The second law of photochemistry, which is guilty only in terms of classical optics, states that "one quantum of light is absorbed per molecule which emits light or is chemically altered after the light absorption" (Stark, 1908; Einstein, 1912). Einstein introduced the concept of *quantum yield*, Φ, which can be adapted to photoinactivation of cells, Φ_{in}, as

$$\Phi_{in} = \frac{\text{number of cells photoinactivated}}{\text{number of photons absorbed by the cell-bound chromophore}}. \qquad (2)$$

Usually values for Φ_{in} are used to compare efficiencies of photoinactivation at different wavelengths or to compare Φ_{in} for different sensitizers. In such cases only relative values are necessary. When cells are exposed to monochromatic light of the wavelength λ_1, the relative quantum yield of photoinactivation, $\Phi_{\text{in, rel}}(\lambda_1)$, can be expressed as

$$\Phi_{\text{in, rel}}(\lambda_1) = \frac{\text{number of cells photoinactivated}}{\text{OD}(\lambda_1) \times I_0(\lambda_1) \times t}, \tag{3}$$

where $\text{OD}(\lambda_1)$ is the absorption of the chromophore at λ_1, $I_0(\lambda_1)$ is the fluence rate given in number of photons per time interval and t is the time of exposure. This relationship is of practical use only for fluences that inactivate significantly less than 100% of the cells. Furthermore, Eq. (3) holds only for small absorbances and low cell densities such that

$$I_{\text{abs}} = \text{const.} \times \text{OD} \times I_0,$$

i.e.

$$I_{\text{abs}} = I_0 - I = I_0(1 - 10^{-\text{OD}}) = I_0(1 - \text{e}^{-0.4\text{OD}}) \cong I_0(1 - 1 + 0.4\,\text{OD}).$$

Thus,

$$I_{\text{abs}} \cong (0.4 \times \text{OD} \times I_0),$$

where I_0, I_{abs}, and I describe the incident, absorbed and transmitted light, respectively. Light penetration at large absorbances can be corrected for (see Section 3.4.3).

Fluence-response curves often deviate from linearity in semilog plots. Therefore, Φ_{in} for different treatments should usually be compared at the same level of survival. Thus,

$$\Phi_{\text{in, rel}, S} = \frac{S}{\text{OD}(\lambda_1) \times I_{0,S}(\lambda_1) \times t}, \tag{4}$$

where S is the surviving fraction at λ_1.

Example

Cells are treated with the photosensitizers A and B. Fifty per cent of those treated with A and a fluence rate of $7\,\text{W cm}^{-2}$ at 400 nm for $t_A = 5$ min are inactivated. The same level of inactivations (50%) is obtained when treating the cells with B and a fluence rate of $5\,\text{W cm}^{-2}$ at 600 nm for $t_B = 10$ min. The optical density of A in the cells (1 cm light path of the cuvette) is 0.06 at 400 nm, and that of B is 0.08 at 600 nm. When the fluence rates are corrected for the relationship between wavelength and photon energy (see Section 3.4.3) we then have

$$\frac{\Phi_{\text{in}}(\text{A, 400 nm})}{\Phi_{\text{in}}(\text{B, 600 nm})} = \frac{\text{OD(B)} \times I(600\,\text{nm}) \times t_B \times 600}{\text{OD(A)} \times I(400\,\text{nm}) \times t_A \times 400}$$

$$= \frac{0.08 \times 5 \times 10 \times 600}{0.06 \times 7 \times 5 \times 400} = \frac{2400}{840} = 2.9.$$

Thus, with respect to sensitizing cells to photoinactivation A is 2.9 times more efficient than B.

The absolute number of absorbed photons by a cell bound photosensitizer can be measured in the following way. The energy of a single quantum of light is given by the equation

$$E = \frac{hc}{\lambda}, \tag{5}$$

where h is Planck's constant (6.62×10^{-34} J s), c is the speed of light (3×10^8 m/s) and λ the wavelength. Thus, the number of incident photons per cm^2, N_i, is

$$N_i = \frac{I_{i\lambda} \times t}{E_\lambda}, \tag{6}$$

where $I_{i\lambda}$ is the fluence rate (in W/m^2) of the incident light at wavelength λ, t is time of exposure and E_λ is the energy of a photon at the wavelength λ. The number of absorbed photons, N_a, per cells is given by

$$N_a = N_i N_c \sigma, \tag{7}$$

where N_c is the number of photosensitizer molecules per cell and σ is the molecular cross section of the photosensitizer given by

$$\sigma = \frac{2300\, \varepsilon}{N_A}, \tag{8}$$

where N_A is Avogadro's number (6×10^{23} molecules/mol) and ε the molecular extinction coefficient (in l/mole × cm). Molecular extinction coefficients are usually lower in biological material than in organic solvents. Biologically relevant extinction coefficients can be estimated by measuring the optical density of the dye in the cells and the total amount of dye in the cell suspension. Additionally, the light path must be estimated. This can be done by measuring the optical density of a dye which does not bind to the cells, in the presence and absence of cells. The extinction coefficient can then be estimated from Eq. (1).

3.4.3. ACTION SPECTRA

The absorption spectrum of a substance does not necessary give the full information about the wavelength dependency of its photochemical activity. For example, molecules may absorb infrared light without causing any electronic excitation. This is due to the low energy of the infrared light which can excite only vibrational and rotational modes. The only effect is release of heat. In cells the chromophore may be in different states of aggregation, and the absorption spectrum is caused by a mixture of monomeric and aggregated species. As will be discussed below, aggregated species have a low quantum yield for photoinactivation of cells. In order to determine the optimal wavelength for inducing a phototoxic effect, an action spectrum has to be determined. An *action spectrum* is a plot of the relative effectiveness of light of different wavelengths versus the wavelength.

To make an action spectrum dose-response curves must be made for each wavelength and a plot of the inverse value of (the relative) number of incident photons (N_s) needed to reach a given effect (for instance inactivation of 90% of cells), vs. the wavelength can be made. The effectiveness, E_s, can then be described as

$$E_s = \frac{1}{N_s} \tag{9}$$

at a dose where S% of the cells survive. The relative number of incident photons (N) is

$$N = I_0(\lambda) \times t \times \lambda, \tag{10}$$

where $I_0(\lambda)$ is the fluence rate of the light at the wavelength λ, t is the time of exposure and λ is the wavelength. The wavelength is included to correct the inverse relationship between the wavelength and the energy of the photon. At the same fluence, i.e. $I_0(\lambda) \times t$, twice as many photons are emitted at 800 nm as at 400 nm. The relative quantum efficiency is given by

$$\Phi_{\text{in, rel}, s} = \frac{1}{N_s \times \text{OD}}, \tag{11}$$

where OD is the absorbance of the chromophore in the cells (see also Eq. (4)).

At OD values higher than about 0.1 inner filter effects should be paid attention to. The fluence rate of the light follows the equation

$$I = I_0\, 10^{-\varepsilon c x_n} = I_0\, \mathrm{e}^{-\ln 10 \varepsilon c x_n}, \tag{12}$$

where x_n is the path length of the light (see Fig. 1). The mean fluence rate (I_{mean}) is

$$I_{\text{mean}} = \frac{I_0}{x_1}\int_0^{x_1} \mathrm{e}^{-\ln 10 \varepsilon c x}\, \mathrm{d}x = \frac{I_0}{x_1 \ln 10 \varepsilon c}(1 - \mathrm{e}^{-\ln 10 \varepsilon c x_1})$$

$$= \frac{I_0}{\ln 10 \times \text{OD}}(1 - 10^{-\text{OD}}). \tag{13}$$

The penetration of light through the solution will depend on the absorbance of the solution at the selected exposure wavelength and the action spectrum must be corrected by the factor $1/(\ln 10 \times \text{OD})\,(1 - 10^{-\text{OD}})$ according to Eq. (13). The effects of light scattering on light penetration and absorption will not be discussed in this chapter.

Example

An enzyme solution is mixed with $TPPS_4$ in a circular cuvette, placed on a rotating and mixing device and exposed to monochromatic light from a xenon lamp equipped with a monochromator. The inactivation of 50% of the enzymatic activity has been determined at each wavelength as well as the absorption spectrum of the solution. The calculations of the action spectrum is described in Table 1 and the results are presented in Fig. 2.

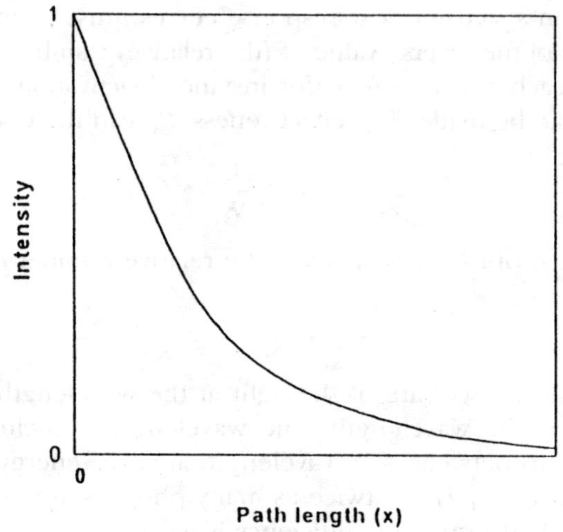

Figure 1 The intensity of light at different depths in a homogenous solution of the chromophore. The penetration depth is the distance over which the space irradiance falls off with a factor e^{-1}.

Table 1 The calculations of the action spectrum is based on the optical density (OD) of the solution at the different wavelength (nm), correction of the mean light intensity reaching $TPPS_4$ $[(1/OD) \times (1-10^{-OD})]$, and the inverse of the dose needed for inactivating 50% of the enzymatic activity (Rel. E_{obs}). Rel. E_{obs}, effectiveness, $E_{OD\ corr}$, corrected for differences in transmission; $E_{OD,\ nm\ corr}$, $E_{OD,corr}$ corrected for wavelength differences in photon energy; and E_{norm}, normalization of $E_{OD,\ nm\ corr}$

(nm)	OD	$(1/OD) \times (1-10^{-OD})$	*Rel.* E_{obs}	$E_{OD\ corr}$	$E_{OD,\ nm\ corr}$	E_{norm}
405	0.39	1.51	1.38	0.91	0.86	0.63
410	0.56	1.30	1.51	1.16	1.11	0.81
415	0.77	1.06	1.51	1.42	1.37	1.00
420	0.77	1.06	1.44	1.36	1.33	0.97
430	0.29	1.59	1.0	0.63	0.63	0.46

Action spectra for photoinactivation of cells in monolayer can be obtained using a continuous spectrum source, such as a xenon lamp, and a monochromator or narrow-band interference filters. The intensity of the light source can be measured by means of a thermopile (which has a flat wavelength response curve) or a photodiode with known wavelength characteristics. The thermopile must be protected against infrared emission, while the photodiode, which is a more light-sensitive and less heat-sensitive device, must be calibrated against a thermopile. A device to determine action spectra by exposing confluent layers of cells to a spot of monochromatic light moving with increasing speed over the culture flask has been described (Moan *et al.*, 1984). Both monolayer and suspension cells may also be exposed to light in solution and seeded out for survival measurements afterwards (see Chapter 1.3).

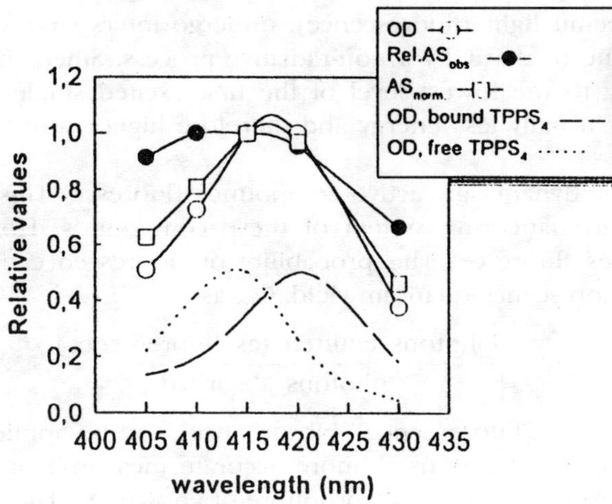

Figure 2 Absorption spectrum of $TPPS_4$ in the protein solution (OD), action spectrum (Rel. AS_{obs}) as the inverse of the dose needed for 50% enzyme inactivation, and action spectrum (AS_{norm}) corrected for penetration of light through the solution and differences in photon energy, all normalized to unity at 415 nm.

3.4.4. CONVOLUTION INTEGRALS

The quantum yield for photoinactivation of cells by different photosensitizers or the same sensitizer at different intracellular concentrations can be compared even after exposure to non-monochromatic light sources. The relative quantum yield is determined by

$$\Phi_{\text{in, rel}, S} = \frac{S}{K \times t \times \int_{\lambda_1}^{\lambda_2} \text{OD}(\lambda) \times I_0(\lambda) \times \lambda \, \text{d}\lambda}, \tag{14}$$

where OD(λ) is the absorption at the wavelength λ and $I_0(\lambda)$ is the fluence rate of the excitation light at the wavelength λ, t is the time of exposure and K is a constant. Equation (14) is valid only when OD is small ($\approx < 0.1$). For higher OD's we have

$$\Phi_{\text{in, rel}, S} = \frac{S}{K \times t \times \int_{\lambda_1}^{\lambda_2} (1 - 10^{-\varepsilon c x_1}) \times I_0(\lambda) \times \lambda \, \text{d}\lambda}, \tag{15}$$

where x_1 is the length of the light path.

3.4.5. FLUORESCENCE SPECTRA

A molecule excited to a singlet state will pass to the lowest vibrational level of the lowest excited singlet state by vibrational relaxation. The excited molecule can then either emit light (fluorescence), undergo intersystem crossing to the lowest triplet state or decay by a non-radiative process. Since energy is usually lost in dropping to the lowest level of the first excited singlet state, emitted fluorescence has usually less energy and therefore higher wavelength than the excitation light.

Nearly all photodynamically active compounds fluoresce. This is due to the relatively rigid aromatic ring system of these compounds. However, not all excited molecules fluoresce. The probability of fluorescence emission is described as the fluorescence quantum yield, Φ_{fl}, as

$$\Phi_{fl} = \frac{\text{photons emitted (as fluorescence)}}{\text{photons absorbed}}. \tag{16}$$

Relative numbers, i.e. [fluorescence] : [absorbance], can be applied for comparative studies of dilute solutions. A more accurate measurement of Φ_{fl} can be performed by comparison with a fluorophore of known Φ_{fl}. The quantum yield, $\Phi_{fl,A}$ of a sample A is

$$\Phi_{fl,A} = \frac{F_A \Phi_{fl,B} OD_B}{F_B OD_A} \tag{17}$$

in which $\Phi_{fl,B}$ is the quantum yield of the standard, F_A and F_B are the integrated fluorescence intensities of the sample and the standard, respectively, and OD_A and OD_B are the absorption of each solution at the exciting wavelength. The solutions are usually adjusted so that $OD_A = OD_B < 0.1$. As a standard fluorescein, quinine sulfate or proflavin can be used (see Parker, 1968 and Eaton, 1988 for more details). Measurements on cells should be carried out as described in Section 3.4.1. Most fluorescence spectrometers give corrected excitation spectra up to about 600 nm. To obtain corrected excitation spectra above 600 nm, see Chapter 3.5. for suggestions.

When measuring Φ_{fl}, one should be aware of the inner filter effect of the solution. Fluorescence is usually measured perpendicularly to the excitation light (Fig. 3). The mean length of the light path is $I_1 + I_2$ (see Fig. 3), while for the inner filter effect I_1 should usually be considered to a first approximation as the length of the light path. As an example let us assume that the OD is 0.1 in a solution when measured in a cuvette with 0.5 cm length of the light path. In a 3×3 mm fluorescence cuvette the mean light path is 1.5 mm and the reduction in transmission will be $1 - 10^{-0.1 \times 1.5/5} \times 100 = 6.7\%$. If the fluorescence cuvette has an inner size of 1 cm the transmission will be reduced by $1 - 10^{-0.1 \times .5/5} \times 100 = 21\%$.

In spectrofluorometers the monochromatic light is usually obtained by means of a reflection grating. These grating monochromators introduce in addition to the chosen wavelength also 2nd order light, e.g. when the excitation light is set at 450 nm there will also be some 225 nm and some 900 nm light in the excitation beam. This light can easily be eliminated by appropriate cut-off filters on the excitation or emission side of the sample. It should also be emphasized that practically all spectrofluorometers present uncorrected fluorescence emission spectra.

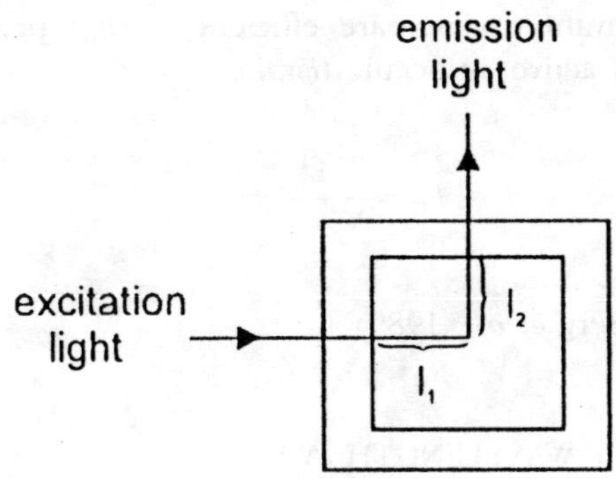

Figure 3 Cross section of a fluorescence cuvette and the light path through the cuvette.

3.4.6. APPLICATIONS OF FLUORESCENCE SPECTRA FOR OPTIMIZATION OF WAVELENGTH

In cells, as well as in solutions, both Φ_{fl} and fluorescence spectra of chromophores are dependent on the microenvironment and more so than absorption spectra. Typically, radiationless processes compete with fluorescence and thereby reduce Φ_{fl}, a phenomenon called *quenching*. In cells and other biological systems, quenching is due to collision processes (resulting in exchange of energy or to chemical reactions) or resonance energy transfer. Energy transfer from amino acids (mainly tryptophan) in proteins to cell bound porphyrins is observed as a quenching of tryptophan fluorescence and generation of porphyrin fluorescence from cells excited at the absorption band of tryptophan (Moan, 1985). Chromophores used in PDT tend to aggregate in cells. The absorption spectrum of aggregated species are usually broader and sometimes wavelength shifted, relative to that of the monomeric species (Moan *et al.*, 1987). Aggregates have a low Φ_{fl}. Absorption- and fluorescence excitation spectra of such chromophores in cells are therefore often different due to the mixture of monomeric and aggregated species in the cells (Moan *et al.*, 1987). Measurements have shown that action spectra for cell photosensitization of several photosensitizers follow the fluorescence excitation spectra of the dyes and not the absorption spectra (see Section 3.4.8 and Chapter 3.5). Furthermore, the efficiency of a photosensitizer in photoinactivation of cells is directly related to the amount of fluorescing dye in the cells but not to the amount of absorbing dye (Moan *et al.*, 1992b). These indications suggest that to a first and good approximation one may assume that only the fluorescing molecules are able to stimulate formation of singlet oxygen upon exposure to light. Thus, estimation of the optimal wavelength for photodynamic treatment should include measurements of fluorescence excitation spectra of the dye in a biologically relevant environment. For photosensitizers with similar photophysical properties or for the same photosensitizer at different intracellular concentrations it is relevant to compare efficiencies (E_{fl}) per fluorescing, supposedly photochemically active, molecule (F), i.e.

$$E_{\mathrm{fl}} = \frac{1}{N_s \times F}, \tag{18}$$

equivalent to Eq. (10) (Berg *et al.*, 1989).

3.4.7. OPTIMIZATION OF WAVELENGTH *IN VIVO*

Photosensitizers are used for a variety of purposes in biology and medicine; photochemotherapy of cancer and psoriasis being the best known examples. In order to optimize wavelengths of photosensitization at the very surface of tissue one can simply measure the fluorescence excitation spectrum of the photosensitizing drug (see Section 3.4.6) by means of a fiberoptic accessory adapted to an ordinary commercial fluorescence spectrofluorimeter (Moan *et al.*, 1994; Heyerdahl *et al.*, 1993). However, in photochemotherapy of cancer, the crucial point is to kill the tumor cells at the bottom of the tumor, where the space irradiance can be more than an order of magnitude lower than at the tissue surface. Under such conditions the penetration spectrum of light into tissue needs to be taken into account (Moan *et al.*, 1996). To a first approximation one may assume that the space irradiance ($E(x, \lambda)$) of light decreases exponentially in tissue:

$$E(x, \lambda) = E_0 \mathrm{e}^{-x/\delta(\lambda)}, \tag{19}$$

where E_0 is proportional to the fluence rate falling on the tissue surface, x is the depth below the tissue surface and $\delta(\lambda)$ is the penetration depth of light into tissue (see legend to Fig. 1). The action spectrum at the base of a tumor, $x = x_1$, can be approximated by the following product:

$$E(x_1, \lambda) = \mathrm{const}.\, E(0, \lambda)\, \mathrm{e}^{-x_1/\delta(\lambda)}, \tag{20}$$

where $E(0, \lambda)$ is the fluorescence excitation spectrum of the sensitizer at the tissue surface, and $E(x_1, \lambda)$ is a relative value for the quantum yield of inactivation of tumor cells at a depth x_1, measured per quantum of light incident on the tissue surface.

A direct, but very resource-consuming method to optimize the exposure wavelength would be to determine the fluence, $I_E(\lambda) \times t$, necessary to obtain a given effect, for instance a tumor growth delay of 5 days, and then determine the wavelength giving the maximum value of $1/[I_E(\lambda) \times t]$. Such an approach has been followed by Gomer (Gomer *et al.*, 1984) and Star (Star *et al.*, 1990). See Chapter 3.5 for a more detailed discussion of *in vivo* action spectroscopy.

Table 2 Summary of data from the literature concerning absorption peaks and the concomitant extinction coefficients (ε), fluorescence excitation peaks, and peak of the action spectra for several photosensitizers at the clinically relevant wavelength region

Dye	*Abs. peak* (nm)	ε ($M^{-1} cm^{-1}$)	*Fluor. excitation peak* (nm)	*Peak action spectrum* (nm)	*Solution*	*References**
1st genertion sensitizers						
HpD/DHE				630	Cells	
	630				TMW	Kessel, 1986.
HpD	622				5% FCS	Gomer *et al.*, 1984.
	630				cells	Gomer *et al.*, 1984.
				627.5–630	cells (1 h inc.)	Gomer *et al.*, 1984.
				630–632.5	cells (12 h inc.)	Gomer *et al.*, 1984.
				627	cells	Whitehurst *et al.*, 1993; Star *et al.*, 1990.
				625	*in vivo* (ear damage)	
			625		*in vivo*	Gijsbers *et al.*, 1987.
	625				*in vivo*	Potter *et al.*, 1994.
	625	≈3,000			PBS	Richter *et al.*, 1987.
Phthalocyanines						
$AlPcS_4$	674	190,000			methOH	Brasseur *et al.*, 1987b.
	678	72,000				Brasseur *et al.*, 1985.
	675		675	675	medium + serum cells	Western and Moan, 1988.
$AlPcS_{2a}$	≈672		≈672	≈672	cells	Moan *et al.*, 1992.
	685			685	*in vivo*	Cubeddu *et al.*, 1995.
$AlPcS_1$	669				methOH	Berg *et al.*, 1989.
	≈675		≈675	≈675	cells	Moan *et al.*, 1992.
AlPcS	674				aqueous sol	
	678				BSA	Ben-Hur and Rosenthal, 1986a.
	674	190,000			methOH	Brasseur *et al.*, 1988.
AlPc	≈671				ethOH	
	680 + 641				aq. BSA	Ben-Hur and Rosenthal, 1986b.
				680	cells	Ben-Hur *et al.*, 1992.
	675				cells	Paardekooper *et al.*, 1994.
	680				DMSO	

Table 2 *(Continued)*

Dye	*Abs. peak* (nm)	ε ($M^{-1} cm^{-1}$)	*Fluor. excitation peak* (nm)	*Peak action spectrum* (nm)	*Solution*	*References**
ZnPc	≈680				chloroform : metOH	Biolo *et al.*, 1991.
	676				aq. cetrimide	Ben-Hur *et al.*, 1987.
	670				cells	Firey *et al.*, 1988.
	666		666		ethOH	Valduga *et al.*, 1987.
	673	241,000			pyridine	Reddi *et al.*, 1990.
	670		670		LDL	Valduga *et al.*, 1987.
	674		674		cells	unpublished observations.
$ZnPcS_4$			670		methOH	Griffiths *et al.*, 1994.
			680 + 695		cells	Griffiths *et al.*, 1994.
				≈692	*in vivo*	Griffiths *et al.*, 1994.
	677	110,000			aq. CTAB	Spikes and Bommer, 1986.
	663				PBS	Spikes and Bommer, 1987.
ZnPcS	668	180,000			methOH	Brasseur *et al.*, 1988.
$GaPcS_2$	674	210,000			methOH	Brasseur *et al.*, 1987a.
$GaPcS_4$	674	210,000			methOH	Brasseur *et al.*, 1987b.
	678	37,000			medium + serum	Brasseur *et al.*, 1985.
Naphtalocyanines						
AlNcS	771	160,000			methOH	Paquette *et al.*, 1990.
iso-BOSiNc	774	557,000			THF	Cuomo *et al.*, 1990.
SiNc(OPEGM-1900)	784	220,000			ethanol	Bellemo *et al.*, 1992.
SiNc	786				ethanol	Bellemo *et al.*, 1992.
ZnNc	760				DMF	Shopova *et al.*, 1994.
	756	170,000			DMF	Wöhrle *et al.*, 1993.
Chlorins						
m-THPC	650	22.400			methanol	Bonnett *et al.*, 1987.
	≈655		≈655	≈655	cells	Ma *et al.*, 1994.
chlorin e_6	660	59.000				Oseroff *et al.*, 1986.
	≈665		≈655	≈655	cells	Western and Moan, 1988.
MACE	664	38,000			10% FCS	Roberts *et al.*, 1988.
	664				cells	

DACE	664	23,000			10% FCS	Roberts *et al.*, 1988.
	664				cells	
Bacteriochlorins						
m-THPBC	735	91.000			methanol	Bonnett *et al.*, 1987.
Bacteriochlorin A	764				methOH	van Best *et al.*, 1993.
	765	320,000			PBS	Beems *et al.*, 1987.
CA-BC derivatives	708–747	29,823–			ethOH	Kessel *et al.*, 1993.
		53,343			ethOH	
Benzoporhyrins						
MgTBP	630				S. areus	Ehrenberg *et al.*, 1993.
ZnTBP	640				S. aureus	Ehrenberg *et al.*, 1993.
BPD-MA	688	≈34,000			ethOH	Waterfield *et al.*, 1994.
	692				liposomes	Waterfield *et al.*, 1994.
				684–694	cells	Waterfield *et al.*, 1994.
				687–690	normal skin	Waterfield *et al.*, 1994.
				685–693	tumor	Waterfield *et al.*, 1994.
	692	13,000			aqueous sol.	Richter *et al.*, 1987.
	689		689		cells	unpublished observations.
Others						
PPIX (from ALA)				635	cells	Diddens, 1993.
Acridine orange	470				SDS (dimer)	Miyoshi *et al.*, 1988.
	495				SDS (monomer)	
methyl-Pheophorbide-a	666	45,000			CH_2Cl_2	Pandey *et al.*, 1991.
HEDP	660				0.1% Tween-80	Ho *et al.*, 1990.
(pheophorbide-a derivative)				665	*in vivo*	
Verdin	701	11,631			NS	Morgan *et al.*, 1987a.
	695				CH_2Cl_2	Morgan *et al.*, 1987c.
Nile blue A	623	75,300			methanol : acetic acid	Lin *et al.*, 1991.
m-THPP	648	3,600			FCS/DMSO	Berenbaum *et al.*, 1986.
	≈646		≈641	≈641	cells	Western and Moan, 1988.
hypericin	599	43,000			DMSO or medium	Andreoni *et al.*, 1994.
Hypocrellin A	580	≈18,000			ethOH	Hu *et al.*, 1994.

Table 2 *(Continued)*

Dye	*Abs. peak* (nm)	ε ($M^{-1}cm^{-1}$)	*Fluor. excitation peak* (nm)	*Peak action spectrum* (nm)	*Solution*	*References**
Hypocrellin A-Al	592	26,800			ethOH	
hematoporphyrin	621	5,180			dioxane	Falk, 1964.
	608				aq. sol (monomer)	Smith *et al.*, 1989.
	620				aq. sol (aggregate)	Smith *et al.*, 1989.
EtNBS	652	68,600			methanol	Cincotta *et al.*, 1994.
CdTX	770 (broad)				S. aureus	Ehrenberg *et al.*, 1993.
CdTX	767.5	410,000			methOH	Kreimer-Birnbaum, 1989.
Sapphyrin	669	17,000			$CHCl_3$	Judy *et al.*, 1991.
	711	100,000				
mesochlorin-Hp-	640	120,000			TMW	Kessel, 1986.
ester				640	cells	
$SnET2Cl_2$	659	300,000			CH_2Cl_2	Morgan *et al.*, 1988a.
(purpurin)	659				chremophore	Morgan *et al.*, 1987b.
				655 + 670	cells	Morgan *et al.*, 1988b.
MC540	570 (mono) 532 (di)			570	erythrocytes	Singh *et al.*, 1991.
Mesoporphyrin	620				ethOH	Kessel and Kohn, 1980.
	620				cells	
CP	786		739		ethOH	Kessel, 1991.
CP-Se/O	660	200,000			NS	Modica-Napolitano *et al.*, 1990.
CP-Se/S	710	200,000			NS	
	730	200,000			NS	
EDKC	700	120,000			PBS	Valdes-Aguilera *et al.*, 1987.
	706	230,000			methOH	
	712				RBC membranes	
Porphycene	633	420,000			toluene	Aramendia *et al.*, 1986.
Victoria blue-BO	616	50,000			NS	Modica-Napolitano *et al.*, 1990.

Table 2 (*Continued*)

Abbreviations: BPD-MA, benzoporphyrin derivative monoacid ring A; CA-BC, bacteriochlorin derivatives; CP, chalcogenapyrylium dye; DACE, diaspartyl chlorin e_6; EDKC, N,N′-bis (2-ethyl-1,3-dioxyl-ene) kryptocyanine; EtNBS, 5-ethylamino-9-diethylaminobenzo[a]phenoxazinium chloride; HEDP, 2(1-O-hexyl)ethyl-desvinyl-methyl pheophorbide a; Hp, hematoporphyrin; MACE, monoaspartyl chlorin e_6; MC540, merocyanine 540; $MePcS_n$, metallo (Al, Ga or Zn) phthalocyanine with n sulfonate groups; Nc, naphthalocyanine; $SnET2Cl_2$, Sn(IV) etiopurpurine dichloride; TBP, tetrabenzoporphyrin; m-THPBC, meso-tetra(hydroxyphenyl) bacteriochlorin; m-THPP, meso-tetra(hydroxyphenyl) porphine; TX, texaphyrin; TMW, THF : methOH : aqueous phosphate; BSA, bovine serum albumin; THF, tetrahydrofuran; DMF, dimethylformamide; NS, not specified; FCS, foetal calf serum; RBC, red blood cells.

*Andreoni *et al.*, 1994, *Photochem. Photobiol.*, **59**: 529–533; Aramendia *et al.*, 1986, *Photochem. Photobiol.* **44**: 555–559; Beems *et al.*, 1987, *Photochem. Photobiol.*, **46**: 639–643; Bellemo *et al.*, 1992, *Cancer Lett.*, **65**: 145–150; Ben-Hur and Rosenthal, 1986a, *Photochem. Photobiol.*, **43**: 615–619; Ben-Hur and Rosenthal, 1986b, *Lasers Med. Sci.*, **1**: 79–86; Ben-Hur *et al.*, 1987, *Cancer Lett.*, **38**: 215–222; Ben-Hur *et al.*, 1992, *Int. J. Radiat. Biol.*, **61**: 767–772; Berenbaum *et al.*, 1986, *Br. J. Cancer*, **54**: 717–725; Berg *et al.*, 1989, *Photochem. Photobiol.*, **49**: 587–594; Biolo *et al.*, 1991, *Photochem. Photobiol.*, **53**: 113–118; Bonnett *et al.*, 1987, *Biochem. J.*, **261**: 277–280; Brasseur *et al.*, 1985, *Photochem. Photobiol.*, **42**: 515–521; Brasseur *et al.*, 1987a, *Photochem. Photobiol.*, **45**: 581–586; Brasseur *et al.*, 1987b, *Photochem. Photobiol.*, **46**: 739–744; Brasseur *et al.*, 1988, *Photochem. Photobiol.*, **47**: 705–711; Cincotta *et al.*, 1994, *Cancer Res.*, **54**: 1249–1258; Cubeddu *et al.*, 1995, Proceedings of the 5th Int. Photodyn. Ass. Biennal Meeting, *SPIE*, **2371**: 172–176; Cuomo *et al.*, 1990, *Br. J. Cancer*, **62**: 966–970; Diddens, 1993, Workshop in Photodynamic Therapy and Diagnostics: Present State and Future Developments, Lübeck; Ehrenberg *et al.*, 1993, *Lasers Med. Sci.*, **8**: 197–203; Falk, 1964, Porphyrins and Metalloporphyrins (Vol.2), Amsterdam, Elsevier; Firey *et al.*, 1988, *Photochem. Photobiol.*, **48**: 357–360; Gijsbers *et al.*, 1987, *Lasers Life Sci.*, **1**: 29–48; Gomer *et al.*, 1984, *Photochem. Photobiol.*, **39**: 365–368; Griffiths *et al.*, 1994, *J. Photochem. Photobiol.*, **24**: 195–199; Ho *et al.*, 1990, *SPIE* Vol.1203 Photodynamic Therapy: Mechanisms II, pp. 224–232; Hu *et al.*, 1994, *J. Photochem. Photobiol.*, 219–227; Judy *et al.*, 1991, *Photochem. Photobiol.*, **53**: 101–107; Kessel, 1986, *Cancer Res.*, **46**: 2248–2251; Kessel and Kohn, 1980, *Cancer Res.* **40**: 303–307; Kessel, 1991, *Photochem. Photobiol.*, **53**: 73–76; Kessel *et al.*, 1993, *Photochem. Photobiol.*, **58**: 200–203; Kreimer-Birnbaum, 1989, *Seminars in Hematology*, **26**: 157–173: Lin *et al.*, 1991, *Cancer Res.*, 1109–1116; Ma *et al.*, 1994, *Int. J. Cancer*, **57**: 883–888; Moan *et al.*, 1992, *Photochem. Photobiol.*, **56**: 171–175; Modica-Napolitano *et al.*, *Cancer Res.*, **50**: 7876–7881; Morgan *et al.*, 1987a, *SPIE*, Vol. 847 New Directions in Photodynamic Therapy, 166–171; Morgan *et al.*, 1987b, *SPIE*, Vol. 847 New Directions in Photodynamic Therapy, 172–178; Morgan *et al.*, 1987c, *Photochem. Photobiol.*, **46**: 441–444; Morgan *et al.*, 1988a, *Cancer Res.*, **48**: 194–198; Morgan *et al.*, 1988b, *SPIE* Vol. 847 New Directions in Photodynamic Therapy, 172–178; Myoshi *et al.*, 1988, *Photochem. Photobiol.*, **47**: 685–688; Oseroff *et al.*, 1986, *PNAS*, **83**: 8744–8748; Paardekooper *et al.*, 1994, *Photochem. Photobiol.*, **59**: 161–166; Pandey *et al.*, 1991, *Photochem. Photobiol.*, **53**: 65–72; Paquette *et al.*, 1990, *Photochem. Photobiol.*, **51**: 313–317; Potter *et al.*, 1994, 5th Meeting Int. *Photodyn. Ass. Abstract* **46**; Reddi *et al.*, 1990, *Br. J. Cancer*, **61**: 407–411; Richter *et al.*, 1987, *JNCI*, **79**: 1327–1332; Roberts *et al.*, 1988, *JNCI*, **80**: 330–336; Shopova *et al.*, 1994, *J. Photochem. Photobiol.*, **23**, 35–42; Singh *et al.*, 1991, *Photochem. Photobiol.*, **53**: 493–500; Smith *et al.*, 1989, *Photochem. Photobiol.*, **49**: 49–52; Spikes and Bommer, 1986, *Int. J. Radiat. Biol.*, **50**: 41–45; Spikes and Bommer, 1987, *Photochem. Photobiol.*, **45S**, p.79S; Star *et al.*, 1990, *Photochem. Photobiol.*, **52**: 547–554; Valdes-Aguilera *et al.*, 1987, *Photochem. Photobiol.*, **45**: 337–344; Valduga *et al.*, 1987, *J. Inorg. Biochem.*, **29**, 59–65; van Best *et al.*, 1993, *Lasers Med. Sci.*, **8**: 157–162; Waterfield *et al.*, 1994, *Photochem. Photobiol.*, **60**: 383–387; Western and Moan, 1988, Light in Biology and Medicine Vol.1, Plenum Press, pp. 85–89; Whitehurst *et al.*, 1993, *Lasers Med. Sci.*, **8**, 259–267; Wöhrle *et al.*, 1993, *J. Photochem. Photobiol.*, **21**: 155–165.

3.4.8. FLUORESCENCE EXCITATION AND ABSORPTION PEAKS AND PEAKS OF ACTIONS SPECTRA OF PHOTOSENSITIZERS

Table 2 summarizes data from the literature concerning absorption peaks, ε, fluorescence peaks, and peaks of the action spectra for several photosensitizers in the clinically relevant wavelength region. As seen from the table, the peak of the action spectra does not always coincide with the absorption peak of the sensitizer in solution and even not in the same biological environment. This is for example seen with MC540 where the absorption spectrum has two peaks (532 and 570 nm) while the action spectrum has only one peak (570 nm) (Singh *et al.*, 1991). This correlates well with photochemical action of the monomeric species of MC540. Absorption and fluorescence excitation spectra of photosensitizers in cells are often different. This is most likely due to the fact that aggregated material has a very low fluorescence quantum yield compared to monomers. In many cases, e.g. 3-THPP, 3-THPC, Chlorin e_6, $AlPcS_4$, $AlPcS_{2a}$, $AlPcS_1$, HpD and PII, the action spectrum was found to correlate well with the fluorescence excitation spectrum but not with that of the absorption spectrum although the peak of the action spectrum may coincide with both spectra ((Moan and Sommer, 1984; Moan *et al.*, 1992a; Western and Moan, 1988; Williams and Runge, 1987; Ma *et al.*, 1994), Table 2). Thus, the photochemical effect seems to be mainly due to the monomeric fraction of the photosensitizers in the biological environments. Griffiths *et al.* (1994) found two fluorescence excitation peaks of equal intensity (680 and 695 nm) of $ZnPcS_4$ in culture cells, a 670 nm fluorescence excitation peak in methanol while 692 nm light was more efficient than 680 and 670 nm light in inducing tumor retardation. Similarly, the peak of the action spectrum for $AlPcS_{2a}$ in cells in culture has been found to be located at 672 nm, while the peak *in vivo* is found to be located at 685 nm (Table 2). Such studies emphasize the importance of determining action spectra both in cells in culture and *in vivo* and has been discussed in more detail in Chapter 3.5.

REFERENCES

Bensasson, R. V., Land, E. J., and Truscott, T. G. (1993): Excited states and free radicals in biology an medicine. Contributions from flash photolysis and pulse radiolysis. Oxford University Press, Oxford, pp. 24–63.

Berg, K., Bommer, J. C., and Moan, J. (1989): Evaluation of sulfonated aluminum phthalocyanines for use in photochemotherapy. A study on the relative efficiencies of photoinactivation. *Photochemistry and Photobiology* **49**: 587–594.

Draper, J. W. (1841): On some analogies between phenomena of chemical rays and those of radiant heat. *Philos. Mag.* **19**: 195–210.

Eaton, D. F. (1988): Reference materials for fluorescence measurements. *Journal of Photochemistry and Photobiology* **2**: 523–531.

Einstein, A. (1912): Thermodynamic foundations of the law of photochemical equivalents. *Ann. Physik.* **37**: 832–838.

Gomer, C. J., Doiron, D. R., Rucker, N., Razum, N. J., and Fountain, S. W. (1984): Action spectrum (620–640 nm) for hematoporphyrin derivative induced cell killing. *Photochemistry and Photobiology* **39**: 365–368.

Griffiths, J., Cruse-Sawyer, J., Wood, S. R., Schofield, J., Brown, S. B., and Dixon, B. (1994): On the photodynamic therapy action spectrum of zinc phthalocyanine tetrasulphonic acid *in vivo*. *Journal of Photochemistry and Photobiology, B – Biology* **24**: 195–199.

Grotthus, T. (1815): Über einen neuen Lichtsauger nebst einigen allegemeinen Betrachtungen über die Phosphoreszenz und die Farben. *J. Chem. Physik* **14**: 133–192.

Heyerdahl, H., Warloe, T., Peng, Q., Svanberg, K., Moan, J., Steen, H., Svaasand, L., and Giercksky, K. (1993): Dosimetry and light distribution systems for photodynamic therapy at the Norwegian Radium Hospital. In: Photodynamic Therapy of Cancer, G. Jori, J. Moan, and W. Star, eds. Proc. SPIE, Vol. 2078 Bellingham, pp. 27–36.

Ma, L., Moan, J., and Berg, K. (1994): Evaluation of a new photosensitizer, meso-tetra-hydroxyphenyl-chlorin, for use in photodynamic therapy: a comparison of its photobiological properties with those of two other photosensitizers. *Int. J. Cancer* **57**: 883–888.

Moan, J., Høvik, B., and Sommer, S. (1984): A device to determine fluence-response curves for photoinactivation of cells *in vitro*. *Photobiochemistry and Photobiophysics* **8**: 11–17.

Moan, J. (1985): Porphyrin photosensitization of cells. In: Photodynamic Therapy of Tumors and Other Diseases. G. Jori and C. Perria, eds. Libreria Progetto, Padova, pp. 101–112.

Moan, J., Peng, Q., Evensen, J. F., Berg, K., Western, A., and Rimington, C. (1987): Photosensitizing efficiencies, tumor- and cellular uptake of different photosensitizing drugs relevant for photodynamic therapy of cancer. *Photochemistry and Photobiology* **46**: 713–721.

Moan, J., Berg, K., Bommer, J. C., and Western, A. (1992a): Action spectra of phthalocyanines with respect to photosensitization of cells. *Photochemistry and Photobiology* **56**: 171–175.

Moan, J., Berg, K., Steen, H. B., Warloe, T., and Madslien, K. (1992b): Fluorescence and photodynamic effects of phthalocyanines and porphyrins in cells. In: Photodynamic Therapy: basic principles and clinical applications. B. W. Henderson and T. J. Dougherty, eds. Marcel Dekker, Inc. New York, pp. 19–36.

Moan, J., Høydalsvik, E., Peng, Q., Ma, L., Warloe, T., and Heyerdahl, H. (1994): Measurements of sensitizer fluorescence in patients by means of an ordinary fluorescence spectrometer. In: 5th International Photodynamic Association Biennial Meeting. D. A. Cortese, ed. Bellingham, pp. 516–521.

Moan, J., Iani, V., and Ma, L. (1996): Choice of the proper wavelength for photochemotherapy. In: Photochemotherapy: Photodynamic Therapy and Other Modalities. Ehrenberg, B., Jori, G. and Moan, J., eds. Proc. SPIE, Vol. 2625. pp. 544–549.

Moan, J. and Sommer, S. (1984): Action spectra for hematoporphyrin derivative and Photofrin II with respect to sensitization of human cells *in vitro* to photoinactivation. *Photochemistry and Photobiology* **40**: 631–634.

Parker, C. A. (1968): Photoluminescence of Solutions. Elsevier, Amsterdam, pp. 266–267.

Singh, R. J., Feix, J. B., Pintar, T. J., Girotti, A. W., and Kalyanaraman, B. (1991): Photodynamic action of merocyanine 540 in artificial bilayers and natural membranes: action spectra and quantum yields. *Photochemistry and Photobiology* **53**: 493–500.

Star, W., Versteeg, J., van Putten, W., and Marijnissen, H. (1990): Wavelength dependence of hematoporphyrin derivative photodynamic treatment effects on rat ears. *Photochemistry and Photobiology* **52**: 547–554.

Star, W. M. (1995): *In vivo* action spectra, absorption and fluorescence excitation spectra of photosensitizers for photodynamic therapy. *Journal of Photochemistry and Photobiology, B – Biology* **28**: 101–102.

Stark, J. (1908): Further remarks upon thermal and chemical absorption in the band spectrum. *Z. Physik* **9**: 889–894.

van de Hulst, H. C. (1981): Light Scattering by Small Particles. Dover Publications, Inc. New York,

Western, A. and Moan, J. (1988): Action spectra for photoinactivation of cells in the presence of tetra(3-hydroxyphenyl)porphyrin, chlorin e_6 and aluminium phthalocyanine tetrasulphonate. In: Light in Biology and Medicine. R. H. Douglas, J. Moan, and F. Dall' Acqua, eds. Plenum Press, New York, pp. 85–89.

Williams, R. D. and Runge, T. C. (1987): Photodynamic therapy of human bladder cancer cells *in vitro* correlated with cellular fluorescence levels of Photofrin-II. *Photochemistry and Photobiology* **46**: 733–737.

3.5. ACTION SPECTRA OF DYES RELEVANT FOR PHOTODYNAMIC THERAPY

JOHAN MOAN, KRISTIAN BERG and VLADIMIR IANI

Action spectroscopy has been designed to find the chromophores responsible for given reactions, such as photosynthesis, in complex biological systems, e.g. leaves and human skin. In such systems, all of the incident light is usually absorbed but only a fraction of it leads to biological reactions other than heating. The action spectrum for a given process is then simply

$$E(\lambda) = N^{-1}(\lambda), \tag{1}$$

where $N(\lambda)$ is the number of incident photons needed at the wavelength λ to produce a given effect, for instance 90% cell killing, or, in the case of erythema, a given redness of the skin. To identify the chromophore for the process one has to compare the action spectrum $E(\lambda)$ with absorption spectra of substances known to be present in the biological system. However, the action spectrum may be distorted in comparison with the absorption spectrum because the active molecules may be shielded by absorbing inert molecules. Let us, as an example, consider photocarcinogenesis and assume that the action spectrum for producing cancer cells is identical with the absorption spectrum of DNA. In skin the living and dividing cells are shielded by nondividing cells and cell debris (stratum granulosum and stratum corneum) through which the radiation has to penetrate before it reaches the living and dividing cells. The real action spectrum for photocarcinogenesis would then be the DNA absorption spectrum corrected for the absorption in the dead skin layers (Moan *et al.*, 1989). The situation is somewhat similar in photodynamic therapy: To cure a tumor, light has to penetrate to the tumor cells at the base of it, and the real action spectrum for tumor eradication is the action spectrum for photoinactivation of cells corrected for the wavelength dependency of light penetration to the base of the tumor. To determine the relevant action spectrum is the only way to optimize the wavelength for therapy. The relevant action spectrum can be obtained in two ways; either by direct action spectroscopy on tumors of the given size, which is impossible in humans and difficult even in animals since the endpoint has to be tumor eradication, or by determining the action spectrum for killing cells and the spectrum for penetration of light through the tumor. Since photodynamic tumor eradication is often due to vascular effects, one might instead of using the action spectrum of cell photoinactivation, use the action spectrum for vascular damage in the upper dermis. This spectrum can be approximated by the spectrum for induction of skin reddening, which can be objectively measured. Other spectra that can be used as approximations for the action spectrum of cell photoinactivation are fluorescence excitation spectra and action spectra for photodegradation of the sensitizer in the skin (see below).

3.5.1. ACTION SPECTRA FOR SINGLE CELLS

As discussed in Chapter 3.4, fluorescence excitation spectra are good approximations for action spectra of cell photoinactivation in the presence of photosensitizers. In all cases studied by us (Photofrin, HpD, $AlPcS_4$, $AlPcS_2$, $AlPcS_1$, Chlorin e_6, 3THPP and 3-THPC (for abbreviations, see legend to Table 2 in Chapter 3.4)) the action spectra for cell photoinactivation coincide with the fluorescence excitation spectra, but not with the absorption spectra of the dyes in the cells (Moan and Sommer, 1984; Western and Moan, 1988; Moan *et al.*, 1992; Ma *et al.*, 1994). This is certainly due to aggregation: While aggregates absorb light, they neither fluoresce nor generate singlet oxygen with significant yields. However, one should distinguish between aggregates, such as those present in HpD and Photofrin, which are probably to a large extent kept together by covalent bonds, and aggregates formed in concentrated solutions of pure substances such as hematoporphyrin. In the latter case it seems that singlet oxygen can be formed in significant amounts upon photoexcitation of the aggregates (Moan, 1984).

Some authors have presented action spectra as the fraction of inactivated cells after fixed exposure at different wavelengths. This is an adequate approach to find the optimal wavelength, but the resulting "action spectrum" cannot be used for comparison with absorption and fluorescence excitation spectra to determine the state of aggregation of the dyes in the cells. However, if a survival curve relevant for the dye and the cells is known, extrapolations can easily be made to obtain the number of photons ($N(\lambda)$) that would be needed at different wavelengths to kill a given fraction of the cells, and thus obtain the action spectrum according to Eq. (1). This is a valid approach if bleaching of the dye is insignificant; otherwise corrections have to be introduced.

Most fluorescence spectrometers give corrected excitation spectra up to about 600 nm. However, above 600 nm the spectra are essentially uncorrected. The reason for this is that rhodamine, which is used for quantum counting of the excitation light, has a very low absorption above 600 nm. This is unfortunate for the application of fluorescence excitation spectroscopy in the study of second and third generation photosensitizers for photochemotherapy. Most of these dyes have their main absorption in the wavelength region 600–800 nm. To obtain corrected excitation spectra in such cases one can follow three procedures: (1) One can record the absorption and fluorescence spectrum of a dye that is known to be monomeric and that absorbs light in the wavelength region in question. We have used DMSO solutions of $AlPcS_4$ in a low concentration ($OD < 0.1$) for this purpose. This dye in SDS micelles can also be used. The correction curve for the spectrometer is then simply obtained as the ratio of the absorption spectrum to the fluorescence excitation spectrum. (2) One can use an external, tunable monochromatic light source (a dye laser or a xenon lamp fitted to a monochromator) to excite the fluorescence and measure it with a fluorescence spectrometer in the bioluminescence or phosphorescence mode. The fluence rate of the exposure light can be measured with a thermopile or a photodiode with known wavelength characteristics. (3) One can uncouple the inbuilt correction system of the spectrometer, record the spectra and correct them manually. The wavelength dependence of the excitation light can be measured as described above.

3.5.2. *IN VIVO* ABSORPTION SPECTRA

The *in vivo* absorption spectra of dyes seem to be similar to the spectra in cells *in vitro* (Cubeddu *et al.*, 1994). Due to protein binding, these spectra are usually red-shifted compared to the corresponding spectra in aqueous solutions. Absorption spectra of dyes in cells can be conveniently measured by means of an ordinary spectrophotometer equipped with an integrating sphere or by the use of scattering quartz plates placed behind the cuvettes (Moan *et al.*, 1992).

Measurements of absorption spectra *in vivo* are far more complicated. A method applying fibre optics is described by Cubeddu *et al.* (1994). In a similar way approximative spectra can be obtained by means of a spectrofluorimeter equipped with fibre optics. The emission fibre is positioned parallel to the excitation fibre, at a distance of 0.5–1 cm, against the tissue. Then the emission and excitation monochromators are scanned simultaneously, all the way positioned at the same wavelength. *In vivo* absorption spectra can be estimated by calculating the ratio of such spectra taken before and after dye injection. A couple of absorption spectra obtained in this way are shown below.

A more precise method, applicable for some localizations on humans and animals and on biopsies, is sketched in Fig. 1. Light from a xenon lamp or a halogen lamp is guided via a perspex cylinder to the tissue. On the other side of the tissue a light collecting fibre can be positioned at known distances x from the end of the perspex cylinder. Provided this distance x is significantly smaller than the diameter of the perspex cylinder, one can obtain quite good approximations for the penetration spectra of light into tissue as well as for absorption spectra of dyes in the tissues by this method. As shown in Fig. 2 the light intensity collected by the fibre decreases in an exponential manner, and the penetration depth can be calculated from the slopes at all wavelengths within the lamp spectrum according to Eq. (17) in Chapter 3.4. Depending on the scattering conditions and the blood content of the samples, penetration spectra can be quite different. For instance, the penetration depth of light at 630 nm into a human ear is about 2.6 mm (Fig. 2) while that into a human basal cell carcinoma is about 1.6 mm (Fig. 3).

3.5.3. ACTION SPECTRA *IN VIVO*

In vivo action spectroscopy is difficult and time consuming. Therefore, very few *in vivo* action spectra have been published, see Table 2 in Chapter 3.4.

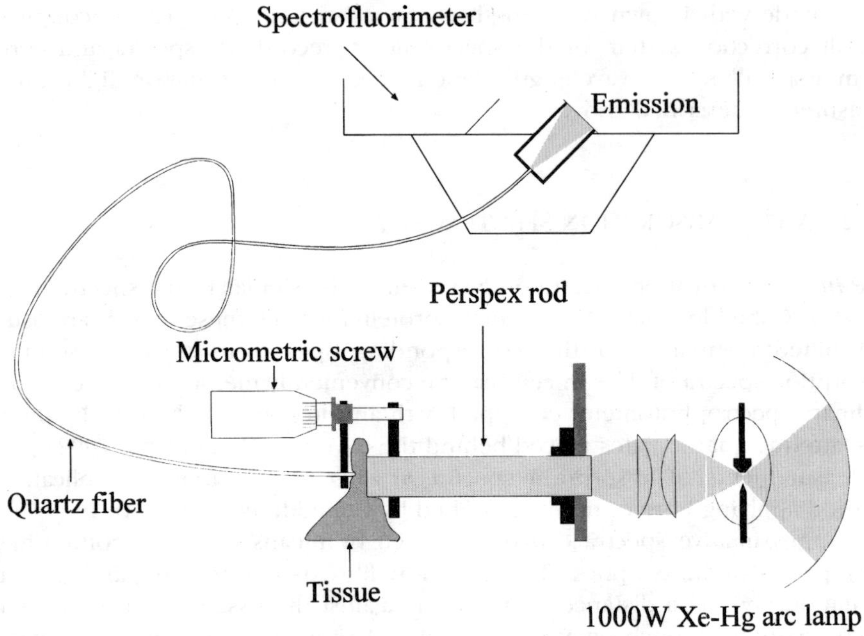

Figure 1 An experimental setup for measurements of optical penetration spectra in tissue and for absorption spectra of dyes *in vivo*.

The most important version of an action spectrum is that for tumor eradication. One such spectrum has been published (Waterfield *et al.*, 1994). The closest approximations to such a spectrum is that for the depth of tumor necrosis and that for tumor growth delay. Two spectra of this type – the only ones found in the literature so far – are shown below (Griffiths *et al.*, 1994; Farrell *et al.*, 1992). These spectra are influenced by two factors, one related to cell inactivation (i.e. the action spectrum for inactivation of cells at the surface) and one related to light penetration to deeper parts of the tumor. A good approach to obtain the action spectrum of photosensitized damage to skin and vascular structures is that of Star *et al.* (1990). These investigators studied the effects of photodynamic therapy with hematoporphyrin derivative on rat ears, quantified four parameters (ear thickness, erythema, escar and loss of tissue), and established a combined score. Since rat ears are thin (~ 0.4 mm) this score is probably describing effects close to the skin surface, and not so much dependent upon light penetration into deeper layers of the tissue. Surface spectra can also be approximated by action spectra for photodegradation (bleaching) of the dye in skin. Since both processes, photodegradation as well as tissue damage, are mainly caused by photosensitized production of singlet oxygen, this approximation is probably valid. Data for protoporphyrin IX (Pp IX) are shown in Fig. 3.

From surface spectra one can calculate the spectra at deeper layers, using known spectra for the optical penetration depth. For Pp IX in a human basal cell

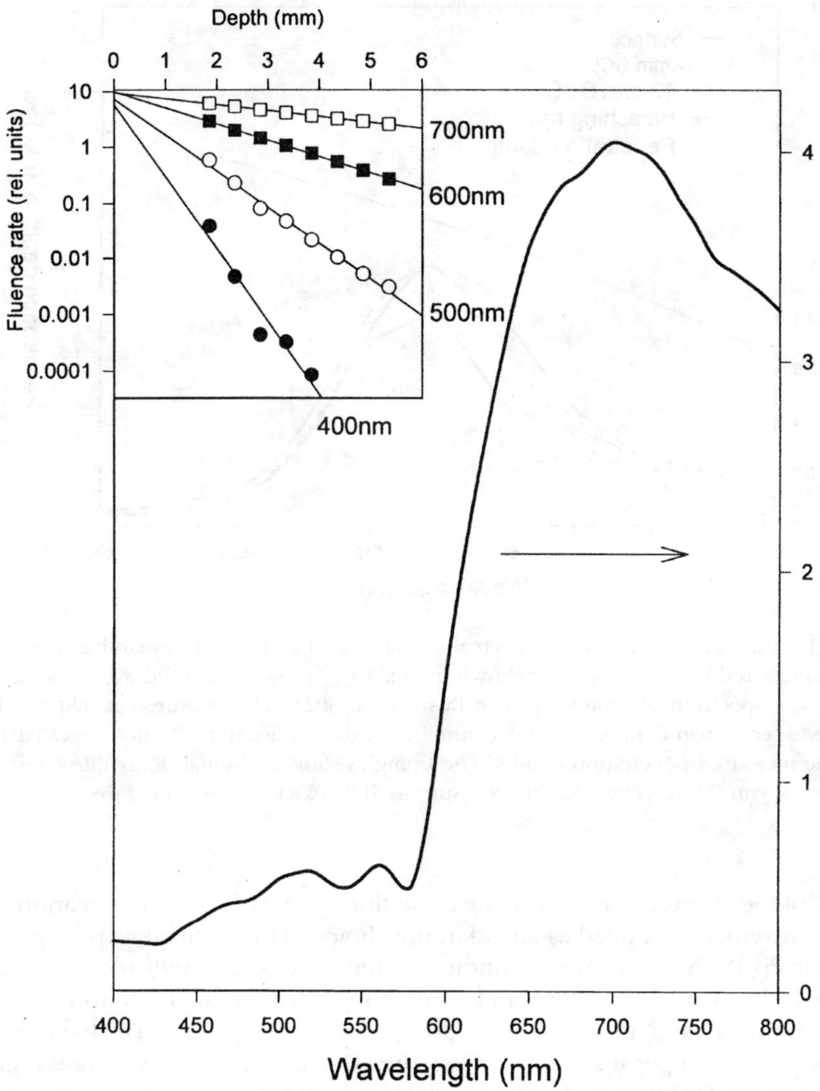

Figure 2 Experimental data obtained on a human ear tip *in vivo*, using the experimental setup shown in Fig. 1. The fluence rate of light transmitted a distance x through the tissue from the perspex cylinder to the fiber follows the relationship $I = I_0 \exp(-x/d)$ where d is the optical penetration depth.

carcinoma (BCC) the spectrum (620–650 nm) is redshifted by about 1 nm when going from the surface to a depth of 12 mm (Fig. 3).

A simple, approximative method to determine the action spectrum for inactivation of cells at a given depth below the skin surface, is to measure fluorescence excitation spectra of the dye in cells and to mount different thicknesses of tissue

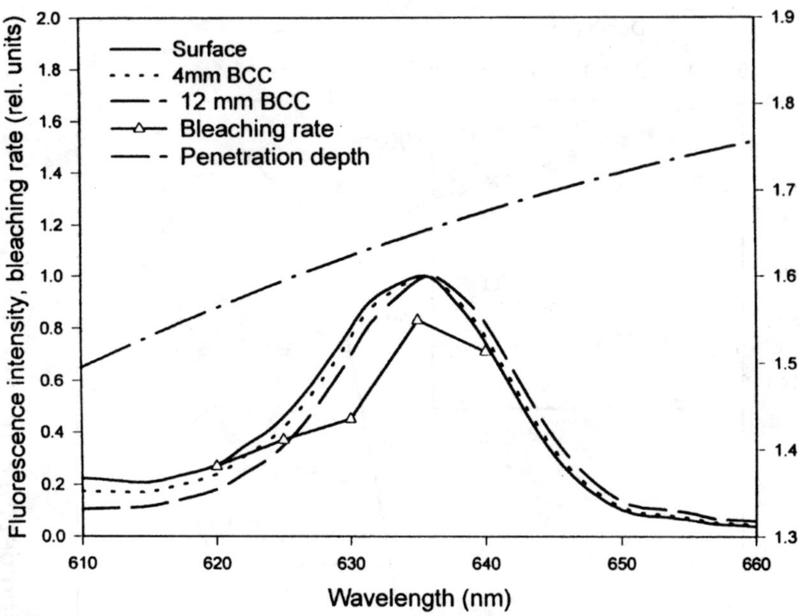

Figure 3 The optical penetration spectrum of light into an excised human basal cell carcinoma measured by the equipment shown in Fig. 1 (—·—·—). The full drawn curve is the fluorescence spectrum of protoporphyrin IX in NHIK 3025 cells measured at 690 nm. The excitation spectrum at depths of 4 and 12 mm below the surface of the tumor are calculated using the measured penetration depths. The triangles show the initial decay rate constants of the porphyrin fluorescence during exposure to 100 mW/cm^2 light from a dye laser.

in front of the cuvette to attenuate the excitation beam (Fig. 4). Such an approach can be conveniently applied as an aid in the choice of the optimal wavelength for PDT. For Pp IX in mouse tissue, photons within the wavelength region around 400 nm as well as around 510 nm, are more efficient than photons in the commonly used band around 335 nm down to about 2 mm (Fig. 4). However, to all cells located deeper than 2 mm below the skin surface, the wavelength region around 635 nm is best suited.

3.5.4. EXAMPLES OF ACTION SPECTRA FROM THE LITERATURE

As our first example we will consider the classical PDT photosensitizer Photofrin (Fig. 5). It is well known that this drug is composed of more than one porphyrin component, and one may, therefore, expect to find different spectra under different conditions. The two *in vivo* spectra both have their maximum at 625 nm (Star *et al*., 1990; Farrell *et al*., 1992) as has the fluorescence excitation spectrum of Photofrin in aqueous solution containing 10% human serum

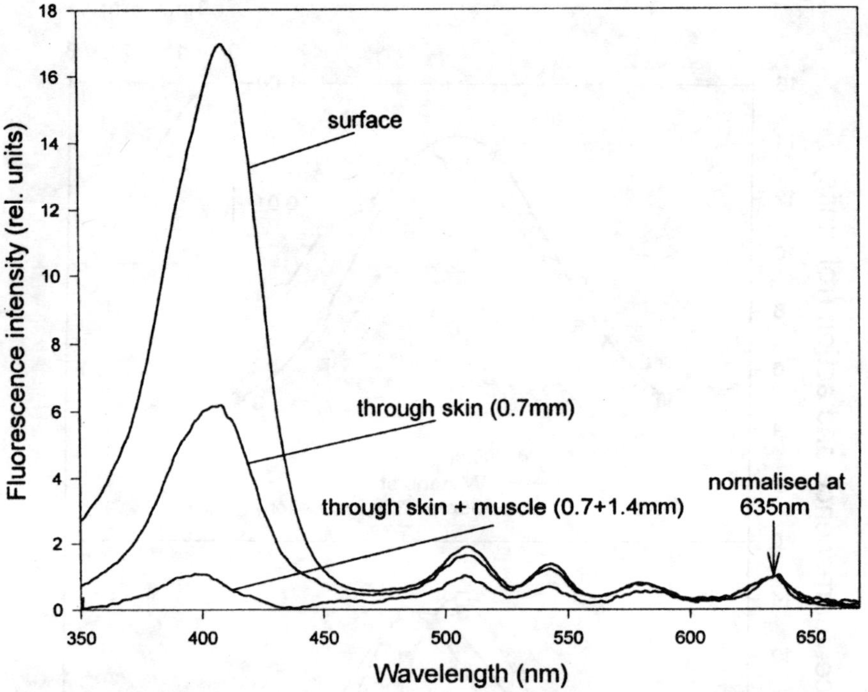

Figure 4 Fluorescence excitation spectra of protoporphyrin IX in PBS containing 10% human serum measured by means of a Perkin Elmer LS 50B fluorescence spectrometer with the emission wavelength set at 690 nm, 10 nm slit widths and with biopsies of mouse skin and mouse skin + muscle placed in the excitation beam in front of the cuvette.

(Fig. 5). The absorption spectrum of the dye in cells as well as its action spectrum in cells, has maximal value at about 627–630 nm (Gomer *et al.*, 1984; Kessel, 1986; Whitehurst *et al.*, 1993).

For the new photosensitizer benzoporphyrin derivative monoacid ring A (BPD MA) all spectra (absorbance in cells, absorbance in mouse tissue *in vivo*, fluorescence excitation in cells, photoinactivation of cells, and cure of mouse tumors) show a maximal value close to 690 nm (Waterfield *et al.*, 1994, present work, Fig. 6). The similarity of the shape of the absorption spectrum and the fluorescence excitation spectrum of the dye in cells, indicates that it is mainly present in the monomeric form.

The action spectrum for tumor growth delay sensitized by zinc phthalocyanine tetrasulphonic acid ($ZnPcS_4$) is very different from its fluorescence excitation spectrum in cells (Fig. 7, Griffiths *et al.*, 1994). This discrepancy cannot be explained by the spectrum of light penetration in tissue (Fig. 2) and deserves further attention.

Disulphonated aluminium phthalocyanine ($AlPcS_2$) has been studied by our group (Moan *et al.*, 1992) as well as by Cubeddu *et al.* (1994) (Fig. 8). The

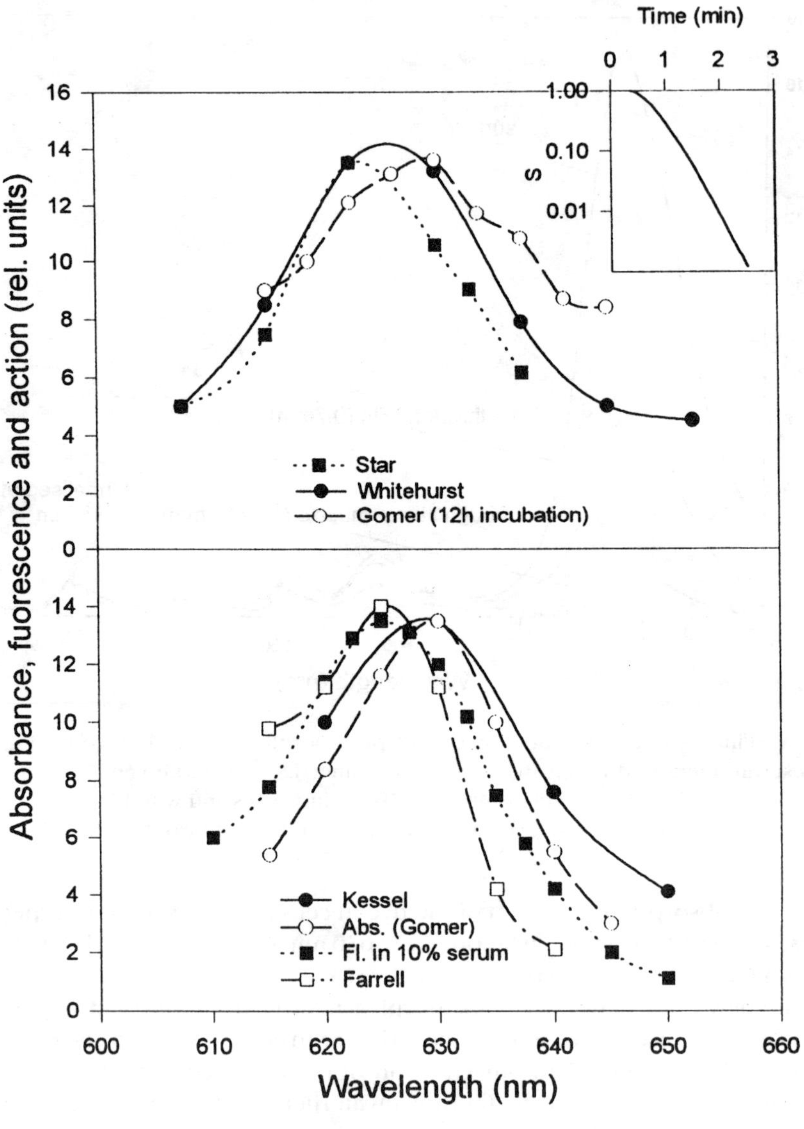

Figure 5 Spectra of Photofrin. The fluorescence excitation spectrum ($I_{em} = 690$ nm) for the drug in 10% human serum is prepared by the authors. The other spectra are calculated using data from Star *et al.* (1990) (*in vivo*, rat ears), Farrell *et al.* (1992) (*in vivo*, rat liver), Gomer *et al.* (1984) (cells in culture), Kessel (1986) (cells in culture), Whitehurst *et al.* (1993). The latter spectrum was calculated as described in the text, using the survival curve from the work of Whitehurst *et al.* (inset, upper right).

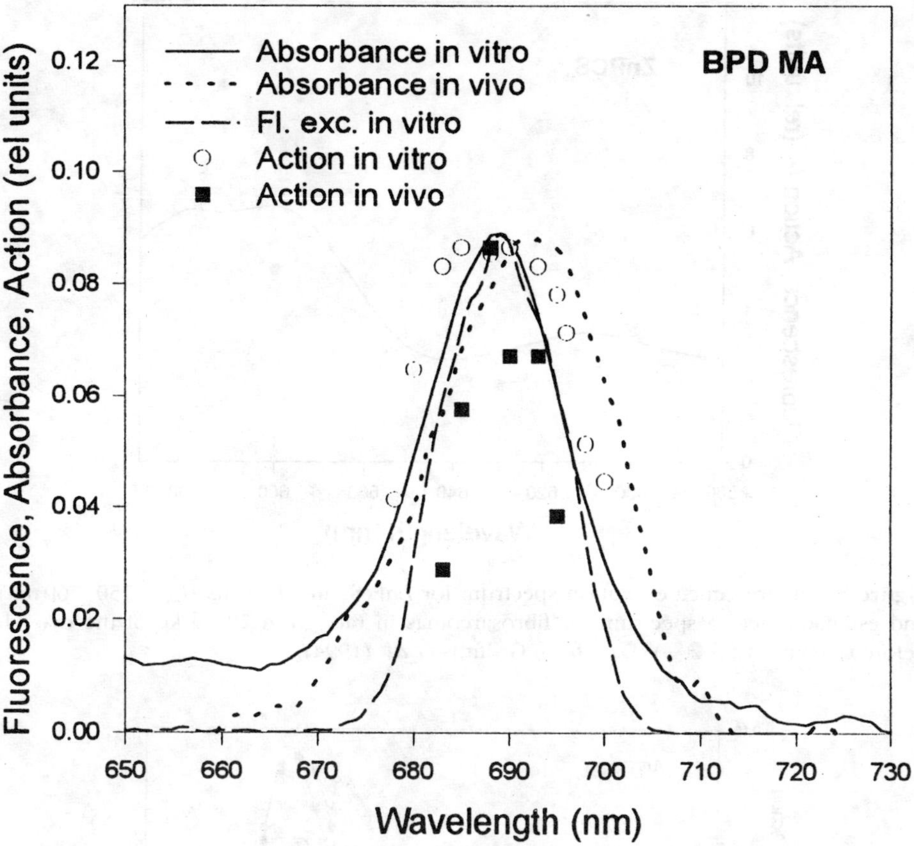

Figure 6 Spectra of the Q band of BPD MA (benzoporphyrin derivative monoacid ring A). ——: absorption spectrum in NHIK 3025 cells *in vitro*; — — —: fluorescence excitation spectrum of the dye in NHIK 3025 cells *in vitro*, $I_{em} = 750$ nm; ·····: absorption spectrum in mouse skin 4 h after i.p. injection of 5 mg/kg measured with fiber optics and a synchronously scanned fluorescence spectrometer. The separation between the excitation fiber and the emission fiber was 5 mm. ○: action spectrum calculated from the data given by Waterfield *et al.* (1994). ■: action spectrum for eradication of mouse tumors (Waterfield *et al.*, 1994). BPD MA was obtained from QLT, Vancouver, Canada.

absorption spectrum of $AlPcS_2$ *in vivo* has a peak at about 685 nm (present work, and Cubeddu *et al.*, 1994) coinciding with the absorption spectrum of the drug in L1210 ascites cells (Cubeddu *et al.*, 1994). However, in an earlier work we found that the fluorescence excitation spectrum, the absorption spectrum and the action spectrum for sensitizing cells of the line NHIK 3025 (human carcinoma cell) all showed a peak at 670 nm (Fig. 8). The reason for this discrepancy is not known. The lipophilic unsulphonated phthalocyanine (ZnPc) delivered to cells in liposomes was investigated in the present work, using the same cell line

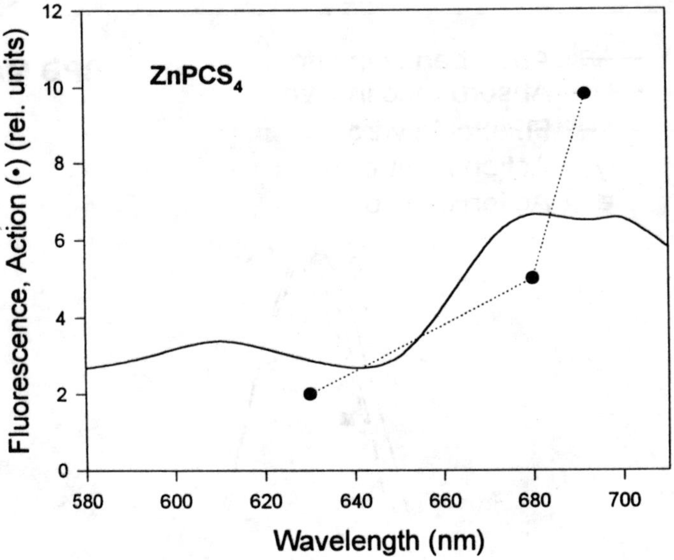

Figure 7 Fluorescence excitation spectrum for $ZnPcS_4$ in 3T3 cells ($I_{em} = 750–760$ nm) and estimated action spectrum for fibrosarcomas in rats given 20 mg/kg of the dye 3 h before irradiation (···●···). Data from Griffiths *et al*. (1994).

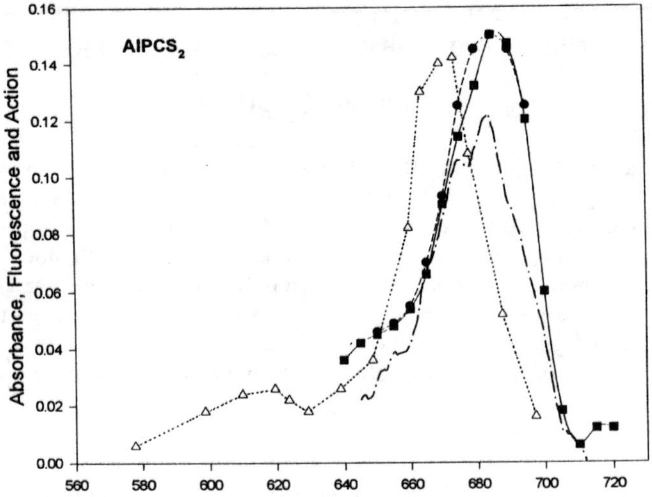

Figure 8 *In vivo* and *in vitro* spectra for $AlPcS_2$. —■— and —●—: Absorption spectra *in vivo* (L1210 tumors in mice) and in cells *in vitro*, respectively (Cubeddu *et al*., 1994). -·-·-·-: *in vivo* absorption spectrum in nude mice measured 2 h after i.p. injection of the dye, 5 mg/kg. The measurements were carried out as described under Fig. 6. ···Δ··· action spectrum for cell photoinactivation (NHIK 3025 cells) (Moan *et al*., 1992).

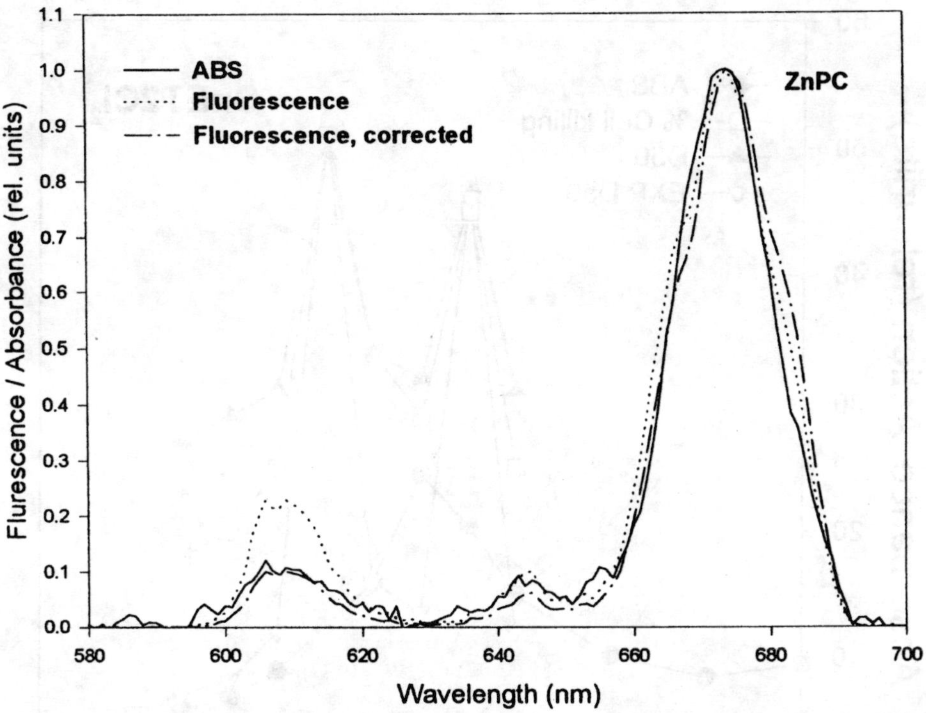

Figure 9 Absorption (—) and fluorescence excitation spectrum (I_{em} = 710 nm, slit 5 nm) of ZnPc in NHIK 3025 cells incubated for 18 h with the drug (5 mg/ml) in medium containing 10% serum. The correction of the fluorescence excitation spectrum is described in the text. Liposome-bound ZnPc was obtained from Ciba-Geigy, Basel, Switzerland.

as mentioned above (NHIK 3025, Fig. 9). The corrected fluorescence excitation spectrum had a shape close to that of the absorption spectrum of the drug in cells, indicating that the drug was present mainly as monomers in the cells. The peak of these spectra was located at 673 nm, i.e. close to that of $AlPcS_2$. Figure 9 demonstrates the necessity to correct excitation spectra in the wavelength region above 600 nm whenever instruments applying rhodamine as quantum counters are used.

Spectra for tin etiopurpurin ($SnET2Cl_2$) are shown as the last example, Fig. 10 (Morgan *et al.*, 1987). For this drug the absorption is very different from the action spectrum for cell photoinactivation. This figure demonstrates that the shape of action spectrum is dependent on the way it is presented, either as per cent of the cells inactivated by a constant exposure, or, more correctly, according to the basic definition of the action spectrum, Eq. (1).

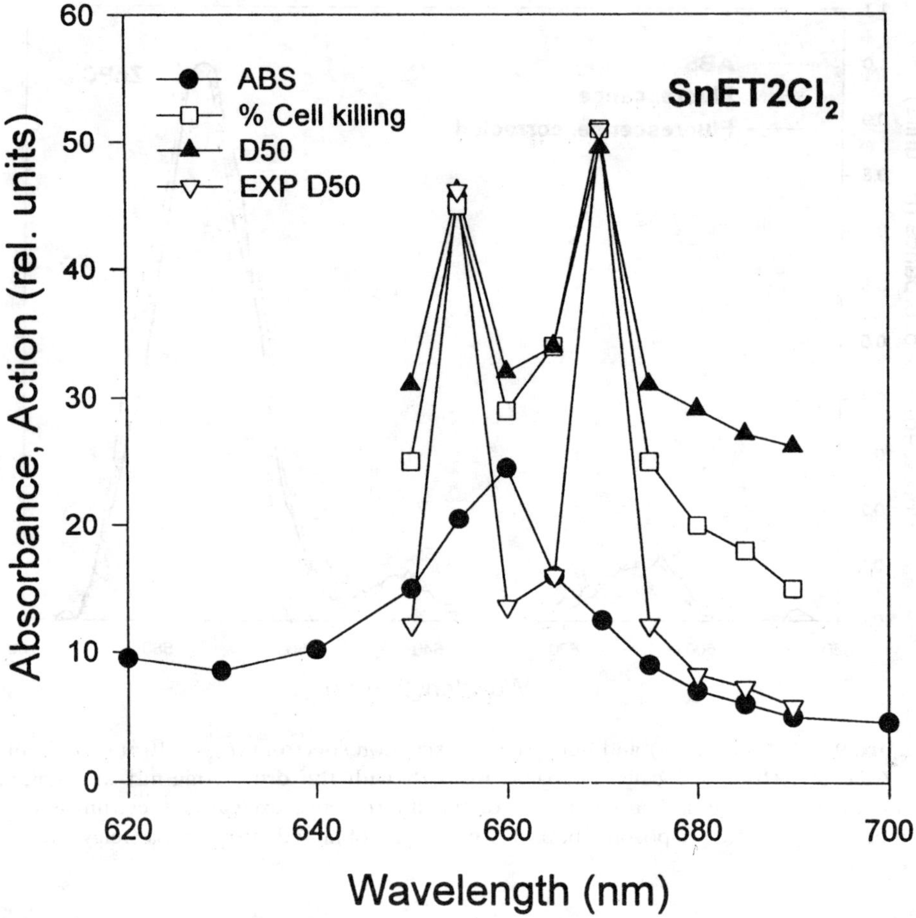

Figure 10 Spectra for $SnET2Cl_2$ calculated using the data of Morgan *et al.* (1987). —●—: absorption spectrum; —□—: % inactivation at a constant dose; —∇—: action spectrum assuming an exponential survival curve; —▲—: action spectrum assuming a shouldered survival curve (see inset in Fig. 5).

REFERENCES

Cubeddu, R., Canti, G., Pifferi, A., Taroni, P., and Valentini, G. (1994): *In vivo* and *in vitro* absorption spectrum of disulphonated aluminum phthalocyanine in tumor-bearing mice. Proceedings of the 5th Int. Photodynamic Association Biennal Meeting, *SPIE* **2371**, pp. 172–176.

Farrell, T. J., Olivo, M. C., Patterson, M. S., Wrona, H., and Wilson, B. C. (1992): Investigation of the dependence of tissue necrosis on irradiation wavelength and time post injection using a photodynamic threshold dose model. In: Photodynamic Therapy and

Biomedical Lasers. Spinelli, P., Dal Fante, M., and Marchesini, R., eds. Elsevier Science Publishers B.V. Amsterdam, pp. 830–834.

Gomer, C. J., Doiron, D. R., Rucker, N., Razum, N. J., and Fountain, S. W. (1984): Action spectrum (620–640 nm) for hematoporphyrin derivative induced cell killing. *Photochemistry and Photobiology* **39**, 365–368.

Griffiths, J., Cruse-Sawyer, J., Wood, S. R., Schofield, J., Brown, S. B., and Dixon, B. (1994): On the photodynamic therapy action spectrum of zinc phthalocyanine tetrasulphonic acid *in vivo*. *Journal of Photochemistry and Photobiology, B – Biology* **24**, 195–199.

Kessel, D. (1986): Localization and photosensitization of murine tumors *in vivo* and *in vitro* by a chlorin-porphyrin ester. *Cancer Research* **46**, 2248–2251.

Ma, L., Moan, J., and Berg, K. (1994): Evaluation of a new photosensitizer, meso-tetrahydroxyphenyl-chlorin, for use in photodynamic therapy: a comparison of its photobiological properties with those of two other photosensitizers. *International Journal of Cancer* **57**, 883–888.

Moan, J. (1984): The photochemical yield of singlet oxygen from porphyrins in different states of aggregation. *Photochemistry and Photobiology* **39**, 445–449 (Abstract).

Moan, J., Dahlback, A., Larsen, S., Henriksen, T., and Stamnes, K. (1989): Ozone depletion and its consequences for the fluence of carcinogenic sunlight. *Cancer Research* **49**, 4247–4250.

Moan, J., Berg, K., Bommer, J. C., and Western, A. (1992): Action spectra of phthalocyanines with respect to photosensitization of cells. *Photochemistry and Photobiology* **56**, 171–175.

Moan, J. and Sommer, S. (1984): Action spectra for hematoporphyrin derivative and Photofrin II with respect to sensitization of human cells *in vitro* to photoinactivation. *Photochemistry and Photobiology* **40**, 631–634.

Morgan, A. R., Garbo, G. M., Keck, R. W., and Selman, S. H. (1987): Tin(IV) Etiopurpurin dichloride: An alternative to DHE? In: *SPIE* Vol. 847. New Directions in Photodynamic Therapy. Bellingham, pp. 172–178.

Star, W., Versteeg, J., van Putten, W., and Marijnissen, H. (1990): Wavelength dependence of hematoporphyrin derivative photodynamic treatment effects on rat ears. *Photochemistry and Photobiology* **52**, 547–554.

Waterfield, E. M., Renke, M. E., Smits, C. B., Gervais, M. D., Bower, R. D., Stonefield, M. S., and Levy, J. G. (1994): Wavelength-dependent effects of benzoporphyrin derivative monoacid ring A *in vivo* and *in vitro*. *Photochemistry and Photobiology* **60**, 383–387.

Western, A. and Moan, J. (1988): Action spectra for photoinactivation of cells in the presence of tetra(3-hydroxyphenyl) porphyrin, chlorin e_6 and aluminum phthalocyanine tetrasulphonate. In: Light in Biology and Medicine. Douglas, R. H., Moan, J., and Dall'Acqua, F., eds. Plenum Press, New York, pp. 85–89.

Whitehurst, C., Byrne, K., and Moore, J. V. (1993): Development of an alternative light source to lasers for photodynamic therapy: 1. Comparative *in vitro* dose response characteristics. *Lasers in Medical Science* **8**, 259–267.

3.6. A NOVEL TISSUE-INSERTED OPTICAL OXYGEN MICROSENSOR: ON-LINE DETERMINATION OF EFFECTIVE PHOTODYNAMIC THERAPY IN SOLID MELANOTIC MELANOMA TUMORS

JUDITH ZILBERSTEIN, VARDA ROSENBACH-BELKIN,
AVIGDOR SCHERZ and YORAM SALOMON

Successful application of anticancer therapy in general and in photodynamic therapy mediated by type II processes (PDT II) in particular depends strongly on the oxygen content within the tumor before and during treatment. Application of a novel oxygen sensor allowed, for the first time, continuous measurements of temporal variations (in the second time range) of the oxygen partial pressure (p_{O_2}) within a tumor for several hours during PDT. Mouse M2R melanotic melanoma tumors implanted in CD1 nude mice were treated with bacteriochlorophyll-Serine (Bchl-Ser) (a new photodynamic reagent) and subsequently subjected to pulsed illumination ($900 > \lambda > 700$ nm) at a fluence rate of 12 mW/cm^2. Illumination led to total depletion of oxygen with a rate of 0.58 μM $(O_2) \times s^{-1}$ up to a depth of 8–9 mm from the tumor surface. Integration of the new sensor in PDT experiments enables *in vivo* analysis of the basic mechanisms underlying photoinduced cytotoxicity as well as the development of treatment protocols in which drug levels and light fluence will be optimized and light pulses will be synchronized with oxygen recovery rates.

INTRODUCTION

In type II photodynamic therapy (PDT II) (Foote, 1987), a photosensitizer drug, light and oxygen are used to cause photochemically induced cell death. In this modality of cancer treatment, singlet oxygen molecules ($^1O_2$) are generated via energy transfer from sensitizing dye molecules that are administered to the tumor and then excited by visible (VIS) or near infrared (NIR) radiation (Foote, 1987; Dougherty, 1992; Fiedor *et al.*, 1993). It is generally believed that tumor destruction in PDT II is accomplished through *in situ* generation of $^1O_2$ with consequent combustion/destruction of cellular constituents (Keene *et al.*, 1986; Weishaupt *et al.*, 1976). Tumor tissue may often be heterogeneous with respect to O_2 distribution and may thus contain cells at varying levels of oxygenation (Lartigau *et al.*, 1992; Vaupel, 1991). Cells in hypoxic tumor regions are thought to be relatively resistant to radio-, chemo- and type II photodynamic therapies thus limiting anticancer treatment to well oxygenated zones (Henderson and Fingar, 1989; Hirst, 1989; Moulder and Rockwell, 1987). Therefore the knowledge of oxygenation levels in the tumor may be extremely important in selecting the treatment strategy and in predicting treatment efficiency.

The novel technology for oxygen sensing was used to monitor bacteriochlorophyll-serine (Bchl-Ser) based PDT, recently developed in our laboratories.

The new sensitizer was made water soluble by conjugation to serine (Ser) but can also be conjugated to peptides and proteins, notably antibodies for specific cell/tissue targeting purposes (Fiedor, 1994; Scherz and Salomon, 1992; Scherz *et al*., 1994). When compared to Photofrin II the clinically used hematoporphyrin derivative (HpD), Bchl-based PDT agents, have superior spectral properties: $\lambda_{max} = 770–780$ nm and higher extinction coefficient (10^5 mole^{-1} cm^{-1}), eliminating the need for strong laser sensitization, much higher ($> \times 200$) phototoxicity, low dark toxicity and much faster clearance rates (< 24 h) (Rosenbach-Belkin *et al*., 1996). The photodynamic activity of Bchl-Ser in treatment of M2R mouse melanotic melanoma *in vivo* has been previously shown by us (Fiedor, 1994; Scherz and Salomon, 1992; Scherz *et al*., 1994; Rosenbach-Belkin *et al*., 1996; Zilberstein *et al*., 1994a, 1995).

Since type II PDT involves light induced utilization of molecular oxygen, the progress of PDT can be monitored by following light dependent oxygen consumption in the photosensitizer-treated-tumor. Electrochemical measurements of oxygen depletion in course of *in vitro* PDT with other sensitizers, have been previously reported (Gottfried *et al*., 1988; Kimel *et al*., 1989; Murasecco *et al*., 1985). In these studies dissolved oxygen levels were monitored during light irradiation of solutions containing photosensitizers and suitable acceptor compounds. Follow-up of the oxygen levels, using a transcutaneous oxygen electrode, based on polarographic measurements, during *in vivo* PDT was also demonstrated (Tromberg *et al*., 1990), and oxygen microelectrodes were used to measure oxygen partial pressure (p_{O_2}) before and after HpD based PDT (Reed *et al*., 1989). Nonetheless, the precision and time resolution of this and similar measurements that attempted to monitor the kinetics of oxygen consumption during PDT were relatively low due to inherited drawbacks of the polarographic assays; first, oxygen consumption by the electrode and the electrical current involved in this detection technique led to low accuracy of the measurements especially at low oxygen tensions, where the ratio of signal to noise is low, resulting in uncertainty of the results (Stone *et al*., 1993). Second, the stability of the electrode could be affected by cathode contamination. Moreover the use of transcutaneous electrodes requires heating of the skin surface to 44°C in order to accelerate oxygen diffusion, imposing an undesirable impact of the probe itself. The nature of the electrode also limits its spatial resolution and its applications are limited to subcutaneous tumors (Tromberg *et al*., 1990). Other methods for measuring tissue oxygen and related parameters consist of more complex procedures that usually involve analyses of tissue biopsies. Oxygen level determinations in these cases are based on several different principles that include: nitroimidazole binding assays, hemoglobin saturation assays, magnetic resonance spectroscopy, electron spin resonance spectroscopy, phosphorescence imaging, and an assay for tumor interstitial pressure (Stone *et al*., 1993). The major shortcoming of these methods is that none provides instantaneous on-line information about the influence of treatment on tumor oxygenation with a high spatial resolution.

The new technique is using an optical fiber (180 μm diameter) that was designed for monitoring oxygen partial pressure (p_{O_2}) in blood (Bromberg *et al.*, 1996; Zilberstein, 1994b). This Blood Gas Monitor (BGM) correlates the oxygen pressure with the quenched fluorescence of pyrene immobilized on a solid support. The sensor consists of two light guides; one is used to excite the pyrene molecules and the other to collect their fluorescence. Since the latter is very sensitive to the presence of oxygen molecules (Wolfbeis, 1984), the level of pyrene fluorescence monitors the presence of oxygen molecules down to very low local concentrations. Furthermore, temporal changes in p_{O_2} are immediately sensed with a high time resolution. The new sensor does not consume oxygen and is protected from poisoning (Bromberg *et al.*, 1995). Measurements of the blood oxygen level with the BGM technology were proven accurate and reliable. In 82 determinations of p_{O_2} conducted *in vitro* in fresh heparinized human blood samples the accuracy of the obtained values was ± 1.2 mmHg as compared to two commercial ABL 330 Radiometer blood gas analyzing instruments currently in clinical use with an intersensor precision of 2.6–2.9 mmHg (Bromberg *et al.*, 1996).

These properties made the pyrene coated optical sensor most promising for measuring *in vivo* p_{O_2} variations in tumors during PDT (Zilberstein *et al.*, 1996). Here, the novel technique is used to monitor the oxygen levels in implanted M2R melanoma tumors during Bchl-Ser based PDT.

MATERIALS AND METHODS

Photosensitizer

Bchl-Ser was prepared from the natural pigment Bchl a by chemical modification of its macrocycle at the C-17 propionic residue and conjugation to a serine molecule (Fiedor, 1994; Scherz *et al.*, 1992, 1994; Rosenbach-Belkin *et al.*, 1996). The Bchl-Ser was kept dry under argon in the dark at $-20°C$ until used.

Animals

Photodynamic treatments and oxygen measurements were performed on CD1 male (30–35 g) nude mice.

Tumor Model

M2R cells were maintained as monolayer as previously described (Gerst, 1986). For tumor implantation the cells were scraped and suspended in normal saline 1×10^6 cells/0.025 ml and subcutaneously injected to the back of the mice as previously described (DeJordy *et al.*, 1992). In approximately 2–3 weeks, the melanotic tumors appear as dark and solid confined structures with an average diameter of 8–12 mm.

Anesthesia

Mice were anaesthetized by i.p. injection of 5 mg/kg Ketamine (Rhone Merieux, Lyon, France) +1 mg/kg Xylazine, (Bayer, Leverkusen, Germany) (40 µl) which has a minimal effect on the blood flow and consequently the oxygen levels within the treated tissue are less affected. This dose is sufficient to keep the animal under anesthesia for about 30–40 min. Additional injections of 10–20 µl were performed as needed allowing several hours of anesthesia, up to 8 h.

Photodynamic Treatment

Administration of drug: Mice were treated with 200 µg of Bchl-Ser in 0.05 ml (alcohol 95% : saline 1 : 1) injected under anesthesia into the tumor. The injection was performed by inserting a Gauge #28 × 1/2 needle through the skin and drug delivery into the tumor sufficiently close to the oxygen measurement site.

Light irradiation: A home-built light source equipped with 100 W white halogen lamp, a RG-700 cut-off filter and a 10 cm water layer provided irradiation at $900\,\text{nm} > \lambda > 700\,\text{nm}$ with an average power 12 mW/cm^2. No heating effects were observed at the site of illumination. The diameter of the irradiation spot was 1.2 cm covering the examined area within the tumor.

Oxygen Microsensor

The BGM is an on-line, real-time system that provides continuous monitoring of blood gases (developed by OST, Israel). The oxygen sensor technology is based on fluorescence measurements of a pyrene derivative which is quenched in a concentration dependent manner by molecular oxygen (Stern-Volmer relation, Wolfbeis *et al.*, 1984). This instrument provides linear read-out of fluorescence in the range of 0–150 mm Hg p_{O_2} (0–21% atmospheric O_2). The pyrene molecules are attached to the porous tip at the distal end of the fused silica fiber (180 µm diameter) and the response time of the oxygen sensor is diffusion limited (Zilberstein *et al.*, 1994b; Bromberg *et al.*, 1996). The porous glass tip is coated with a thin gold layer to insulate the sensor from interference by external light and covered with anticoagulant membrane to avoid clot formation upon contact with blood.

Oxygen Measurements

(a) *Calibration*: Calibration in the range of 28–57 mm Hg is done before each measurement, using distilled water equilibrated at 37°C with 4% and 8% and 100% oxygen mixture with nitrogen. At the end of the measurements, the oxygen sensor is put back in the calibration solution, to ensure read out stability during the examination period.

(b) *In vivo oxygen measurements*: The oxygen sensor was inserted through a hypodermic needle (gauge #22) a few millimeters into the studied tissue of the anaesthetized mouse. Oxygen levels were recorded under dark conditions until a stable p_{O_2} baseline was established. The tumor was then illuminated for a few minutes, to ensure that the oxygen level readout is not affected by light. At this stage the Bchl-Ser was injected directly into the tumor and allowed to distribute in the tissue. The site of injection was selected in proximity to the site of measurement. The tumor was then irradiated for different time intervals as described. The p_{O_2} levels were continuously displayed on the computer screen during the period of examination as mmHg p_{O_2} versus time.

RESULTS

Determination of p_{O_2} During PDT

In the experiment depicted in Fig. 1, oxygen levels in a melanotic M2R tumor were monitored under similar PDT conditions used for tumor eradication as previously described (Zilberstein *et al.*, 1995, 1994a) except that the light fluence was 12 mW/cm^2 instead of 100 mW/cm^2.

Following anesthesia of the mouse the oxygen sensor was inserted into the tumor and p_{O_2} levels were recorded until a stable baseline reading around 20 mm Hg was established. The tumor was then illuminated several times with the sensitizing light source to ensure that the measuring system is light tight. For this purpose the light was turned on and off several times inducing no detectable changes in tumor p_{O_2}.

Bchl-Ser was then injected directly into the tumor and p_{O_2} was recorded in the dark for about 2 h allowing free distribution of the pigment in the tumor. Administration of the pigment did not affect baseline p_{O_2} values. At this time the tumor was illuminated by an alternating light/dark schedule (Fig. 1). Approximately every 10 min (Fig. 1 at arrow) the tumor was illuminated inducing a fast decline in the p_{O_2}. When the p_{O_2} approached zero values the light was turned off and the system was allowed to reoxygenate. This sequence of light/dark cycles was repeated over a long period of time (5 h) demonstrating the dynamic response of the sensor. A segment of the experiment between 130 and 180 min is shown (Fig. 1).

Examination of the p_{O_2} profile of this experiment revealed that the rate of light dependent oxygen depletion was always faster than the rate of reoxygenation observed when the light was switched off. A single exponential fit of a typical depletion/reoxygenation profile of one light/dark cycle in such a PDT experiment is shown in Fig. 2. We calculated the rate of change in p_{O_2} and the half-life time ($t_{1/2}$) of the depletion and reoxygenation processes. While $t_{1/2}$ of oxygen depletion in the light/dark cycle was around 24 s the $t_{1/2}$ of the oxygen recovery phase was much longer, around 60 s. The oxygen depletion and reoxygenation rates were 0.58 and 0.15 µM (O_2) $\times$ s^{-1} respectively.

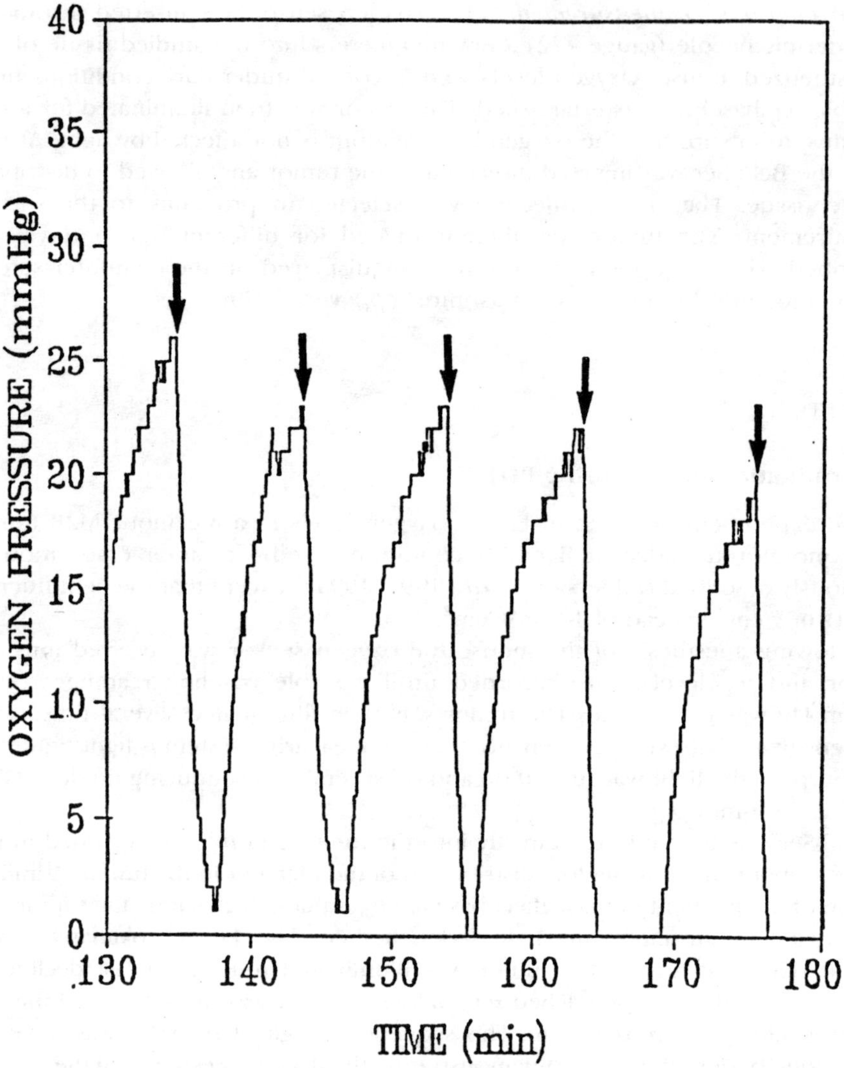

Figure 1 Measurements of p_{O_2} in melanoma tumor during PDT: The sensor was inserted into the tumor of the anesthetized mouse and baseline level p_{O_2} was recorded for several hrs. After testing the light tightness of the sensor by turning the light on and off Bchl-Ser was injected into the tumor and about 2 h later the light was turned "on" (arrow) and "off" when the p_{O_2} values approached zero. This light/dark cycle was repeated several times approximately every 10 min.

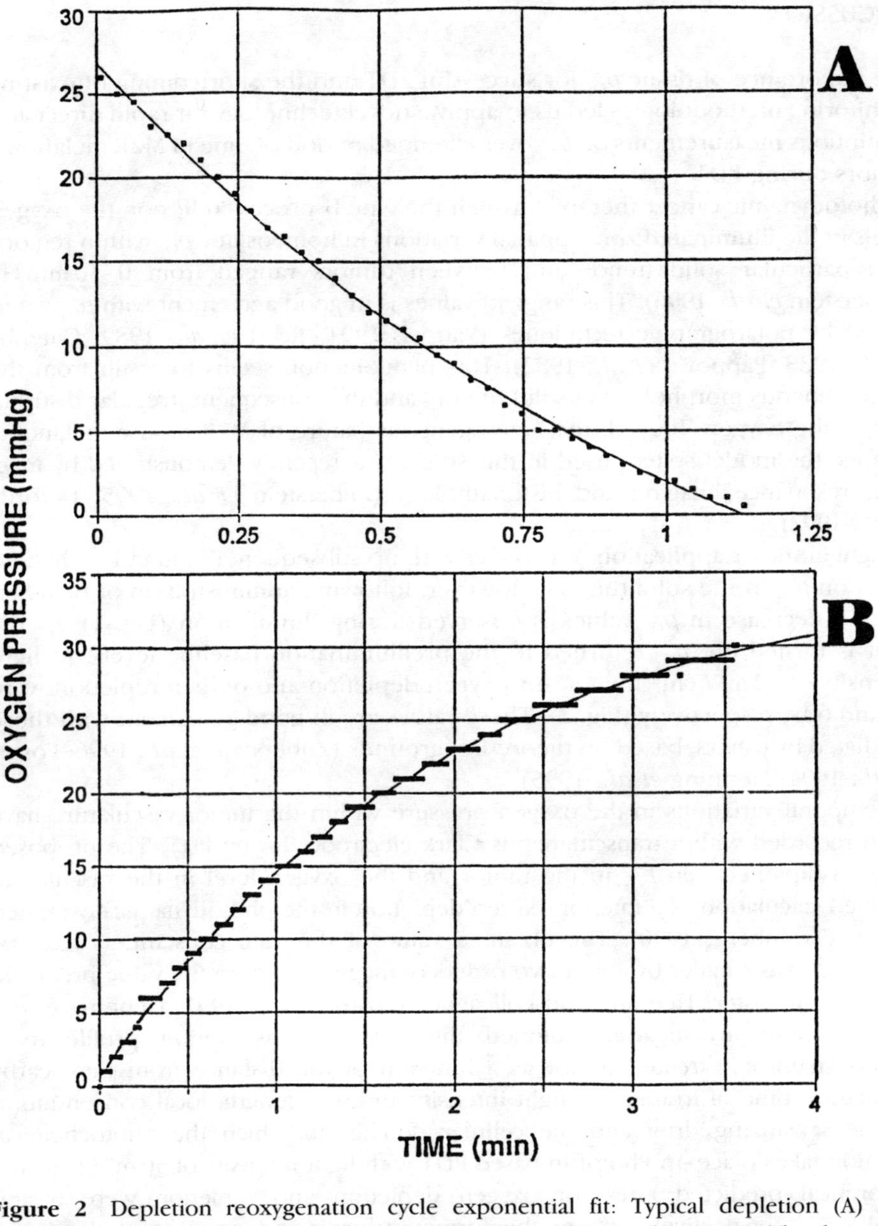

Figure 2 Depletion reoxygenation cycle exponential fit: Typical depletion (A) and reoxygenation (B) profiles of a light/dark cycle that is illustrated in Fig. 1. The data were fitted to a single exponential function (adj. $r^2 = 0.993$).

DISCUSSION

The importance of tissue p_{O_2} for successful PDT and the shortcoming of existing monitoring methodologies led us to apply a novel technology for rapid direct and continuous measurements of p_{O_2} over extended period of time in M2R melanoma tumors during PDT.

Photodynamic cancer therapy through the type II process relies on the oxygen levels in the illuminated zone. Spatial variations in homeostatic p_{O_2} within regions of a particular solid tumor and between tumors ranged from 0–30 mm Hg (Zilberstein *et al.*, 1996). This range of values is in good agreement with p_{O_2} determined by polarographic techniques (Vaupel, 1991; Reed *et al.*, 1989; Gatenby *et al.*, 1988; Pappov'a *et al.*, 1982). This phenomenon seems to result from the heterogeneous morphology of solid tumors and the consequent irregular distribution of the oxygen. Indeed, the heterogeneous nature of M2R mouse melanoma tumors, the model system used in this study, was recently demonstrated by magnetic resonance imaging and histopathology (Zilberstein *et al.*, 1995; DeJordy *et al.*, 1992).

Light alone or application of Bchl-Ser with no subsequent illumination, had no effect on p_{O_2} in the solid tumors. However, following administration of Bchl-Ser, a rapid decrease in p_{O_2} values is observed during illumination (Fig. 1). As the light is turned off, p_{O_2} returned to the preillumination baseline levels. At light intensity of 12 mW/cm^2 the $t_{1/2}$ for oxygen depletion and oxygen repletion were 24 and 60 s, respectively (Fig. 2). These values are in good agreement with those predicted by others, based on theoretical grounds (Zilberstein *et al.*, 1996; Foster *et al.*, 1991; Henning *et al.*, 1995).

Temporal variations in the oxygen pressure within the tumor vasculature have been recorded with a transcutaneous Clark electrode during PDT. The proposed relationships between p_{O_2} in the tumor and the oxygen level in the vasculature enabled calculation of a rate for oxygen depletion in the photodynamically treated tumor (Tromberg, 1990). The obtained value of this rate constant, $\sim 10^{-3}\,\mu M\ O_2 \times s^{-1}$, was smaller by about two orders of magnitude from the value predicted recently by Foster, Henning and colleagues (Foster *et al.*, 1991; Henning *et al.*, 1995). These investigators outlined the oxygen consumption profile in a photodynamically treated tumor as a function of the distance from the nearby capillaries, time of irradiation, light intensity and wavelength, local concentration of the sensitizing drug and the cellular domain in which the photochemical reaction takes place. In Photofrin based PDT with light intensity of 50 mW/cm^2, the theoretical predicted rates for oxygen depletion and repletion were 6 and $1\,\mu M \times s^{-1}$, respectively, where the former value is independent of the initial oxygen concentration in the treated tumor. According to Henning and his colleagues this implies that irradiation for 30 s should be followed by a dark period of 60 s to obtain a maximal PDT effect (Henning *et al.*, 1995). These predictions were basically confirmed by our measurments with the new oxygen sensor.

Optimal type II PDT according to our results would be delivered by pulsed illumination where the light period is adjusted to the radiation fluence and local sensitizer concentration. Under light intensity of 50 mW/cm^2 the rate of oxygen depletion is in the order of μM × s^{-1} provided that the local concentration of the sensitizer is above the saturation level. Oxygen repletion is completed with a half-life time of 60 s provided that the tumor vasculature is not damaged. Taken together, the optimum light regime for PDT most probably consists of alternate 30 s/60 s on/off pulses as recently predicted by Henning *et al.* (1995) and measured in the present study.

The use of the optical microsensor during *in vivo* PDT allows on-line measurement of the influence of PDT on tissue oxygen levels. These changes can reflect on the blood flow, clearance of the sensitizer, mechanism of cytotoxicity and effective depth of treatment. Knowledge of these parameters may be helpful in elucidating the fine details of PDT *in vivo*, in estimating the expected effectiveness of PDT in the region of interest and in developing PDT drugs or treatment protocols.

We wish to add that in addition to the above we also found good agreement between values of resting homeostatic p_{O_2} in normal healthy mouse tissues measured by the new technology (Zilberstein *et al.*, 1996) and those reported by others in various animal models using different methodologies (Gatenby *et al.*, 1988; Pappov'a *et al.*, 1982; Gustafsson *et al.*, 1994; Harrison, *et al.*, 1990; Dewhirst *et al.*, 1992; Kahandelwal *et al.*, 1993; Brezis *et al.*, 1994a, b).

ACKNOWLEDGEMENTS

Y.S. is the incumbent of the Charles and Tillie Lubin Chair of Biochemical Endocrinology; J.Z., in partial fulfillment of the Ph.D. thesis the Feinberg Graduate School of the Weizmann Institute of Science. We wish to thank OST Ltd. Haifa Israel for providing the oxygen sensor instrument. This study was supported in part by grants from: The Lynne and William Frankel Fund for the Diagnosis and Treatment of Ovarian and Breast Cancer, The Jaffe Family Foundation and Yeda Research and Development Co. Ltd. Israel and the Ministry of Science and Technology, Israel, the Commission of the European Communities. The authors are in debt to S. Zuckerman for her generous support of this research. The authors wish to thank R. Benjamin and M. Kopelowitz for their excellent secretarial assitance.

REFERENCES

Brezis, M., Agmon, Y., and Epstein, F. H. (1994a): Determination of internal oxygenation I. Effect of diuretics. *Am. J. Physiol.* **267**, F1059–F1062.

Brezis, M., Heyman, S. N., and Epstein, F. H. (1994b): Determination of internal oxygenation II. Hemodynamic effect. *Am. J. Physiol.* **267**, F1063–F1068.

Bromberg, A., Zilberstein, J., Riesemberg, S., Benor, I. E., Silberstein, E., Zimnavoda, J., Frishman, G., and Krietzman, A. (1996): Optical fiber sensors for blood gases and pH, based on porous glass tips. *Sensor and Actuators* **B31**, 181–191.

DeJordy, J. O., Bendel, P., Horowitz, A., Salomon, Y., and Degani, H. (1992): Correlation of MR Imaging and histologic findings in mouse melanoma. *J. Magn. Reson. Imag.* **2**, 695–700.

Dewhirst, M. W., Ong, E. T., Klitzman, B., Secomb, T. W., Vinuya, R. Z., Dodge, R., Brizel, D., and Gross, J. F. (1992): Perivascular oxygen tensions in a transplantable mammary tumor growing in a dorsal flap window chamber. *Radiat. Res.* **130**, 171–182.

Dougherty, T. J. (1992): Photochemistry in the treatment of cancer. *Advances in Photochem.* **17**, 275–311.

Fiedor, L., Gorman, A. A., Hamblett, I., Rosenbach-Belkin, V., Salomon, Y., Scherz, A., and Tregub, I. (1993): A pulsed laser and pulse radiolysis study of amphiphilic chlorophyll derivatives with PDT activity toward malignant melanoma. *Photochem. Photobiol.* **58**, 506–511.

Fiedor, L. (1994): Modified chlorophylls as models for primary photosynthesis and photosensitizers for photodynamic therapy of cancer. Ph.D. Thesis, The Weizmann Institute of Science, Rehovot, Israel.

Foolte, C. S. (1987): Light activated pesticides. *American Chem. Soc. Symposium Ser.* **1**, 22–38.

Foster, T., Murant, R., Bryant, R., Knox, R., Gibson, S., and Hilf, R. (1991): Oxygen consumption and diffusion effects in photodynamic therapy. *Radiat. Res.* **126**, 296–303.

Gatenby, R. A., Kessler, H. B., Rosenblum, J. S., Coia, L. R., Moldofsky, P. J., Hartz, W. H., and Broder J. G. (1988): Oxygen distribution in squamous cell carcinoma metastases and its relationship to outcome of radiation therapy. *Int. J. Radiate. Oncol. Biol. Phys.* **14**, 831–838.

Gerst, J. E., Sole, J., Mather, J. P., and Salomon, Y. (1986): Regulation of adenylate cyclase by β-melanotropin in M2R melanoma cell line. *Mol. Cell. Endocrinol.* **46**, 137–147.

Gottfried, V., Peled, D., Winkelman, J. W., and Kimel, S. (1988): Photosensitizers in organized media: singlet oxygen production and spectral properties. *Photochem. Photobiol.* **48**, 157–163.

Gustafsson, U., Sjoberg, F., Lewis, D. H., and Thorborg, P. (1994): Effect of hypoxic hypoxia and ritanserin on capillary flow and oxygenation in rabbit skeletal muscle. *Acta Physiol. Scand.* **150**, 39–45.

Harrison, D. K., Kessler, M., and Knauf, S. (1990): Regulation of capillary blood flow and oxygen supply in skeletal muscle in dogs during hypoxia. *J. Physiol.* **420**, 431–446.

Henderson, B. W. and Fingar, V. H. (1989): Oxygen limitation of direct tumor cell kill during photodynamic treatment of murine tumor model. *Photochem. Photobiol.* **49**, 299–304.

Henning, J., Fournier, R., and Hampton, A. (1995): A transient mathematical model of oxygen depletion during photodynamic therapy. *Radiat. Res.* **1442**, 221–226.

Hirst, D. G. (1989): Tumor hypoxia implication for therapy. *Int. J. Radiat. Biol.* **56**, 207–213.

Kahandelwal, S. R., Randad, R. S., Lin, P. S., Meng, H. P., Pittman, R. N., Kontos, H. A., Choi, S. C., Abraham, D. J., and Scmidt-Ullrich, R. (1993): Enhanced oxygenation *in vivo* by allosteric inhibitors of hemoglobin saturation. *Am. J. Physiol.* **265**, H1450–H1453.

Keene, J. P., Kessel, D., Land, E. J., Redmond, R. W., and Truscott, T. G. (1986): Direct detection of singlet oxygen sensitized by hematoporphyrin and related compounds. *Photochem. Photobiol.* **43**, 1037–1041.

Kimel, S., Tromberg, B. G., Roberts, W. G., and Berns, M. W. (1989): Singlet oxygen generation of porphyrins, chlorins, and phthalocyanines. *Photochem. Photobiol.* **50**, 175–183.

Lartigau, E., Vitu, L., Haie-Meder, C., Cosset, M. F., Delapierre, M., Gerbaulet, A., Eschwege, F., and Guiichard, M. (1992): Feasibility of measuring oxygen tension in uterine cervix carcinoma. *Eur. J. Cancer* **28**, 1354–1357.

Moulder, J. P. and Rockwell, S. (1987): Tumor hypoxia: Its impact on cancer therapy. *Cancer Metastasis Rev.* **5**, 313–341.

Murasecco, P., Oliveros, E., Braun, A. M., and Monnier, P. (1985): Quantum yield measurements of hematoporphyrin derivative sensitized singlet oxygen production. *Photochem. Photobiol.* **9**, 193–201.

Pappov'a, N., Siracka, E., Vacek, A., and Durkovsky, J. (1982): Oxygen tension and prediction of the radiation response. Polarographic study in human breast cancer. *Neoplasm.* **29**, 669–674.

Reed, M. W. R., Mullins, A. P., Anderson, G. L., Miller, F. N., and Wieman, T. J. (1989): The effect of photodynamic therapy on tumor oxygenation. *Surgery* **106**, 94–99.

Rosenbach-Belkin, V., Chen, L., Fiedor, L., Tregub, I., Pavlotsky, F., Brumfeld, V., Salomon, Y., and Scherz, A. (1996): Serine conjugates of chlorophyll and bacteriochlorophyll: Photocytotoxicity *in vitro* and tissue distribution in mice bearing melanoma tumors. *Photochem. Photobiol.* **64**, 174–181.

Scherz, A., Feodor, L., and Salomon, Y. (1992): Chlorophyll and bacteriochlorophyll derivatives, their preparation and pharmacological compositions comprising them. Israel Patent Application #102645.

Scherz, A., Salomon, Y., and Fiedor, L. (1994): Chlorophyll and bacteriochlorophyll derivatives, preparation and pharmaceutical compositions comprising them as photosensitizers for photodynamic therapy. Yeda Research and Development Co., Ltd., (Weizmann Institute of Science) Eur. Pat. Appl. EP 584,552 (Cl. A61K47/48), 02 Mar 1994, Chem. Abs. **120**, 386.

Stone, H. B., Brown, J. M., Philips, L. T., and Sutherlands, R. M. (1993): Oxygen in human tumor: Correlation between methods of measurements and response to therapy. *Radiat. Res.* **136**, 422–434.

Tromberg, B. J., Orenstein, A., Kimel, S., Barker, S. J., Hayatt, J., Nelson, J. S., and Berns, M. W. (1990): *In vivo* tumor oxygen tension measurements for the evaluation of the efficiency of photodynamic therapy. *Photochem. Photobiol.* **52**, 375–385.

Vaupel, P., Schlenger, K., Knoop, C., and Hockel, M. (1991): Oxygenation of human tumors: Evaluation of tissue distribution in breast cancer by computerized O_2 tension measurements. *Cancer Res.* **51**, 3316–3322.

Weishaupt, K. R., Gomer, C. J., and Dougherty, T. J. (1976): Identification of singlet oxygen as the cytotoxic agent in photoinactivation of a murine tumor. *Cancer Res.* **36**, 2326–2329.

Wolfbeis, O. S., Offenbacher, H., and Marsoner, H. (1984): A fast responding fluorescence sensor for oxygen. *Mikrochim. Acta [Wien]* **I**, 153–158.

Zilberstein, J., Scherz, A., Bromberg, A., Bendel, P., Neeman, M., and Salomon, Y. (1994a): Chlorophyll based PDT of melanoma: follow up by MRI and by tissue inserted oxygen sensor. In abstract book of the conference: The Tumor Microenvironment: Its Characterization, Modification and Clinical Implication Faculty of Medicine, University of Granada, Granada, Spain.

Zilberstein, J., Bromberg, A., and Berkovic, G. (1994b): Fluorescence study of pyrene chemically bound to controlled-pore glass. *J. Photochem. Photobiol. A: Chemistry* **77**, 69–81.

Zilberstein, J., Scherz, A., Bromberg, A., Bendel, P., Neeman, M., and Salomon, Y. (1995): Mechanisms involved in chlorophyll based photoinduced cell damage: photodynamic therapy of melanoma. In: Proceedings of the Society of Magnetic Resonance Nice, France. **3**, 1681–1681.

Zilberstein, J., Bromberg, A., Franz, A., Rosenbach-Belkin, V., Kritzmann, A., Pfefermann, R., Salomon, Y., and Scherz, A. (1997): Light dependent oxygen consumption in bacteriochlorophyll-serine treated melanoma tumors: an on line determination using a tissue-inserted oxygen microsensor. *Photochem. Photobiol.* **65**, 1012–1019.

3.7. COMPARING *IN VITRO* AND *IN VIVO* PHOTOTOXICITIES

QIAN PENG, JOHAN MOAN and M. KONGSHAUG

Measurement of the effects of light exposure on photosensitizer-containing tissues or cultivated cells can provide information concerning the photophysical, biochemical and biological mechanisms associated with the phototoxicity. However, the exercise of drawing conclusions from data obtained *in vitro* regarding possible events *in vivo* should be made with due care: photochemical events are more complicated *in vivo*, owing to the possible influence from systemic and local factors, such as the pathophysiology of intratumoral vascular and interstitial microenvironments. In particular, both neoplastic and non-neoplastic cells may contribute to the overall photochemical effect on the tumor. Even so, several determinants of phototoxicity are operating both *in vitro* and *in vivo* systems. These determinants include drug structure, light fractionation, dye photodegradation, oxygen, pH, temperature, etc. In this chapter, we summarize data, in a selective manner, as to how these determinants affect phototoxicity. There is not much such information available for 2nd and 3rd generation photosensitizers (drugs with well defined chemical structure/composition, longer wavelengths of light absorption, and often short persistence in tissues). Therefore, we also include some early findings obtained with the 1st generation photosensitizers, such as hematoporphyrin derivative and its related version, Photofrin. In several respects, all these groups of photosensitizers behave in a similar manner, and Photofrin is still the most important photosensitizer in clinical use.

3.7.1. *IN VIVO–IN VITRO* PROTOCOL

In one noteworthy approach, tumors are photochemically treated, followed by immediate killing of the animal and removal of the tumors. Single cell suspensions are then made from the excised tumors by means of enzymatic or mechanical methods, and finally tumor cell survival is measured *in vitro* in terms of total cell yield per g tumor tissue, plating efficiency of recovered cells, cell clonogenicity, etc. (Henderson, 1990; van Bruggen *et al.*, 1992). Provided that indirect effects on the cell survival from tumor vasculature and/or stroma can be neglected at short times after light exposure, such an experiment can give information concerning the direct photochemical effect on the tumor cells. Such direct effects obtained *in vitro* may be compared with the corresponding phototoxicity conferred on the tumor. However, the possibility that some of the sublethally damaged cells might be further damaged or killed by the isolation procedure as such should be noted.

Furthermore, the vascular and/or stromal effects can be studied by comparing the cell survival after a given PDT-dose for different time intervals between light exposure and tissue removal under otherwise similar conditions. However, the interpretation of the results is complicated since other factors will not remain constant. Thus, there will be a time-dependent photochemical effect upon stromal and vascular components, and also the concentration and localization pattern of the drug and possible toxic products in the tumor may vary with time.

Alternatively, the illumination can be performed *in vitro* after the removal of tumor cells from photosensitizer-doped tumors in mice (Henderson *et al.*, 1985). In such a manner, one attempts at examining the tumor cell-localizing ability *in vivo* and the corresponding phototoxicity of the sensitizer under *in vitro* conditions. In contrast to the protocol of light exposure of the tumor *in situ*, exposure of the removed cells allows control of factors such as pH and oxygen concentration, and the limited tissue-penetrating ability of light is of no concern. However, one should be aware that the preparation of a single cell suspension may affect the intracellular photosensitizer content and distribution.

Henderson and Bellnier (1989) have found that in the family of sulfonated aluminum phthalocyanines ($AlPcS_n$) $AlPcS_2$ is more efficient in sensitizing the RIF tumor cells to photoinactivation than $AlPcS_4$. A similar trend was also obtained from experiments *in vitro* using V79 cells (Brasseur *et al.*, 1988; Berg *et al.*, 1989), Colo 26 cells (Chan *et al.*, 1991) and LOX cells (Peng *et al.*, 1996a). Moreover, similar findings were achieved in various tumor models (Boyle *et al.*, 1992; Chatlani *et al.*, 1992; van Leengoed *et al.*, 1993; Peng *et al.*, 1995a), although these were obtained by other protocols *in vivo*.

One should realize that combined application of these two complementary protocols may offer a great possibility of comparing the direct photochemical effects on the same type of neoplastic cells *in vitro* and *in vivo*, although no such information is available so far.

3.7.2. DRUG STRUCTURE–FUNCTION RELATIONSHIPS

Phototoxicity of drugs *in vitro* and *in vivo* may be studied with respect to drug structural parameters, such as polarity (as measured by, for example, octanol/water partition coefficients or HPLC retention times) and variations in structural features (Berg *et al.*, 1990b; Chan *et al.*, 1991; Peng *et al.*, 1996b). Whilst drugs with pronouncedly different structures do not adhere to a simple relationship between their polarity and phototoxicity, simple correlations between these parameters have been noticed for more structurally similar drugs (Kongshaug *et al.*, 1989, 1990). For a given class of drugs, decreasing polarity is often associated with increasing phototoxicity in both *in vitro* and *in vivo* experiments. This holds for linear dialkyl ether derivatives of hematoporphyrin (see Fig. 1; Evensen *et al.*, 1987; Moan *et al.*, 1988; Rimington *et al.*, 1988), sulfonated derivatives of phthalocyanines (Brasseur *et al.*, 1988; Berg *et al.*, 1989; Chan *et al.*, 1991; Peng *et al.*, 1996a; Peng and Moan, 1995a) or tetraphenyl porphines (Berg *et al.*, 1990a; Peng *et al.*, 1994). This is the general trend. However, of two similar purpurins, the more polar one showed the largest phototoxicity both *in vitro* and *in vivo* (Kessel, 1989). Moreover, several diporphyrins and dichlorins showed a poor correlation between their phototoxicity *in vitro* and the corresponding toxicities *in vivo*

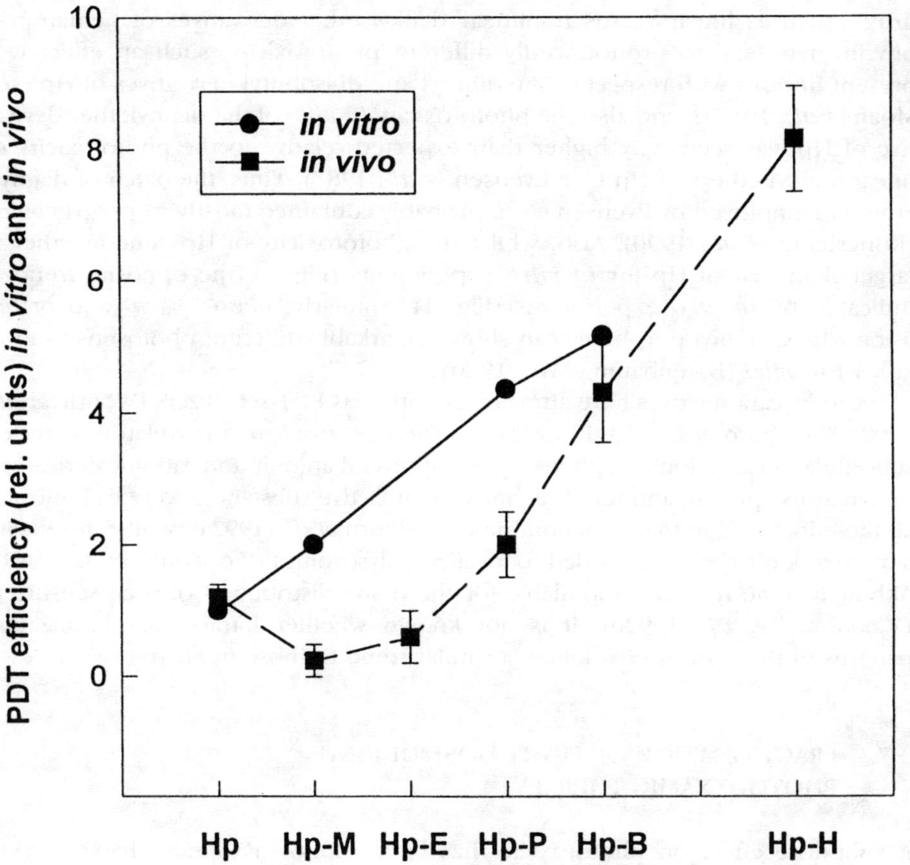

Figure 1 PDT efficiency for linear Hp dialkyl ethers *in vitro* refers to NHIK 3025 cells in culture (adopted from Moan *et al*., 1987a); *in vivo* results refer to C3H mouse mammary carcinoma (adopted from Evensen *et al*., 1987). Hp, hematoporphyrin; Hp-M, Hp dimethyl ether; Hp-E, Hp diethyl ether; Hp-P, Hp dipropyl ether; Hp-B, Hp dibutyl ether; Hp-H, Hp dihexyl ether.

(Kessel *et al*., 1991a). Furthermore, aluminum (or zinc) phthalocyanine monosulfonate is more apolar than the corresponding disulfonate, yet the former shows a lower phototoxicity than the latter both *in vitro* and *in vivo* (Brasseur *et al*., 1988; Berg *et al*., 1989; Peng and Moan, 1995). A similar finding holds for mono- and di-substituted tetraphenylporphines (Kessel *et al*., 1987; Berg *et al*., 1990a; Peng *et al*., 1994). Two sulfonate groups in adjacent positions equip the photosensitizer with a high degree of amphiphilicity and this may significantly affect the cellular/tissue uptake and phototoxicity of the photosensitizer *in vitro* (Kessel *et al*., 1987; Paquette *et al*., 1988) and *in vivo* (Berg *et al*., 1990a; Peng *et al*., 1994). Furthermore, subtle structural differences which do not affect the polarity of the drugs, such as linear versus nonlinear dialkyl ether derivatives of hematoporphyrin, may lead to pronouncedly different phototoxicity: such an effect was present *in vitro* with respect to the dibutyl and di-isobutyl derivatives of Hp (see Moan *et al.*, 1987a), and also the phototoxicity *in vivo* of the diamylether derivative of Hp was seemingly higher than expected relative to the phototoxicity of linear dialkyl ethers of Hp (see Evensen *et al.*, 1987). Thus, the batch of diamylether Hp employed by Evensen *et al.* probably contained mostly isopentyl chains (Kongshaug *et al.*, 1990). Also, whilst the phototoxicity of Hp-dimethylether is larger than that of Hp for *in vitro* experiments (Fig. 1), the opposite trend is indicated by *in vivo* experiments (Fig. 1). Similarly, *meso-*, *para-* and *ortho-*tetrahydroxyphenyl porphines can show remarkably different photosensitization at least *in vivo* (Barenbaum *et al.*, 1986).

Recently, cationic dyes have attracted attention as PDT sensitizers (Wöhrle *et al.*, 1990; Woodburn *et al.*, 1991, 1992a, b). There is, *in vitro*, a correlation between subcellular localization and phototoxicity of several anionic and cationic derivatives of hematoporphyrin, and the three most photoactive substances were cationic and all these localized in the mitochondria (Woodburn *et al.*, 1992a), whilst those with a more anionic character tended to localize in lysosomes (Woodburn *et al.*, 1991). Although some results are available for the tissue distribution of such sensitizers (Woodburn *et al.*, 1992b), it is not known whether intracellular localization patterns of the dyes *in vivo* follow a similar trend to those *in vitro*.

3.7.3. FRACTIONATION OF LIGHT DOSE DURING PHOTODYNAMIC THERAPY

A split-dose effect on phototoxicity has been found in Chinese hamster cells *in vitro* using Zinc tetrahydroxyphthalocyanine as a photosensitizer (Ben-Hur *et al.*, 1988). Moreover, Berg *et al.* (1992) demonstrated *in vitro* that an initial small light dose increased the photosensitivity of $TPPS_4$-loaded NHIK 3025 human carcinoma cells to a second exposure. This increase (60–150%) was interpreted in terms of a light-induced increase in the fluorescence yield of cell-bound $TPPS_4$. Similarly, in earlier experiments, the hematoporphyrin (Hp)-induced photo-destruction of NHIK 3025 cells *in vitro* was more efficient for fractionation of the light dose than for the delivery of the dose in a single exposure (Moan and Christensen, 1979). This might be related to their finding that the first part of the split dose induced a membrane damage that led to an increased cellular uptake of Hp (Moan and Christensen, 1979). Similar results were also obtained with HpD (Moan and Christensen, 1981). Moreover, an increased uptake of Photofrin was found in the CaD2 mouse mammary carcinoma model subsequent to the delivery of an initial small light dose, but the photochemical efficiency of fractionation versus no fractionation was not determined (Ma *et al.*, 1992). Dougherty *et al.* (1979) reported some encouraging clinical results using fractionated HpD-PDT of regional chest wall recurrences of breast cancer. A split-dose (delivering the light dose in two fractions) was recently found to improve the efficacy of PDT of tumor-bearing animals using as photosensitizers either hematoporphyrin oligomers (Pe *et al.*, 1994), Photofrin (Gibson *et al.*, 1990; Foster *et al.*, 1991) or 5-aminolevulinic acid (ALA) (van der Veen *et al.*, 1994; Hua *et al.*, 1995; Messmann *et al.*, 1995). van der Veen *et al.* (1994) found that the first light exposure did not severely damage the vascular functions. This might be related to the observed photobleaching of ALA-induced protoporphyrin IX (PpIX). PpIX fluorescence reappeared, and this allowed the second light dose to induce complete vascular stasis in the tumor. In these experiments the relatively long time interval between the drug administration and the second light exposure (1.5 h) would allow further conversion of ALA into PpIX. By contrast, in the other experiments the interval was too short to allow significant PpIX synthesis (Messmann *et al.*, 1995). Presumably, reoxygenation of the tumor tissue might be involved during PDT in this case (Messmann *et al.*, 1995). Foster *et al.* (1991) found that the possible effect of oxygen depletion in Photofrin-PDT of an animal tumor model could be partially overcome by appropriate modulation of the light fractionation. The initial non-lethal portion of split-dose might induce vasoconstriction of the tumor tissue, followed by vasodilatation and hyperemia, and finally stasis may occur (Star *et al.*, 1986). The stage of vasodilatation might permit reoxygenation of the injured tissue. Oxygen is an essential mediator of the photochemical effect. Moreover, the vasodilatation and hyperemia could possibly lead to increased tumor uptake of photosensitizers from the circulation (Ma *et al.*, 1992; van der Veen *et al.*, 1994).

However, Bellnier and Lin (1985) found that a split-dose regimen was less efficient in sensitizing cultured EJ human urinary bladder carcinoma cells to photoinactivation than a single light dose in the presence of HpD, and that the initial part of the split-dose did not induce significant change in intracellular HpD levels. They suggested that the cells had developed an increased tolerance to photosensitized damage after prior PDT. *In vivo* Evensen and Moan (1988) demonstrated that fractionation of the light dose gave a lower phototoxicity than the application of a single light exposure in HpD-PDT of C3H mouse mammary carcinoma. They speculated that the first light exposure might severely destroy the tumor vascular system and thus result in an increased fraction of hypoxic cells. Such hypoxic cells would be rather resistant to the second light exposure. Thus, the factors affecting oxygen depletion and reoxygenation in split-dose-treated tumors might depend on the type of biological systems and the particular PDT protocols applied (Foster *et al.*, 1993).

3.7.4. PHOTODEGRADATION DURING PHOTODYNAMIC THERAPY

Photodegradation of HpD and Photofrin occurs both *in vitro* in NHIK 3025 cells (Moan *et al.*, 1984; Moan, 1986, 1988) and *in vivo* in SMT-F mouse mammary carcinoma and human melanoma transplanted into mice (Moan *et al.*, 1984; Moan, 1986, 1988; Mang *et al.*, 1987). Thus, one reason why some photosensitizers show a low phototoxicity below certain threshold concentrations could be due, in part, to photodegradation; in such conditions, exposure to an increasing light dose does not need to increase the phototoxicity because of photodegradation. A threshold tissue concentration of the photosensitizer, sulfonated aluminum phthalocyanine (AlSPc) may exist (Barr *et al.*, 1987). Such thresholds combined with photodegradation and the circumstance that photosensitizers often show a substantially increased uptake in tumor tissue relative to that in the surrounding normal tissue, offer a possibility of improving the selectivity of PDT by reducing the damage to normal tissue (Moan, 1985; Mang *et al.*, 1987; Barr *et al.*, 1990). To this end, the concentration of the photosensitizer in the surrounding normal tissue should be at a certain level so as to have a relatively low phototoxicity in the normal tissue. Photobleaching would protect the normal tissue towards toxicity and simultaneously increase the portion of light reaching the tumor. For a highly preferential tumor uptake of the photosensitizer, such an increased light dose might lead to efficient tumor damage. This would occur provided that the photobleaching of the sensitizer in the tumor would not be too counterproductive relative to its ability to induce phototoxicity. Some systems are known which *in vitro* and *in vivo* exhibit increased phototoxicity with increasing light exposure at sufficiently high concentrations of the photosensitizer (Henderson *et al.*, 1983; Gibson and Hilf, 1985; Cowled and Forbes, 1985; Gossner *et al.*, 1994). However, Moesta *et al.* (1995) found that there was a lack of reciprocity between photosensitizer concentration and light dose in terms of phototoxicity in pancreatic adenocarcinoma cell lines. In these cases photodegradation might have been too counterproductive. It seems to be commonly overlooked that the photodegradation of a given photosensitizer may depend on its local milieu. For example, efficient scavenging of singlet oxygen ($^1O_2$) by other components than the photosensitizer could protect it against photobleaching. Thus, depending on microenvironmental circumstances, the photobleaching of a given photosensitizer at a given concentration could be smaller, equal or larger in a given tumor than in the surrounding normal tissue.

3.7.5. OXYGEN-DEPENDENT PHOTODYNAMIC THERAPY

Several early studies *in vitro* have indicated that photocytotoxicity with HpD was most likely induced via $^1O_2$ (Weishaupt *et al.*, 1976; Moan *et al.*, 1979). The photoinactivation of the sensitized cells decreased with decreasing oxygen concentration, and no cellular photodestruction was observed when the atmosphere above the medium overlying the cells was pure N_2 (LeeSee *et al.*, 1984; Moan and Sommer, 1985). Also, the photosensitizing effect with most 2nd generation photosensitizers is likely $^1O_2$-mediated at least in the *in vitro* situation (Moan *et al.*, 1987b; Kimel *et al.*, 1989). Interestingly, photochemical results obtained for the liver of rats have correlated well with those found in studies *in vitro*: The lipid-rich microsomal membranes and the heme-protein cytochrome P-450 were potentially targets of $^1O_2$-mediated photochemical reaction in hepatic cells of rats pretreated with HpD *in vivo*, followed by long-wave ultraviolet light exposure *in vitro* (Das *et al.*, 1985). The oxygen-dependent phototoxicity in the RIF mouse tumor model using dihematoporphyrin ether (Henderson and Fingar, 1987) followed a similar trend as found in the NHIK 3025 cells *in vitro* (Moan and Sommer, 1985). Similarly, there was no phototoxicity of HpD-mediated PDT on human retinoblastoma cells transplanted into the anterior chamber of the nude mouse eye due to the absence of tumor vascularity in this model (White *et al.*, 1988), nor on normal anoxic (clamped) mouse skin (Gomer and Razum, 1984).

3.7.6. EFFECT OF LOW pH DURING PHOTODYNAMIC THERAPY

The pH in the interstitium is significantly lower in many tumors than in non-neoplastic tissues. This may arise via anaerobic glycolysis: being usually poorly vascularised, tumors have to provide a significant amount of their energy via anaerobic glycolysis, leading to production of lactic acid and low pH (Eden *et al.*, 1955; Gullino *et al.*, 1965). The effect of low pH in the tumor interstitium on the uptake of HpD by tumor tissue has recently attracted much interest (Moan *et al.*, 1987b; Pottier, 1990; Barrett *et al.*, 1990). Hematoporphyrin and related dyes may attain a reduced charge by protonation and thus become more lipophilic when the pH in their surroundings is reduced from 7.4 to 6.5. There was an increase in the binding of HpD to lipid films with decreasing pH (Rich *et al.*, 1992) and an increased cellular uptake of the dyes in cells in culture (Moan *et al.*, 1980, 1987b; Moan and Christensen, 1981; Bohmer and Morstyn, 1985). The low pH-induced enhanced uptake of the dye was associated with a more efficient photoinactivation of the cells following light exposure (Moan *et al.*, 1980). The extracellular pH in tumor tissue may also be lowered by multiple injections of glucose in tumor-bearing animals (Eden *et al.*, 1955; Calderwood and Dickson, 1982; Jain *et al.*, 1984; Thistlethwaite *et al.*, 1987; Volk *et al.*, 1993). Pretreatment with multiple i.p. injections of glucose resulted in an increase in the porphyrin fluorescence of tumor tissues 48 h after an i.v. injection of HpD in the rhabdomyosarcoma-bearing rats (Thomas and Girotti, 1989) and 4 h after an i.p. administration of Photofrin in the human tumor LOX xenograft (Peng *et al.*, 1991a). The uptake of the dyes by the liver and normal tissues surrounding the tumor remained unchanged (Thomas and Girotti, 1989; Peng *et al.*, 1991a). Thus, glucose-induced acidosis may be tumor-specific (Volk *et al.*, 1993). Consistently, glucose administration combined with PDT produced a larger percentage cure of C3HBA tumor-bearing mice than PDT alone (Nelson *et al.*, 1992).

3.7.7. EFFECT OF TEMPERATURE DURING PHOTODYNAMIC THERAPY

In many clinical treatments, using a standard regime of PDT, local heating of the tissue due to absorption of light energy is inevitable. In fact, both hyperthermia and hypothermia may significantly enhance HpD-induced phototoxicity in *in vitro* and *in vivo* experiments, although attention has been primarily paid to hyperthemia as an adjuvant. Increased temperature can enhance the phototoxicity in paramecia (Giese and Crossman, 1946). Christensen *et al.* (1984) found that hyperthermia (42.5°C and 45°C) given shortly after PDT led to a synergistic phototoxic effect on NHIK 3025 cells *in vitro*. *In vivo* hyperthermia, generated by local microwave application, increased the response of the SMT-F tumors to HpD-PDT (Waldow and Dougherty, 1984). Similarly, CO_2 laser-induced hyperthermia combined with porphyrin-PDT resulted in a synergistic effect of about 40% with respect to damaging the vascular structure in a chick chorioallantoic membrane model (Kimel *et al.*, 1992). Moreover, Kinsey *et al.* (1983) demonstrated *in vivo* that the rise in temperature was dependent upon the fluence rate of the light applied. When a fluence rate of 200 mW/cm^2 was used the HpD-induced phototoxicity was at least partially due to the effect of hyperthermia. However, at 100 mW/cm^2, which induces no hyperthermia, only a 'pure' photosensitizing effect was found. In the case of hypothermia using Hp as a photosensitizer Moan and Christensen (1979) showed that irradiation at 4°C resulted in much more efficient inactivation of NHIK 3025 cells *in vitro* than irradiation at 37°C. Similarly, Jones *et al.* (1983) found that superficial cooling of solid tumors *in vivo* could enhance the tumoricidal effect of HpD-based PDT.

3.7.8. OTHER COMBINATIONS

Ionizing radiation may enhance the cytotoxic effect of PDT on cultured cells (Prinsze *et al.*, 1992; Kavarnos *et al.*, 1994; Berg *et al.*, 1995), although such enhancement is not always present (Belliner and Dougherty, 1986). Augmentation of phototoxicity by ionizing radiation may also occur in *in vivo* tumors (Kostron *et al.*, 1986; Graschew and Shopova, 1986). Chemotherapeutic drugs may also enhance the action of PDT. The combined treatment by mitomycin C (MMC) and PDT produced a greater cytotoxic effect than did the individual treatment modalities both *in vitro* and *in vivo* (Ma *et al.*, 1993, 1995; Baas *et al.*, 1994; van Geel *et al.*, 1995). Treatments such as ionizing radiation and MMC can induce accumulation of the WiDr human colonic carcinoma cells in S and $G_2 + M$ phases of the cell cycle both in cell culture *in vitro* (Berg *et al.*, 1995) and in tumors *in vivo* (Ma *et al.*, 1993, 1995), the phases where they are particularly sensitive to PDT (Christensen *et al.*, 1981).

3.7.9. FINAL REMARKS

The dependence of phototoxicity on a given factor (such as drug structure, fractionation of light exposure, pH, temperature, etc.) shows a similar trend both in cell cultures and in tumors in several cases. This underscores the possibility of continued use of simple cell cultures for experimental elucidation of possible determinants of phototoxicity *in vivo*. However, various findings indicate somewhat different trends *in vitro* and *in vivo*, respectively, of the dependence of phototoxicity on a given parameter. It should be emphasized that even though the effect on phototoxicity of a given parameter may in given conditions follow similar trends *in vitro* and *in vivo*, the mechanisms actually involved in the tumor destruction may obviously be more or less different from those operating on the corresponding neoplastic cells in culture: the phototoxicity *in vivo* may involve contributions from (1) the vascular system, (2) non-neoplastic cells, such as tumor-associated macrophages and their immune reactions such as production of cytokines and (3) components of the extracellular matrix.

In fact, some PDT-relevant information can only be obtained from experiments *in vivo*. For example, the information regarding the distribution of a photosensitizer with respect to its distance from the tumor capillaries (Korbelik and Krosl, 1992). Similarly, the general skin photosensitizing effect of a drug and the determinants involved are best studied *in vivo*, although work *in vitro* on the phototoxicity of endothelial cells in culture, may conceivably shed some light upon factors possibly contributing to skin photosensitivity. Moreover, depending on the type of photosensitizer and tumor system studied, tumor eradication by PDT may be largely due to the photochemical destruction of the tumor vasculature (Henderson and Dougherty, 1992; Moan and Berg, 1992).

Only a small number of the determinants of phototoxicity have been considered herein. Other such determinants include photosensitizer binding to transport proteins and/or the modulatory effects of the use of different drug delivery vehicles, such as low density lipoproteins, liposomes and Cremophor EL. However, the possible influence of such factors have thus been summarized in recent contributions (Mazière *et al.*, 1991; Kongshaug, 1992, 1993; Jori and Reddi, 1993; Kessel and Woodburn, 1993; Nakajima *et al.*, 1995; Moan *et al.*, 1996). Moreover, the intracellular and intratumoral localization patterns of some new photosensitizers seems to be also related to their PDT efficacy in both *in vitro* (Peng *et al.*, 1991, 1996; Woodburn *et al.*, 1991, 1992a) and *in vivo* (Peng *et al.*, 1990, 1995a,b) studies. For instance, the uptake of $AlPcS_2$ and $AlPcS_4$ by the CaD2 mouse mammary carcinoma was similar at given times following administration, but the intratumoral localization patterns of the two dyes were quite different that might lead to a different PDT efficiency of the tumors (Peng and Moan, 1995a). It is still not known whether subcellular localization patterns of the dyes and their phototoxicity *in vivo* follow a similar trend to those *in vitro*.

Much more experimental information is required for the elucidation of photosensitizing determinants/mechanisms under both *in vitro* and *in vivo* conditions, particularly with respect to new generation photosensitizers. Although a variety of new photosensitizers exhibit phototoxicity, to larger or smaller extents, both *in vitro* and *in vivo*, little is yet known as to how such phototoxicity depends on the factors herein discussed. Such photosensitizers include tetra(*m*-hydroxyphenyl) porphine and its chlorin (Berenbaum *et al.*, 1986; Bonnett and Berenbaum, 1989; Peng *et al.*, 1995b), benzoporphyrin derivatives (Richter *et al.*, 1990, 1991), chlorin e_6 (Spikes, 1990), purpurins (Morgan *et al.*, 1987; Kessel, 1989; Morgan and Selman, 1990), phthalocyanines (Ben-Hur and Rosenthal, 1985; Ben-Hur, 1987; van Lier, 1990; Rosenthal *et al.*, 1991; Kessel and Allen, 1992; Biolo *et al.*, 1994; Soncin *et al.*, 1995; Segalla *et al.*, 1995). Hopefully, the experimental protocols for testing 1st generation photosensitizers will be increasingly applied to new generation dyes. Generally, cell types which can grow both *in vitro* and *in vivo* should be increasingly applied so as to make cell culture and tumor systems complementary.

ACKNOWLEDGEMENTS

We thank Prof. Jahn M. Nesland for critically reading the manuscript. This work was supported by The Norwegian Cancer Society.

LITERATURE CITED

Baas, P., Michielsen, C., Oppelaar, H., van Zandwijk, N., and Stewart, F. A. (1994): Enhancement of interstitial photodynamic therapy by mitomycin C and EO9 in a mouse tumor model. *Int. J. Cancer* **56**, 880–885.

Barr, H., Tralau, C. J., MacRobert, A. J., Krasner, N., Boulos, P. B., Clark, C. G., and Bown, S. G. (1987): Photodynamic therapy in the normal rat colon with phthalocyanine sensitisation. *Br. J. Cancer* **56**, 111–118.

Barr, H., Tralau, C. J., Boulos, P. B., MacRobert, A. J., Lewis, M. R., Phillips, D., and Bown, S. G. (1990): Selective necrosis in experimental colon cancer using photodynamic therapy with phthalocyanine photosensitisation. *Gastroenterology* **98**, 1532–1537.

Barrett, A. J., Kennedy, J. C., Jones, R. A., and Pottier, R. H. (1990): The effect of tissue and cellular pH on the selective biodistribution of porphyrin-type photochemotherapeutic agents: A volumetric titration study. *J. Photochem. Photobiol. B: Biol.* **6**, 309–323.

Bellnier, D. A. and Lin, C. W. (1985): Photosensitization and split-dose recovery in cultured human urinary bladder carcinoma cells containing nonexchangeable hematoporphyrin derivative. *Cancer Res.* **45**, 2507–2511.

Bellnier, D. A. and Dougherty, T. J. (1986): Haematoporphyrin derivative photosensitization and gamma-radiation damage interaction in Chinese hamster ovary fibroblasts. *Int. J. Radiat. Biol.* **50**, 659–664.

Ben-Hur, E. and Rosenthal, I. (1985): The phthalocyanines: a new class of mammalian cell photosensitizers with a potential for cancer phototherapy. *Int. J. Radiat. Biol.* **47**, 145–147.

Ben-Hur, E. (1987): Photochemistry and photobiology of phthalocyanines: new sensitizers for photodynamic therapy of cancer. In From photophysics to photobiology (Edited by Fave, A., Tyrell, R., and Cadet, J.). pp. 407–420. Elsevier: New York.

Ben-Hur, E., Rosenthal, I., and Leznoff, C. C. (1988): Recovery of Chinese hamster cells following photosensitization by zinc tetrahydroxyphthalocyanine. *J. Photochem. Photobiol. B: Biol.* **2**, 243–252.

Berenbaum, M. C., Akande, S. L., Bonnett, R., Kaur, H., Ioannou, S., White, R. D., and Winfield, U.-J. (1986): *meso*-Tetra(hydroxyphenyl)porphyrins, a new class of potent tumor photosensitisers with favourable selectivity. *Br. J. Cancer* **54**, 717–725.

Berg, K., Bommer, J. C., and Moan, J. (1989): Evaluation of sulfonated aluminum phthalocyanines for use in photochemotherapy. A study on the relative efficiencies of photoinactivation. *Photochem. Photobiol.* **49**, 587–594.

Berg, K., Bommer, J. C., Winkelman, J. W., and Moan, J. (1990a): Cellular uptake and relative efficiency in cell inactivation by photoactivated sulfonated *meso*-tetraphenylporphines. *Photochem. Photobiol.* **52**, 775–781.

Berg, K., Western, A., Bommer, J. C., and Moan, J. (1990b): Intracellular localization of sulfonated *meso*-tetraphenylporphines in a human carcinoma cell line. *Photochem. Photobiol.* **52**, 481–487.

Berg, K., Madslien, K., and Moan, J. (1992): Retention and phototoxicity of tetra(4-sulfonatophenyl)porphine in cultivated human cells. The effect of fractionation of light. *Photochem. Photobiol.* **56**, 177–183.

Berg, K., Luksiene, Z., Moan, J., and Ma, L. W. (1995): Combined treatment of ionizing radiation and photosensitization by 5-aminolevulinic acid-induced protoporphyrin IX. *Radiat. Res.* **142**, 340–346.

Biolo, R., Jori, G., Soncin, M., Pratesi, R., Vanni, U., Rihter, B., Kenney, M. E., and Rodgers, M. A. (1994): Photodynamic therapy of B16 pigmented melanoma with liposome-delivered Si (IV)-naphthalocyanine. *Photochem. Photobiol.* **59**, 362–365.

Bohmer, R. M. and Morstyn, G. (1985): Uptake of hematoporphyrin derivative by normal and malignant cells: Effect of serum, pH, temperature, and cell size. *Cancer Res.* **45**, 5328–5334.

Bonnett, R. and Berenbaum, M. C. (1989): Porphyrins as photosensitizers. In Photosensitizing compounds: their chemistry, biology and clinical use (Edited by Bock, G. and Harnett, S.). pp. 40–59. Ciba Foundation 146, John Wiley & Sons, Chichester.

Boyle, R. W., Paquette, B., and van Lier, J. E. (1992): Biological activities of phthalocyanines XIV. Effect of hydrophobic phthalimidomethyl groups on the *in vivo* phototoxicity and mechanism of photodynamic action of sulphonated aluminum phthalocyanines. *Br. J. Cancer* **65**, 813–817.

Brasseur, N., Ali, H., Langlois, R., and van Lier, J. E. (1988): Biological activities of phthalocyanines-IX. Photosensitization of V-79 Chinese cells and EMT-6 mouse mammary tumor by selectively sulfonated zinc phthalocyanines. *Photochem. Photobiol.* **47**, 705–711.

Calderwood, S. K. and Dickson, J. A. (1982): Inhibition of tumor blood flow at high blood sugar levels: Effects on tumor pH and hyperthermia. *Natl. Cancer Inst. Monogr.* **61**, 221–223.

Chan, W. S., West, C. M. L., Moore, J. V., and Hart, I. R. (1991): Photocytotoxic efficacy of sulphonated species of aluminium phthalocyanine against cell monolayers, multicellular spheroids and *in vivo* tumours. *Br. J. Cancer* **64**, 827–832.

Chatlani, P. T., Bedwell, J., MacRobert, A. J., and Bown, S. G. (1992): Distribution and photodynamic effects of di- and tetra-sulphonated aluminium phthalocyanines (AlS_2Pc and AlS_4Pc) in normal and neoplastic rat colon. In Photodynamic therapy and biomedical lasers (Edited by Spinelli, P., Dal Fante, M., and Marchesini, R.). pp. 539–544. Elsevier Science, Amsterdam.

Christensen, T., Feren, K., Moan, J., and Pettersen, E. (1981): Photodynamic effects of hematoporphyrin derivative on synchronized and asynchronized cells of different origin. *Br. J. Cancer* **44**, 717–723.

Christensen, T., Wahl, A., and Smedshammer, L. (1984): Effects of haematoporphyrin derivative and light in combination with hyperthermia on cells in culture. *Br. J. Cancer* **50**, 85–89.

Cowled, P. A. and Forbes, I. J. (1985): Photocytotoxicity *in vivo* of hematoporphyrin derivative components. *Cancer Lett.* **28**, 111–118.

Cozzani, I., Jori, G., Bertoloni, G., Milanesi, C., Carlini, P., Sicuro, T., and Ruschi, A. (1985): Efficient photosensitization of malignant human cells *in vitro* by liposome-bound porphyrins. *Chem. Biol. Interact.* **53**, 131–143.

Das, M., Dixit, R., Mukhtar, H., and Bickers, D. R. (1985): Role of active oxygen species in the photodestruction of microsomal cytochrome P-450 and associated monooxygenases by hematoporphyrin derivative in rats. *Cancer Res.* **45**, 608–615.

Dougherty, T. J., Lawrence, G., Kaufman, J. H., Boyle, D., Weishaupt, K. R., and Goldfarb, A. (1979): Photoradiation in the treatment of recurrent breast carcinoma. *J. Natl. Cancer Inst.* **62**, 231–237.

Eden, M., Haines, B., and Kahler, H. (1955): The pH of rat tumor measured *in vivo. J. Natl. Cancer Inst.* **16**, 541–556.

Evensen, J. F., Sommer, S., Rimington, C., and Moan, J. (1987): Photodynamic therapy of C3H mouse mammary carcinoma with haematoporphyrin di-ethers as sensitizers. *Br. J. Cancer* **55**, 483–486.

Evensen, J. F. and Moan, J. (1988): Photodynamic therapy of C3H tumors in mice: Effect of drug/light dose fractionation and misonidazole. *Lasers Med. Sci.* **3**, 1–6.

Foster, T. H., Murant, R., Bryant, R. G., Knox, R. S., Gibson, S. L., and Hilf, R. (1991): Oxygen consumption and diffusion effects in photodynamic therapy. *Radiat. Res.* **126**, 296–303.

Gibson, S. L. and Hilf, R. (1985): Interdependence of fluence, drug dose and oxygen on hematoporphyrin derivative induced photosensitization of tumor mitochondria. *Photochem. Photobiol.* **42**, 367–373.

Gibson, S. L., VanDerMeid, K. R., Murant, R. S., Raubertas, R. F., and Hilf, R. (1990): Effects of various photoradiation regimens on the antitumor efficacy of photodynamic therapy for R3230AC mammary carcinoma. *Cancer Res.* **50**, 7236–7241.

Giese, A. C. and Crossman, E. B. (1946): Sensitization of cells to heat by visible light in presence of photodynamic dyes. *J. Gen. Physiol.* **29**, 193.

Gomer, C. J. and Razum, N. J. (1984): Acute skin response in albino mice following porphyrin photosensitization under oxic and anoxic conditions. *Photochem. Photobiol.* **40**, 435–439.

Gossner, L., Wittke, H., Warzecha, A., Ernst, H., Sroka, R., Hahn, E. G., and Ell, C. (1994): Dose-dependent destruction of human gastrointestinal neoplasms by photodynamic therapy: a quantitative pilot study in athymic nude mice. *Eur. J. Gastroenterol. Hepatol.* **6**, 159–165.

Graschew, G. and Shopova, M. (1986): Photodynamic therapy and gamma-radiation of tumors: Effect of tumor-cell reoxygenation. *Lasers Med. Sci.* **1**, 193–195.

Gullino, P. M., Grantham, F. H., Smith, S. H., and Haggerty, A. C. (1965): Modification of the acid-base status of the internal milieu of tumor. *J. Natl. Cancer Inst.* **34**, 857–869.

Henderson, B. W., Belliner, D. A., Ziring, B., and Dougherty, T. J. (1983): Aspects of the cellular uptake and retention of hematoporphyrin derivative and their correlation with the biological response to PRT *in vitro*. In Porphyrin Photosensitization (Edited by Kessel, D. and Dougherty, T. J.), pp. 129–138. Plenum Press, New York.

Henderson, B. W., Waldow, S. M., Mang, T. S., Potter, W. R., Malone, P. B., and Dougherty, T. J. (1985): Tumor destruction and kinetics of tumor cell death in two experimental mouse tumors following photodynamic therapy. *Cancer Res.* **45**, 572–576.

Henderson, B. W. and Fingar, V. (1987): Relationship of tumor hypoxia and response to photodynamic treatment in an experimental mouse tumor. *Cancer Res.* **47**, 3110–3114.

Henderson, B. W. and Bellnier, D. A. (1989): Tissue localization of photosensitizers and the mechanism of photodynamic tissue destruction. In Photosensitizing compounds: their chemistry, biology and clinical use (Edited by Bock, G. and Harnett, S.). pp. 112–130. Ciba Foundation 146, John Wiley & Sons, Chichester.

Henderson, B. W. (1990): Probing the effects of photodynamic therapy through *in vivo–in vitro* methods. In Photodynamic therapy of neoplastic disease (Edited by D. Kessel), Vol. I, pp. 169–188. CRC Press, Boca Raton.

Henderson, B. W. and Dougherty, T. J. (1992): How does photodynamic therapy work? *Photochem. Photobiol.* **55**, 145–157.

Hoebeke, M. (1995): The importance of liposomes as models and tools in the understanding of photosensitization mechanisms. *J. Photochem. Photobiol. B: Biol.* **28**, 189–196.

Hua, Z., Gibson, S. L., Foster, T. H., and Hilf, R. (1995): Effectiveness of 5-aminolevulinic acid-induced protoporphyrin as a photosensitizer for photodynamic therapy *in vivo*. *Cancer Res.* **55**, 1723–1731.

Jain, R. K., Shah, S. A., and Finney, P. L. (1984): Continuous noninvasive monitoring of pH and temperature in rat Walker 256 carcinoma during normoglycemia and hyperglycemia. *J. Natl. Cancer Inst.* **73**, 429–436.

Jori, G., Tomio, L., Reddi, E., Rossi, E., Corti, L., Zorat, P. L., and Caøzavara F. (1983): Preferential delivery of liposome-incorporated porphyrins to neoplastic cells in tumor-bearing rats. *Br. J. Cancer* **48**, 307–309.

Jori, G., Reddi, E., Cozani, I., and Tomio, L. (1986): Controlled targeting of different subcellular sites by porphyrins in tumor-bearing mice. *Br. J. Cancer* **53**, 615–621.

Jori, G. and Reddi, E. (1990): Strategies for tumor targeting by photodynamic sensitizers. In Photodynamic therapy of neoplastic disease (Edited by D. Kessel), Vol. II, pp. 117–130. CRC Press, Boca Raton.

Jori, G. and Reddi, E. (1993): The role of lipoproteins in the delivery of tumor-targeting photosensitizers. *Int. J. Biochem.* **25**, 1369–1375.

Kavarnos, G., Nath, R., and Bongiorni, P. (1994): Visible-light and X-irradiation of Chinese hamster lung cells treated with hematoporphyrin derivative. *Radiat. Res.* **137**, 196–201.

Kessel, D., Thompson, P., Saatio, K., and Nantwi, K. D. (1987): Tumor localization and photosensitization by sulfonated derivatives of tetraphenylporphine. *Photochem. Photobiol.* **45**, 787–790.

Kessel, D. (1989): Determinants of photosensitization by purpurins. *Photochem. Photobiol.* **50**, 169–174.

Kessel, D., Dougherty, T. J., and Chang, C. K. (1991a): Photosensitization by synthetic diporphyrins and dichlorins *in vivo* and *in vitro*. *Photochem. Photobiol.* **53**, 475–479.

Kessel, D., Morgan, A., and Garbo, G. M. (1991b): Sites and efficacy of photodamage by tin etiopurpurin *in vitro* using different delivery systems. *Photochem. Photobiol.* **54**, 193–196.

Kessel, D. and Allen, R. (1992): Determinants of localization by second-generation PDT sensitizers. In Photodynamic therapy and biomedical lasers (Edited by Spinelli, P., Dal Fante, M., and Marchesini, R.). pp. 526–530. Elsevier Science, Amsterdam.

Kessel, D., and Woodburn, K. (1993): Biodistribution of photosensitizing agents. *Int. J. Biochem.* **25**, 1377–1383.

Kimel, S., Tromberg, B. J., Roberts, W. G., and Berns, M. W. (1989): Singlet oxygen generation of porphyrins, chlorins, and phthalocyanines. *Photochem. Photobiol.* **50**, 175–183.

Kimel, S., Svaasand, L. O., Hammer-Wilson, M., Gottfried, V., Cheng, S., Svaasand, E., and Berns, M. W. (1992): Demonstration of synergistic effects of hyperthermia and photodynamic therapy using the chick chorioallantoic membrane model. *Lasers Surg. Med.* **12**, 432–440.

Kinsey, J. H., Cortese, D. A., and Neel, H. B. (1983): Thermal considerations in murine tumor killing using hematoporphyrin derivative phototherapy. *Cancer Res.* **43**, 1562–1567.

Kongshaug, M., Moan, J., and Brown, S. B. (1989): The distribution of porphyrins with different tumor localizing ability among human plasma proteins. *Br. J. Cancer* **59**, 184–188.

Kongshaug, M., Rimington, C., Evensen, J. F., Peng, Q., and Moan, J. (1990): Hematoporphyrin diethers-V. Plasma protein binding and photosensitizing efficiency. *Int. J. Biochem.* **22**, 1127–1131.

Kongshaug, M. (1992): Review: Distribution of tetrapyrrole photosensitizers among human plasma proteins. *Int. J. Biochem.* **24**, 1239–1265.

Kongshaug, M. (1993): Ph.D thesis. The University of Oslo, Oslo.

Korbelik, M. and Krosl, G. (1994): Cellular levels of photosensitizers in tumors: the role of proximity to the blood supply. *Br. J. Cancer* **70**, 604–610.

Kostron, H., Swartz, M. R., Miller, D. C., and Martuza, R. L. (1986): The interaction of hematoporphyrin derivative, light and ionizing radiation in a rat glioma model. *Cancer* **57**, 964–970.

LeeSee, K., Forbes, I. J., and Betts, W. H. (1984): Oxygen dependence of phototoxicity with haematoporphyrin derivative. *Photochem. Photobiol.* **39**, 631–634.

Ma, L. W., Moan, J., and Peng, Q. (1992): Effect of light exposure on the uptake of Photofrin II in tumors and normal tissues. *Int. J. Cancer* **52**, 120–123.

Ma, L. W., Moan, J., Berg, K., Peng, Q., and Steen, H. B. (1993): Potentiation of photodynamic therapy by mitomycin C in cultured human colon adenocarcinoma cells. *Radiat. Res.* **134**, 22–27.

Ma, L. W., Moan, J., Steen, H. B., and Iani, V. (1995): Anti-tumour activity of photodynamic therapy in combination with mitomycin C in nude mice with human colon adenocarcinoma. *Br. J. Cancer* **71**, 950–956.

Mang, T. S., Dougherty, T. J., Potter, W. R., Boyle, D. G., Sommer, S., and Moan, J. (1987): Photobleaching of porphyrin used in photodynamic therapy and implications for therapy. *Photochem. Photobiol.* **45**, 501–506.

Mazière, J. C., Morliere, P., and Santus, R. (1991): The role of the low density lipoprotein receptor pathway in the delivery of lipophilic photosensitizers in the photodynamic therapy of tumors. *J. Photochem. Photobiol. B: Biol.* **8**, 351–360.

Messmann, H., Mikvy, P., Buonaccorsi, G., Davies, C. L., MacRobert, A. J., and Bown, S. G. (1995): Enhancement of photodynamic therapy with 5-aminolaevulinic acid-induced porphyrin photosensitisation in normal rat colon by threshold and light fractionation studies. *Br. J. Cancer* **72**, 589–594.

Moan, J. and Christensen, T. (1979): Photodynamic inactivation of cancer cells *in vitro*. Effect of irradiation temperature and dose fractionation. *Cancer Lett.* **6**, 331–335.

Moan, J., Pettersen, E. O., and Christensen, T. (1979): The mechanism of photodynamic inactivation of human cells *in vitro* in the presence of hematoporphyrin. *Br. J. Cancer* **39**, 398–407.

Moan, J., Smedshammer, L., and Christensen, T. (1980): Photodynamic effects on human cells exposed to light in the presence of hematoporphyrin. pH effects. *Cancer Lett.* **9**, 327–332.

Moan, J. and Christensen, T. (1981): Cellular uptake and photodynamic effect of hematoporphyrin. *Photobiochem. Photobiophys.* **2**, 291–299.

Moan, J., Christensen, T., and Jacobsen, P. B. (1984): Porphyrin-sensitized photoinactivation of cells *in vitro*. In Porphyrin Localization and Treatment of tumors (Edited by Doiron, D. R. and Gomer, C. J.), pp. 419–442. Alan R. Liss, New York.

Moan, J. (1985): Porphyrin photosensitization of cells. In Photodynamic Therapy of Tumors and Other Diseases (Edited by Jori, G. and Perria, C.), pp. 102–112. Libreria Progetto, Padova.

Moan, J. and Sommer, S. (1985): Oxygen dependence of the photosensitizing effect of hematoporphyrin derivative in NHIK 3025 cells. *Cancer Res.* **45**, 1608–1610.

Moan, J. (1986): Effect of bleaching of porphyrin sensitizers during photodynamic therapy. *Cancer Lett.* **33**, 45–53.

Moan, J., Rimington, C., and Sommer, S. (1987a): Cellular uptake and photosensitizing properties of hematoporphyrin di-ethers with similar chromatographic properties as the tumorlocalizing fraction of hematoporphyrin derivative. *Cancer Lett.* **34**, 283–289.

Moan, J., Peng, Q., Evensen, J. F., Berg, K., Western, A., and Rimington, C. (1987b): Photosensitizing efficiencies, tumor-and cellular uptake of different photosensitizing drugs relevant for photodynamic therapy of cancer. *Photochem. Photobiol.* **46**, 713–721.

Moan, J. (1988): A change in the quantum yield of photoinactivation of cells observed during photodynamic treatment. *Lasers Med. Sci.* **3**, 93–97.

Moan, J., Rimington, C., and Western, A. (1988): Hematoporphyrin ethers-III. Cellular uptake and photosensitizing properties. *Int. J. Biochem.* **20**, 1401–1404.

Moan, J. and Berg, K. (1992): Photochemotherapy of cancer: experimental research. *Photochem. Photobiol.* **55**, 931–948.

Moan, J., Peng, Q., Iani, V., Ma, L. W., Horobin, R. W., Berg, K., Kongshaug, M., and Nesland, J. M. (1996): Biodistribution, pharmacokinetic and *in vivo* fluorescence spectroscopic studies of photosensitizers. *Proc. SPIE.* **2625**, 234–250.

Moesta, K. T., Greco, W. R., Nurse-Finlay, S. O., Parsons, J. C., and Mang, T. S. (1995): Lack of reciprocity in drug and light dose dependence of photodynamic therapy of pancreatic adenocarcinoma *in vitro*. *Cancer Res.* **55**, 3078–3084.

Morgan, A. R., Garbo, G. M., Keck, R. W., and Selman, S. H. (1987): Tin (IV) etiopurpurin dichloride: an alternative to DHE? *Proc. SPIE* **847**, 172–179.

Morgan, A. R. and Selman, S. H. (1990): New tetrapyrroles for photodynamic therapy. In Photodynamic therapy of neoplastic disease (Edited by D. Kessel), Vol. I, pp. 247–262. CRC Press, Boca Raton.

Nakajima, S., Takemura, T., and Sakata, I. (1995): Tumor-localizing activity of porphyrin and its affinity to LDL transferrin. *Cancer Lett.* **92**, 113–118.

Nelson, J. S., Kimel, S., Brown, L., and Berns, M. W. (1992): Glucose administration combined with photodynamic therapy of cancer improves therapeutic efficacy. *Lasers Surg. Med.* **12**, 153–158.

Paquette, B., Ali, H., Langlois, R., and van Lier, J. E. (1988): Biological activities of phthalocyanines. VIII. Cellular distribution in V-79 Chinese hamster cells and phototoxicity of selectively sulfonated aluminum phthalocyanines. *Photochem. Photobiol.* **47**, 215–220.

Pe, M. B., Ikeda, H., and Inokuchi, T. (1994): Tumor destruction and proliferation kinetics following periodic, low power light, haematoporphyrin oligomers mediated photodynamic therapy in the mouse tongue. *Eur. J. Cancer B: Oral. Oncol.* **30B**, 174–178.

Peng, Q., Moan, J., Farrants, G., Danielsen, H. E., and Rimington, C. (1990): Localization of potent photosensitizers in human tumor LOX by means of laser scanning microscopy. *Cancer Lett.* **53**, 129–139.

Peng, Q., Moan, J., and Cheng, L.S. (1991a): The effect of glucose administration on the uptake of Photofrin II in a human tumor xenograft. *Cancer Lett.* **58**, 29–35.

Peng, Q., Farrants, G. W., Madslien, K., Bommer, J. C., Moan, J., Danielsen, H. E., and Nesland, J. M. (1991b): Subcellular localization, redistribution and photobleaching of sulfonated aluminum phthalocyanines in a human melanoma cell line. *Int. J. Cancer* **49**, 290–295.

Peng, Q., Ma, L. W., Berg, K., and Moan, J. (1994): Effect of sulfonation on the photosensitizing efficiency of aluminum phthalocyanine and *meso*-tetraphenylporphine in photodynamic therapy of cancer. *Proc. SPIE* **2078**, 258–267.

Peng, Q. and Moan, J. (1995a): Correlation of distribution of sulfonated aluminum phthalocyanine with their photodynamic effect in tumor and skin of mice bearing CaD2 mammary carcinoma. *Br. J. Cancer* **72**, 565–574.

Peng, Q., Moan, J., Ma, L. W., and Nesland, J. M. (1995b): Uptake, localization and photodynamic effect of *meso*-tetra(hydroxyphenyl)porphine and its corresponding chlorin in normal and tumor tissues of mice bearing mammary carcinoma. *Cancer Res.* **55**, 2620–2626.

Peng, Q., Nesland, J. M., Madslien, K., Danielsen, H. E., and Moan, J. (1996a): Subcellular photodynamic action sites of sulfonated aluminum phthalocyanines in a human melanoma cell line. *Proc. SPIE* **2628**, 102–113.

Peng, Q., Moan, J., and Nesland, J. M. (1996b): Correlation of subcellular and intratumoral photosensitizer localization with ultrastructural features after photodynamic therapy. *Ultrastruct. Pathol.* **20**, 109–129.

Pottier, R. H. (1990): Localization phenomena: pH effects. In Photodynamic therapy of neoplastic diseases (Edited by D. Kessel), Vol. pp. 63–77. CRC Press, Boca Raton.

Prinsze, C., Penning, L. C., Dubbelman, T. M. A. R., and VanSteveninck, J. (1992): Interaction of photodynamic treatment and either hyperthermia or ionizing radiation and of ionizing radiation and hyperthermia with respect to cell killing of L929 fibroblasts, Chinese hamster ovary cells, and T24 human bladder cells. *Cancer Res.* **52**, 117–120.

Rich, M. R., Ferraro, G., and Brody, S. S. (1992): Effects of pH on the binding of hematoporphyrin derivative to monolayer and bilayer membranes. *Biochim. Biophys. Acta* **1104**, 269–272.

Richter, A. M., Waterfield, E., Jain, Ak., Sternberg, E. D., Dolphin, D., and Levy, J. G. (1990): *In vitro* evaluation of phototoxic properties of four structurally related bezoporphyrin derivatives. *Photochem. Photobiol.* **52**, 495–500.

Richter, A. M., Waterfield, E., Jain, Ak., Allison, B., Sternberg, E. D., Dolphin, D., and Levy, J. G. (1991): Photosensitizing potency of structural analogues of benzoporphyrin derivative (BPD) in a mouse tumor model. *Br. J. Cancer* **63**, 87–93.

Rimington, C., Rønnestad, A., Western, A., and Moan, J. (1988): Hematoporphyrin ethers-II. Improvements in method, synthesis of the dihexyl, dicyclohexanyl and diphenyl ethers and their preliminary biological evaluation. *Int. J. Biochem.* **20**, 1139–1149.

Rosenthal, I. (1991): Phthalocyanines as photodynamic sensitizers. *Photochem. Photobiol.* **53**, 859–870.

Segalla, A., Milanesi, C., Jori, G., Capraro, H. G., Isele, V., and Schieweck, K. (1994): CGP 55398, a liposomal Ge (IV) phthalocyanine bearing two axially ligated cholesterol moieties: a new potential agent for photodynamic therapy of tumours. *Br. J. Cancer* **69**, 817–825.

Soncin, M., Polo, L., Reddi, E., Jori, G., Kenney, M. E., Cheng, G., and Rodgers, M. A. (1995): Effect of axial ligation and delivery system on the tumor-localising and photosensitising properties of Ge (IV)-octabutoxy-phthalocyanines.

Spikes, J. D. (1990): New trends in photobiology: Chlorins as photosensitizers in biology and medicine. *J. Photochem. Photobiol. B: Biol.* **6**, 259–274.

Star, W. M., Marijnissen, H. P. A., van den Berg-Blok, A. E., Versteeg, J. A. C., Franken, K. A. P., and Reinhold, H. S. (1986): Destruction of rat mammary tumor and normal tissue microcirculation by hematoporphyrin derivative photoradiation observed *in vivo* sandwich observation chambers. *Cancer Res.* **46**, 2532–2540.

Thistlethwaite, A. J., Alexander, G. A., Moylan, D. J., and Leeper, D. B. (1987): Modification of human tumor pH by elevation of blood glucose. *Int. J. Radiat. Oncol. Biol. Phys.* **13**, 603–610.

Thomas, J. P. and Girotti, A. W. (1989): Glucose administration augments *in vivo* uptake and phototoxicity of the tumor-localizing fraction of hematoporphyrin derivative. *Photochem. Photobiol.* **49**, 241–247.

van Bruggen, N., Chan, W. S., Syha, J., Marshall, J. F., Proctor, E., Williams, S. R., Gadian, D. G., and Hart, I. R. (1992): Cell and tissue response of a murine tumor to phthalocyanine-mediated photodynamic therapy. *Eur. J. Cancer* **28**, 42–46.

van der Veen, N., van Leengoed, H., and Star, W. M. (1994): *In vivo* fluorescence kinetics and photodynamic therapy using 5-aminolaevulinic acid-induced porphyrin: increased damage after multiple irradiations. *Br. J. Cancer* **70**, 867–872.

van Geel, I. P., Oppelaar, H., Oussoren, Y. G., Schuitmaker, J. J., and Stewart, F. A. (1995): Mechanisms for optimising photodynamic therapy: second-generation photosensitisers in combination with mitomycin C. *Br. J.Cancer* **72**, 344–359.

van Leengoed, H. L. L. M., van der Veen, N., Versteeg, A. A. C. A., Ouellet, R., van Lier, J. E., and Star, W. (1993): *In vivo* photodynamic effects of phthalocyanines in a skin-fold observation chamber model: role of central metal ion and degree of sulfonation. *Photochem. Photobiol.* **58**, 575–580.

van Lier, J. E. (1990): Phthalocyanines as sensitizers for PDT of cancer. In Photodynamic therapy of neoplastic disease (Edited by D. Kessel), Vol. I, pp. 279–290. CRC Press, Boca Raton.

Volk, T., Jähde, E., Fortmeyer, H. P., Glüsenkamp, K.-H., and Rajewsky, M. F. (1993): pH in human tumor xenografts: effect of intravenous administration of glucose. *Br. J. Cancer* **68**, 492–500.

Weishaupt, K. R., Gomer, C. J., and Dougherty, T. J. (1976): Identification of singlet oxygen as the cytotoxic agent in photo-inactivation of a murine tumor. *Cancer Res.* **36**, 2326–2329.

White, L., Gomer, C. J., Doiron, D. R., and Szirth, B. C. (1988): Ineffective photodynamic therapy (PDT) in a poorly vascularized xenograft model. *Br. J. Cancer* **57**, 455–458.

Woodburn, K. W., Vardaxis, N. J., Hill, J. S., Kaye, A. H., and Phillips, D. R. (1991): Subcellular localization of porphyrins using confocal laser scanning microscopy. *Photochem. Photobiol.* **54**, 725–732.

Woodburn, K. W., Vardaxis, N. J., Hill, J. S., Kaye, A. H., Reiss, J. A., and Phillips, D. R. (1992a): Evaluation of porphyrin characteristics required for photodynamic therapy. *Photochem. Photobiol.* **55**, 697–704.

Woodburn, K. W., Stylli, S., Hill, J. S., Kaye, A. H., Reiss, J. A., and Phillips, D. R. (1992b): Evaluation of tumor and tissue distribution of porphyrins for use in photodynamic therapy. *Br. J. Cancer* **65**, 321–328.

Wöhrle, D., Iskander, N., Graschew, G., Sinn, H., Friedrich, E. A., Maier, W., Stern, B. J., and Schlag, P. (1990): Synthesis of positively charged phthalocyanines and their activity in the photodynamic therapy of cancer cells. *Photochem. Photobiol.* **51**, 351–356.

3.8. CLINICAL EXPERIENCES AND EXPECTATIONS

DIETER JOCHAM

INTRODUCTION

The broad clinical use of PDT should start – in analogy to other therapeutic modalities – with a clinical validation of the method in comparative studies. Preliminary trials and phase II studies should have to prove the essential effectiveness of the method. Testing of the sensitizer to be used on healthy volunteers in phase I studies is acceptable only for assessment of the pharmacokinetics and for possible side effects of the drug. Any use of photosensitizers in humans presumes the knowledge of the physical and chemical parameters described in the preceding chapters of this book. Because of the complex interactions of the photosensitizers with light as modified by the tissue conditions with its optical and biological properties, animal experiments are an inherent part of preclinical studies.

The history of PDT up to the present with its use of porphyrin derivatives as sensitizers was designed for the use of the working principle only in singular cases (curative trials) or in small series of up to 60 patients per tumor entity without any comparison to standard therapies. Comparative studies were tried. Only palliative designs or questions about the principal effectiveness were concerned, but not for evaluation as compared to a standard therapy.

The biometrical or statistical relevance of the body of data obtained from existing studies has to be critically questioned. The situation described sheds light on the difficulties of obtaining an approval of photosensitizers for clinical use. The availability of comparable clinical data becomes further complicated due to the insufficiently standardized application of light as well as an effective light dosimetry. The actual state of the clinical application or evaluation of the 2nd and 3rd generation photosensitizers shows a general lack of published data. Only a few conference reports and *on dit's* on clinical testing e.g. of benzoporphines, chlorin e_6, Zn-phthalocyanins, and tin etiopurpurin, are available.

THE IDEAL PHOTOSENSITIZER FROM A CLINICAL STANDPOINT

The photosensitizers available at present time show different patterns of distribution in tissue dependent on oral, systemic, or topic application. Most of the more intensively studied photosensitizers allow a tumor therapy only if applied systemically (intravenously) this way attaining a sufficient concentration in tissue. Dependent on water solubility, in hydrophobic photosensitizers in part carrier substances (e.g. liposomes) are applied which with respect to side effects in the organism have to be considered. The therapeutically necessary discrimination between tumor and normal tissue presumes a considerable tumor selectivity so that at complete light induced destruction of the tumor normal tissues are preserved or recover after slight or only short-term stress. The substance should have no dark or intrinsic toxicity as inferred by its chemistry and should leave the organism quickly via gut and/or kidney without uncalculable photoproducts or other intermediates difficult to excrete. Interactions with other medications should be of only minor impact. This should apply as well for the carrier substances as mentioned above.

At present, the optical properties as well of the photosensitizers as of the tissues limit the application of cost effective light sources (conventional, diode lasers, LED's) and the curable tumor types and tumor volumes. Restrictions result further from the photosensitizer-dependent mechanism of damage, i.e. preferably from the vascular vs. at the tumor cell level. 1st generation photosensitizers act primarily by their inclusion into the neovasculature of the tumor and, if present, inside the endothelial cells.

According to these preferences central areas of tumors, especially necrotic regions, show a reduced or lacking storage of photosensitizers. In order to acquire a total destruction of a tumor such photosensitizers have to be preferred which allow direct damage of every living tumor cell. This rule should be obeyed even in cases where a sensitizer is apparently more effective by damaging the tumor vasculature as well as – in part – the tumor cells themselves.

Concluding the aspects discussed above, defined criteria can be found to characterize the *ideal photosensitizer* (1Jocham and Wöhrle, Jan. 1996):

1	Chemically defined substance
2	Absorption maximum in the far red
3.1	No dark toxicity
3.2	High phototoxicity
3.3	No uncalculable photoproducts
4	Limited stability *in vivo* and under irradiation
5.1	Hydrophilicity
5.2	In case of hydrophobicity: clinically safe carrier systems
5.3	Intramolecular polarity to promote cellular uptake
6.1	Tumor-selective cellular storage
6.2	Quick tumor storage (< 2 h)
6.3	Quick excretion (< 1 day)
6.4	No photosensitization of skin, eye, mucous epithelia
7.1	Topic applicability
7.2	No proliferative action
7.3	Wide spectrum of indications
8	Cost effective global availability
9	Admission for clinical application

As the criteria listed above are hardly met by 1st generation photosensitizers, it became obvious that other photosensitizers had to be developed which would more or less fulfill the parameters mentioned.

Before starting to describe this, the actual clinical situation should be depicted so far as *a combination of experimental and clinical studies has contributed to an administrative approval of photosensitizers*.

CLINICAL APPLICATION OF 1st GENERATION PHOTOSENSITIZERS

The historical inauguration of the photodynamic principle goes back to antique times. First publications in modern times to the thematics arose by Finsen (1895) and by Raab and coworkers (1895). In 1903, Jesionek and Tappeiner reported the destruction of a tumor they had previously sensitized topically with eosin. The photodynamic therapy with hematoporphyrin derivative (HpD), the ancestor of the actual 1st generation photosensitizers (e.g. Photophrin™, Photosan™), began in 1976 when Kelly and Snell reported PDT of vesical tumors. Since then numerous types and constellations of tumors have been clinically treated by PDT. PDT has been applied in several thousands of cases. The aim of the treatments was in part curative, in part palliative. During the last years the imputed lack of acceptance of the procedure can be explained first of all on the basis of applications on non-curable, far proceeded tumors, on the other hand on the lack of data based on clinically controlled studies.

The situation has been improved during the last years without a really satisfactory presentation of data. Table 1 presents the clinical indications which Photophrin™ has been approved for in different countries by new. Photophrin™ at the time is the only photosensitizer for which an administration approval has been given.

Further clinical studies with systemically applied Photophrin™ are performed in cooperation with QLT (Vancouver, Canada). Table 2 summarizes these studies. In Germany a prospectively randomized phase III study for the treatment of the superficial vesical carcinoma is being performed in a comparison between PDT vs. BCG (*Bacille Calmette-Guèrin*). This study under the leadership of D. Jocham (Luebeck) requires the recruitment of 200 evaluable cases and a posttreatment observation period of a minimum of 2 years. Results of this study, which is granted by the Ministry of Research and Education (BMBF) of the Federal Republic of Germany and by QLT, will not be due before 1998. Similar long-term

Table 1 Indications for PDT with governmental approval of the photosensitizer Photofrin™ in different countries (state: January, 1996)

Company	*Application*	*Indication*	*Country*
QLT together with Cyanamid	i.v.	bladder	Canada
		lung	Netherlands
		esophagus	Netherlands
QLT together with Sanofi-Wintrop	i.v.	esophagus	USA

Table 2 Active Investigator Studies Using Photofrin™ Cross Referenced to QLT Ind. 25,064

Indication	*Study title*	*Investigator name and site*
Brain	PDT of malignant inoperable brain tumors	Dr. Paul Muller; Dr. Brian Wilson St. Michael's Hospital, University of Toronto, Canada
	Photochemotherapy for malignant brain tumors	Dr. Stephen Powers Milton S. Hershey Medical Centre, Penn State College of Medicine, University Hospital, Hershey, Pennsylvania
	PDT for childhood brain tumors	Dr. Harry Whelan Medical College of Wisconsin, Pediatric Neurology, Milwaukee, Wisconsin
Head and Neck	Evaluation of efficacy of PDT in managing early cancers of the upper aerodigestive tract	Dr. Merill Biel Minneapolis EN&T Clinic, PA, Minneapolis, Minnesota
	A study of the feasibility, toxicity, and response rate of PDT as a treatment for destruction of head and neck squamous cell carcinoma	Dr. B. Wenig Wenske Laser Center, Chicago, Illinois
Eye	PDT for corneal neovascularization	Dr. R. Epstein Rush-Pres-St. Luke's Medical Center, Chicago, Illinois
Esophageal	Pilot protocol for esophageal malignancies treated with PDT – Use of PDT utilizing PHOTOPHRIN™ in patients with esophageal cancer	Dr. James McCaughan Grant Laser Center, Division of Photodynamic Therapy Columbus, Ohio
	Use of PDT utilizing PHOTOFRIN™ in patients with esophageal carcinoma	Dr. B. Overholt Thompson Cancer Survival Center, Knoxville, Tennessee
	A phase III study of the safety and efficacy of PDT utilizing Photofrin™ for treatment of dysplasia or early adenocarcinoma of the esophagus in Barrett's esophagus	
	A centering balloon for PDT of esophageal cancer	
Laryngeal	Prospective open study of the effects of PDT on juvenile laryngotracheobronchial papillomatosis	Dr. Atus Mehta Cleveland Clinic Foundation, Cleveland, Ohio
	Evaluation of efficacy of PDT in managing recurrent juvenile laryngotracheal bronchial papillomatosis	Dr. Merill Biel Minneapolis EN&T Clinic, PA, Minneapolis, Minnesota
	Evaluation of efficacy of PDT in managing early cancers of the larynx	
Lung	The Compassionate use of PDT in conjunction with PHOTOFRIN™ for the treatment of symptomatic primary bronchogenic metastatic endotracheal neoplasms	Dr. R. Allen University of California, Davis Medical Center, Sacramento, California

Table 2 (*Continued*)

Indication	*Study title*	*Investigator name and site*
Lung (continued)	Phase II study of patients with advanced lung cancers	Dr. James McCaughan Grant Laser Center, Div. of Photodynamic Therapy, Columbus, Ohio
	PDT combined with high dose rate brachytherapy for patients with obstructive bronchogenic carcinoma	Dr. G. Loewen Roswell Park Memorial Institute, Buffalo, New York
	Comparative randomized study of the efficacy of photoresection with Nd:YAG laser alone or with Nd:YAG in combination with PDT in the treatment of nonoat cell bronchogenic carcinoma	Dr. J. P. Diaz Jiminéz Durán I. Reynals Hospital, Barcelona, Spain
	Prospective phase II study of inoperable endobronchial bronchocarcinoma with curative aim	Prof. Dr. K. Häussinger Zentralkrankenhaus Gauting der LVA Oberbayern, Germany
Chest wall	Phase II study of patients with cutaneous and subcutaneous breast cancer metastases treated with PHOTOFRIN™ and PDT	Dr. James McCaughan Grant Laser Center, Div. of Photodynamic Therapy, Columbus, Ohio
Breast	A treatment IND protocol for the use of PDT in patients with metastatic cutaneous breast cancer	Dr. S. Edge Roswell Park Memorial Institute, Buffalo, New York
Pleural mesothelioma	Surgery and intracavitary PDT for the treatment of malignant pleural mesothelioma	Dr. H. Takita; Dr. G. Loewen Roswell Park Memorial Institute, Buffalo, New York
	Malignant pleural mesothelioma	Dr. Harvey Pass National Cancer Institute, Rockville, Maryland
Intraoperative abdominal Intraperitoneal Sarcomatosis		Dr. W. F. Sindelar National Cancer Institute. Rockville, Maryland
Bladder	An open label study of PDT in the treatment of transitional superficial cell carcinoma of the urinary tract following recurrence of disease	Dr. U. Nseyo; Dr. F. Hetzel University of West Virginia, Dept. of Urology, Health Science Center Morgantown, West Virginia
	Treatment of superficial carcinoma of the bladder with PDT	Dr. R. Huben Roswell Park Memorial Institute, Buffalo, New York
Gynecology	Photodynamic endometrial ablation and dysfunctional uterine bleeding	Dr. Awadd Wellman Lab.'s of Photomedicine, Boston, Massachusetts
Rectal	Use of PDT utilizing PHOTOFRIN™ in patients with colon cancer	Dr. James McCaughan Grant Laser Center, Div. of Photodynamic Therapy, Columbus, Ohio
Kaposi's Sarcoma	PDT in patients with AIDS related Kaposi's Sarcoma: phase I/II	Dr. Z. Bernstein Roswell Park Memorial Institute, Buffalo, New York

Table 2 (*Continued*)

Indication	*Study title*	*Investigator name and site*
Skin/ Cutaneous	Phase II study of patients with basal and squamous cell skin cancer treated with PDT	Dr. James McCaughan Grant Laser Center, Div. of Photodynamic Therapy, Columbus, Ohio
	A Phase II study of PDT for the treatment of skin carcinoma. A pilot drug dose de-escalation study	Dr. B. Overholt Thompson Cancer Survival Center, Knoxville, Tennessee
	PDT for the treatment of skin carcinoma	
	PDT for the treatment of non-melanoma skin carcinoma	Dr. I. Koehler Wenske Laser Center, Chicago, Illinois
	PDT for the treatment of skin cancer: phase II pilot drug de-escalation study	Dr. B. Wenig Wenske Laser Center, Chicago, Illinois
		Dr. A. Oseroff/B.D. Wilson Roswell Park Memorial Institute, Buffalo, New York
	Information	
Europe	Ad Vermaire, Medical Director Netherlands Tel: ++31-1192-2724 Fax: ++31-1192-2762	
Canada	Cancer Information Line Tel: 879-2323 or 1-800-663-4242	
USA	National Cancer Institute Tel: 1-800-4-CANCER or from Canada Tel: (301)-495-5583	

performances are to be expected for other phase III studies. Details with respect to the design, the number of cases, and the duration of the study result in part from the considerably different clinical frame and questions.

For evaluation of topical applications of Photofrin™, phase II and phase III studies on psoriasis and the cervical neoplasia are currently performed. To conclude present clinical data the following general statements can be made:

PDT with 1st generation photosensitizers (HpD, Photofrin™, Photosan™) at a dosage of 2 mg per kg body weight (bw) allows a curative treatment of tumors in different organ systems so far as the thickness of the tumor layer does not exceed 2–3 mm at the time of irradiation and so far as the complete area or all compartments of the tumor are treated. The clinically relevant superficial dose of irradiation should be 100–150 J/cm^2 at power densities higher than 100 mW/cm^2. More correctly (but clinically impracticable) would be a calculation based on tumor volume.

The individual optical properties of the tumor and the surrounding tissue demand an exact on-line dosimetry of irradiation which is also a prerequisite for comparison of data in the frame of clinical studies. If these noted prerequisites are met, clinical applications of PDT show complete remissions (CR) of tumors in 80–85% of the cases. Long-term success, in some cases over several years, is found in these patients in about 50% of the cases. This situation is true even for tumors which by other modalities of treatment are incurable.

A rationale for this might be the action principle of PDT which differs from other therapeutic modalities. As differentiated according to tumor types the rate of successful therapies may differ considerably from the numbers mentioned above. Pigmented malignant melanomas and osteosarcomas are more or less resistant against PDT with first generation photosensitizers while cervical dysplasia at adequate techniques of irradiation shows nearly 100% success.

ADDITIONAL FIELDS OF PDT APPLICATION

Up to now the application of PDT was directed to the therapy of malignant tumors. The possibility to excite the fluorescence of the photosensitizer in tissue allows development of a diagnosis of early stages of tumors and of its residuals. Only the availability of δ-amino levulinic acid has allowed to obtain a broader application of fluorescent photodynamic diagnosis. Since photosensitizers are stored preferentially either in proliferating cells and tissues or in recently built-up vascularization, there are several instances to apply photodynamic methods just for other indications.

Among these indications are diseases of high incidence with no satisfactory therapeutic possibilities with regard to low efficiency of alternative therapies, the spectrum of side effects, and in some cases high expenses. Here explicitly should be mentioned the myeloproliferative diseases, the synovial proliferations in rheumatic arthritis – an example of a very common disease – angioplasty with its risk of restenosis, and macular degeneration as the most frequent cause of blindness in elderly patients. A successful application of PDT with its special action mechanisms would have – as can easily be seen – considerable economic significance (Table 3).

Table 3 Potential Indications of PDT in Future

Solid Tumors
Purging of Bone Marrow
Psoriasis
HIV-disease
Rheumatoid Arthritis
Arteriosklerosis
Prophylaxis of Restenosis after Angioplasty
Macula degeneration
Therapy of *Streptococcus mutans* infections in caries

CLINICAL EXPERIENCES WITH 2nd AND 3rd GENERATION PHOTOSENSITIZERS

As mentioned in the introduction, results on clinical applications of 2nd and 3rd generation photosensitizers which would allow an evaluation of its efficiency are not available. Table 4 lists new photosensitizers with respect to its producer, the field of application, and the present state of testing. Complementary to the studies listed, there are reports on single cases commenting on the application of 2nd and 3rd generation photosensitizers.

Table 4 Photosensitizers of 2nd and 3rd generation – actual state of clinical application (as modified acc. to J. G. Levy: Photodynamic therapy in focus. Elsevier Science Ltd, 1995)

Company	*Photosensitizer*	*Forms of applications*	*Phase of clinical testing*	*Indications*
DUSA, Pharmaceuticals Mt. Kisco NY, USA,	δ-amino levulinic acid (ALA)	topical oral	phase 1	Psoriasis, Actinic keratosis, Basal cell carcinoma, Gastrointestinal tumors, Psoriasis
MEDAC, Hamburg, Germany	ALA	topical	phase 2 phase 3	Bladder (Diagnosis/Therapy), Lung (Diagnosis), Basal cell carcinoma (Therapy), Bladder (Diagnosis, in planning)
PDT Systems Inc. St. Barbara CA, USA	Tin etiopurpurin (SnET2)	i.v. liposomes	phase 1/2	Skin tumors, Kaposi sarcoma
Scotia Pharmaceuticals Guilford, UK	*meso*-Tetra-hydroxy-phenyl chlorin (MTHPC)	i.v. topical	phase 1/2 phase 1/2	ENT tumors Basal cell carcinoma
Nippon Petrochemical Osaka, Japan	*Mono*-aspartyl chlorin e_6 (NPC-6)	i.v. (emulsion)	phase 1	Skin tumors
Cytopharm-Glaxo NC, USA	porphycenes	topical	preclinical	Psoriasis and other skin diseases
QLT, Vancouver, Canada	Benzoporphin monoacid ring A (BPD)	i.v. liposomes	phase 2	Skin tumors, Psoriasis
QLT/Ciba Vision Zurich, Switzerland	BPD	i.v.	preclinical	Macula degeneration during senescence
QLT/Ciba Geigy Basel, Switzerland	Zinc phthalocyanin	i.v. liposomes	phase 1 preclincial	Lung, Esophagus tumors, Psoriasis

Loh and colleagues investigated by fluorescence microscopy the amount of protoporphyrin IX in patients with inoperable rectum carcinoma after oral administration of δ-amino levulinic acid (ALA) at 30 and 60 mg/kg bw respectively. The tumors stored more of the protoporphyrin IX than the surrounding tissue. The contents of fluorescent substance raised following higher dosage of ALA.

Cairnduff and coworkers used topically applied ALA for the treatment of various skin tumors. 89% of the lesions in *M. Bowen* showed complete remission during 18 months follow-up while only 50% of basal cell carcinoma treatments showed success during 17 months follow-up. Skin metastases at all reacted only insufficiently. The irradiated tumor areals wetted and decomposed during 1 or 2 weeks and healed within 1–2 months.

Svanberg and colleagues treated skin tumors in a total of 26 patients after topical application of ALA in a 20% water-in-oil emulsion (80 basal cell carcinomas in 21 patients, 10 M. Bowen lesions in 3 patients, 4 T-cell lymphomas in 2 patients). The distribution of protoporphyrin IX in comparison to normal skin was 15 : 1 in the case of the basal cell carcinomas and the M. Bowen lesions, in the case of the T-cell lymphomas only 5 : 1.

As well for the therapy of skin tumors PDT with topically applied 9-acetoxy-(2, 7, 12, 17-tetrakis ß-methoxy ethyl) porphycene (ATMPn) has been tried. Studies by Harrer and coworkers on sensitizer penetration in melanoma and in basal cell carcinoma showed an enhanced velocity of penetration of ATMPn in tumors in comparison to normal tissues. Prolonged incubation showed enhanced concentration in melanoma. The topically administered substance reached the basal cell layer of the epidermis. Deeply inserted nests of tumorous tissue were reached by the drug after 6 h of administration.

In 1994, Sokolov and others reported about clinical studies with the photosensitizer Photosens™ which contains a mixture of polysulphonated chloroaluminum phthalocyanins with different degree of substitution. 45 patients with 135 tumor lesions were treated photodynamically. The spectrum of indications comprised tumors of the nasal cavity, the lung, oesophagus, stomach, bladder, vulva, breast, and skin tumors including melanomas and Kaposi sarcomas as well as skin metastases. The cumulative rate of complete remissions after an overall time of postobservation of 12 months was 49.9%. Partial remissions were reported in 34.8% of the lesions. As a non-commented side effect a long-term general photosensitization has to be assumed.

EXPECTATIONS OF THE CLINICIAN FOR THE FUTURE

Despite 20 years of clinical experience, PDT has not progressed beyond the state of clinical experimentation. Only in recent times the necessity of an evaluation according to the rules of clinical prospectively randomized phase II studies has been accepted. Tumor specific concepts of irradiation and dosimetrically reproducible parameters have to be included as essential parts of these studies.

Establishment of PDT as a first-line therapy requires cost effectiveness of the procedure as economic advantages from the side of the photosensitizer as well as of the light sources and light applicators.

The photosensitizers of the future should come as close as possible to the parameters of the "ideal photosensitizer" as mentioned above. Only then can the full potential of the procedure be realized. According to present knowledge, excitation maxima in the longwave red region of the visible spectrum are a central prerequisite for acquiring effects deep inside the tissue in PDT at superficial irradiation.

To what extent monoclonal antibodies (mAb's) as a part of the so-called immunoconjugates will play a role in the hospital will depend on the bioavailability of the conjugates inside the tumor and on the reproducibility of the concept at all. Tumors show a general heteroclonicity, and every concept requiring an individually produced mAb for every individual tumor should be refused.

In face of the poor availability of clinically relevant mAb's that fulfil the criteria mentioned above, a carrier system which does not refer to specific tumoral properties should be preferred.

Furthermore, an essential for the establishment of PDT in the hospital is a broad spectrum of applications of future photosensitizers. The high financial burden for development and clinical evaluation of a substance is justified only if it fulfills this criterion.

According to the experiences of the pharmaceutical industry as referenced by A. D. Cross (Cytopharm Inc., California, USA) only 1 of 16 substances of progressed basic research reaches the stage of principal clinical applicability. From these only 1 out of 4 of the selected substances is further examined in clinical phase II studies. This point of view should be taken into account just on the stage of basic research.

As mentioned repeatedly, prospectively randomized phase III studies should be performed as a basis of broad clinical application in which the PDT principle has to be compared with a standard therapy. A general understanding of this necessity has only developed in the most recent years. Today no real alternative exists in connection with further quality assessment and quality control based upon it. This has to be taken into consideration already in basic research on substance development by consulting early with development representatives of the pharmaceutical industry and with potential applicants.

The next chapter will give some essential aspects of the performance of clinical studies and therapeutical trials.

LITERATURE CITED

Akhlynina, T. V., Rosenkranz, A. A., Jans, D. A., and Sobolev, A. S. (1995): Insulin-mediated intracellular targeting enhances the photodynamic activity of chlorin e6. *Cancer Res.* **55**, 1014–1019.

Anthony, D. J., Profio, A. E., and Balchum, O. J. (1989): Fluorescence spectra in lung with porphyrin injection. *Photochem. Photobiol.* **49**, 583–586.

Bachor, R., Scholz, M., Shea, C. R., and Hasan, T. (1991): Mechanism of photosensitization by microsphere-bound chlorin e6 in human bladder carcinoma cells. *Cancer Res.* **51**, 4410–4414.

Bachor, R., Hautmann, R., and Hasan, T. (1994): Comparison of two routes of photosensitizer administration for photodynamic therapy of bladder cancer. *Urol. Res.* **22**, 21–23.

Bonnett, R. (1995): Photosensitizer of the porphyrin and phthalocyanine series for photodynamics therapy. *Chem. Soc. Rev.* **24 (1)**, 19–33.

Bown, S. G., (1993): Photodynamic therapy in gastroenterology – current status and future prospects. *Endoscopy* **25**, 683–685.

Bremner, J. C. M., Bradley, J. K., Stratford, I. J., and Adams, G. E. (1994): Magnetic resonance spectroscopic studies on "real-time" changes in RIF-1 tumour metabolism and blood flow during and after photodynamic therapy. *Br. J. Cancer* **69**, 1083–1087.

Cairnduff, F., Stringer, M. R., Hudson, E. J., Ash, D. V., and Brown, S. B. (1994): Superficial photodynamic therapy with topical 5-aminolevulinic acid for superficial primary and secondary skin cancer. *Br. J. Cancer* **69**, 605–608.

Dartsch, P. C., Wunderlich, K., and Ben-Hur, E. (1994): Aluminum phthalocyanines-induced photolysis of human vascular wall cells in culture and the effect of fluoride on photodynamic action. *Coronary Artery Disease* **5**, 851–855.

Divaris, D., Kennedy, J. C., and Pottier, R. H. (1990): Phototoxic damage to sebaceous glands and hair follicles of mice after systemic administration of 5-aminolevulinic acid correlates with localized protoporphyrin IX fluorescence. *Am. J. of Pathol.* **136**, 891–897.

Diwu, Z. and Lown, J. W. (1994): Phototherapeutic potential of alternative photosensitizers to porphyrins. *Pharmac. Ther.* **63**, 1–35.

Evrard, S., Aprahamian, M., and Marescaux, J. (1993): Intra-abdominal photodynamic therapy: from theory to feasibility. *Br. J. Surg.* **80**, 298–303.

Fijan, S., Hönigsmann, H., and Ortel, B. (1995): Photodynamic therapy of epithelial skin tumours using delta-aminolevulinic acid and desferrioxamine. *Br. J. Dermatol.* **133**, 282–288.

Fukuda, H., Paredes, S., Del, C., and Batlle, A. (1989): Tumor-localizing properties of porphyrins. *In vitro* studies using the porphyrin precursor, aminolevulinic acid, in free and liposome encapsulated forms. *Drug Design Delivery* **5**, 133–139.

Gollnick, H. P. M., Owsianowski, M., Ramaker, J., Chun, S.C., and Orfanos, C. E. (1995): Extracorporeal photopheresis – A new approach for the treatment of cutaneous T cell lymphomas. Recent results. *Cancer Res.* **139**, 409–415.

Herzog, M., Moser, J., Wagner, B., and Broecker, J. (1994): Shielding effects and hypoxia in photodynamic therapy. *Int. J. Oral Maxillofac. Surg.* **23**, 406–408.

Hillegersberg, R. van., Berg, O. van den., Kort, W. J., Terpstra, O. T., and Wilson., J. H. P. (1992): Selective accumulation of endogenously produced porphyrins in a liver metastasis model in rats. *Gastroenterol.* **103**, 647–651.

Hillegersberg, R. van., Kort W. J., and Wilson., J. H. P. (1994): Current status of photodynamic therapy in oncology. *Drugs* **48**, 510–527.

Hua, Z., Gibson, S. L., Foster, T. H., and Hilf, R. (1995): Effectiveness of δ-aminolevulinic acid-induced protoporphyrin as a photosensitizer for photodynamic therapy *in vivo*. *Cancer Res.* **55**, 1723–1731.

Iinuma, S., Farshi, S. S., Ortel, B., and Hasan, T. (1994): A mechanistic study of cellular photodestruction with 5-aminolevulinic acid-induced porphyrin. *Br. J. Cancer.* **70**, 21–28.

Iinuma, S., Bachor, R., Flotte, T., and Hasan, T. (1995): Biostribution and phototoxicity of 5-aminolevulinic acid-induced PpIX in an orthotopic rat bladder tumor model. *J. of Urol.* **153**, 802–806.

Jocham, D. (1994): Photodynamische Verfahren in der Urologie. *Urol. A* **33**, 547–552.

Kato, H., Imaizumi, T., Aizawa, K., Iwabuchi, H., Yamamoto, H., Ikeda, N., Tsuchida, T., Tamachi, Y., Ito, T., and Hayata, Y. (1990): Photodynamic diagnosis in respiratory tract malignancy using an excimer dye laser system. *J. Photochem. Photobiol. B: Biol.* **6**, 189–196.

Kennedy, J. C. and Pottier, R. H. (1992): Endogenous protoporphyrin IX, a clinically useful photosensitizer for photodynamic therapy. *J. Photochem. Photobiol. B: Biol.* **14**, 275–292.

Kessel, D. and Woodburn, K. (1993): Biodistribution of photosensitizing agents. *Int. J. Biochem.* **25**, 1377–1383.

König, K., Genze, F., and Miller, K. (1993): Photodynamic lasertherapy using aminolevulinic acid and desferrioxamine. *Dermatol. Monatsschrift* **179**, 132–134.

Korbelik, M. and Krosl, G. (1994): Cellular levels of photosensitizers in tumours: the role of proximity to the blood supply. *Br. J. Cancer* **70**, 604–610.

Lam, St. (1994): Photodynamic therapy of lung cancer. *Seminars in Oncology* **21**, 15–19.

Landthaler, M., Rück, A., and Szeimies, R. M. (1993): Photodynamische Therapie von Tumoren der Haut. *Der Hautarzt* **44**, 69–74.

Lui, H, (1994): Photodynamic therapy in dermatology with porfimer sodium and benzoporphyrin derivative: An update. *Seminars in Oncol.* **21**, 11–14 .

Ma, L., Moan, J., and Berg, K. (1994): Evaluation of a new photosensitizer, meso-tetrahydroxyphenyl-chlorin, for use in photodynamic therapy: A comparison of its photobiological properties with those of two other photosensitizers. *Int. J. Cancer* **57**, 883–888.

Malik, Z., Ehrenberg, B., and Faraggi, A. (1989): Inactivation of erythrocytic, lymphocytic and myelocytic leukemic cells by photoexcitation of endogenous porphyrins. *J. Photochem. Photobiol.* **4**, 195–205.

Marcon, N. E. (1994): Photodynamic therapy and cancer of the esophagus. *Seminars in Oncol.* **21**, 20–23.

Mlkvy, P., Messmann, H., Regula, J., Conio, M., Pauer, M., Millson, C. E., MacRobert, A. J., and Bown, S. G. (1995): Sensitization and photodynamic therapy (PDT) of gastrointestinal tumors with 5-aminolevulinic acid (ALA) induced protoporphyrin IX (PPIX). A pilot study. *Neoplasma* **42**, 109–113.

Messmann, H., Mlkvy, P., Buonaccorsi, G., Davies, C. L., MacRobert, A. J., and Bown, S. G. (1995): Enhancement of photodynamic therapy with 5-aminolevulinic acid-induced porphyrin photosensitisation in normal rat colon by threshold and light fractionation studies. *Br. J. Cancer* **72**, 589–594.

Moan, J., Berg, K., Anholt, H., and Madslien, K. (1994): Sulfonated aluminium phthalocyanines as sensitizers for photochemotherapy. Effects of small light doses on localization, dye fluorescence and photosensitivity in V79 cells. *Int. J. Cancer* **58**, 865–870.

Mulroney, C. M., Glück, St., and Ho, A. D. (1994): The use of photodynamic therapy in bone marrow purging. *Seminars in Oncol.* **21**, 24–27.

Orenstein, A., Kostenich, G., Tsur, H., Kogan, L., and Malik, Z. (1995): Temperature monitoring during photodynamic therapy of skin tumors with topical 5-aminolevulinic acid application. *Cancer Letters* **93**, 227–232.

Orth, K., König, K., Genze, F., and Rück, A. (1994): Photodynamic therapy of experimental colonic tumours with 5-aminolevulinic-acid-induced endogenous porphyrins. *J. Cancer. Res. Clin. Oncol.* **120**, 657–661.

Parry, W. L. and Hemstreet, G. P. (1988): Cancer detection by quantitative fluorescence image analysis. *J. Urol.* **139**, 270–274.

Pass, H. I. (1993): Photodynamic therapy in oncology: Mechanisms and clinical use. *J. Nation Cancer Institute* **85**, 443–456.

Peng, Q., Moan, J., Ma, L. W., and Nesland, J. M. (1995): Uptake, localization and photodynamic effect of meso-Tetra (hydroxyphenyl)porphine and its corresponding chlorin in normal and tumor tissues of mice. *Cancer Res.* **55**, 2620–2626.

Peng, Q., Evensen, J. F., Rimington, C., and Moan, J. (1987): A comparison of different photosensitizing dyes with respect to uptake in C3H-tumors and tissues of mice. *Cancer Letters* **36**, 1–10.

Pottier, R. H., Chow, Y. F. A., LaPlante, J. P., Truscott, T. G., Kennedy, J. C., and Beiner, L. A. (1986): Non-invasive technique for obtaining fluorescence excitation and emission spectra *in vivo*. *Photochem. Photobiol.* **44**, 679–687.

Prinz, B. and Plewig, G. (1994): Extrakorporale Photophorese. *Hautarzt* **45**, 746–750.

Ratcliffe, S. L. and Matthews, E. K. (1995): Modification of the photodynamic action of δ-aminolevulinic acid (ALA) on rat pancreatoma cells by mitochondrial benzodiazepine receptor. *Br. J. Cancer* **71**, 300–305.

Rebeiz, N., Rebeiz, C. C., Arkins, S., Kelley, K. W., and Rebeiz, C. A. (1992): Photodestruction of tumor cells by induction of endogenous accumulation of protoporphyrin IX: enhancement by 1,10-phenanthroline. *Photochem. Photobiol.* **55**, 431–435.

Regula, J., MacRobert, A. J., Gorchein, A., Buonaccorsi, G. A., Thorpe, S. M., Spencer, G. M., Hatfield, A. R. W., and Bown, S. G. (1995): Photosensitation and photodynamic therapy of oesophageal, duodenal, and colorectal tumours using 5-aminolevulinic acid induced protoporphyrin IX – a pilot study. *Gut.* **36**, 67–75.

Roeder, B. (1990): Tetrapyrroles: A chemical class of potent photosensitizers for the photodynamic treatment of tumours. *Lasers in Med. Science* **5**, 99–105.

Rosenthal, D. I. and Glatstein, E. (1994): Clinical applications of photodynamic therapy. *Ann. Med.* **26**, 405–409.

Sima, A. F., Kennedy, J. C., Blakeslee, D., and Robertson, D. M. (1981): Experimental porphyric neuropathy: A preliminary report. *J. Canad. Sci. Neurolog.* **8**, 105–114.

Steinbach, P., Kriegmair, M., Baumgartner, R., Hofstädter, F., and Knüchel, R. (1994): Intravesical instillation of 5-aminolevulinic acid: The fluorescent metabolite is limited to urothelial cells. *Urology* **44**, 676–681.

Svanberg, K., Andersson, T., Killander, D., Wang, I., Stenram, U., Andersson-Engels, S., Berg, R., Johansson, J., and Svanberg, S. (1994): Photodynamic therapy of non-melanoma malignant tumours of the skin using topical δ-aminolevulinic acid sensitization and laser irradiation. *Br. J. Dermatol.* **130**, 743–751.

Szeimies, R. M. and Landthaler, M. (1995): Topische photodynamische Therapie in der Behandlung oberflächlicher Hauttumoren. *Hautarzt* **46**, 315–318.

Temeck, B. K. and Pass, H. (1995): Esophagopleural Fistula: A complication of photodynamic therapy. *Southern Med. J.* **88**, 271–274.

Werning, J. W., Stepnick, D. W., Jafri, A., Megerian, C. A., Antunez, A. R., and Zaidi, S. (1995): Metoclopramide enhances the effect of photodynamic therapy on xenografted human squamous cell carcinoma of the head and neck. *Arch. Otolaryngol. Head Neck Surg.* **121**, 783–789.

Whitmore, W. F. and Bush, I. M. (1966): Ultraviolet cystoscopy in patients with bladder cancer. *J. Urol.* **95**, 201–207.

3.9. CLINICAL STUDIES AND THERAPEUTIC TRIALS ACCORDING TO GCP GUIDELINES

DIETER JOCHAM

GCP stands for "good clinical practice", i.e. for guidelines pertaining to the conduct of clinical trials. These guidelines are intended to ensure the gathering of scientifically relevant, reliable data suitable for answering the scientific question posed, while protecting the rights and integrity of trial subjects, i.e. patients. This refers to the planning of trials as well as to their conducting and evaluation.

TRIAL TYPES

In literature, the following terms are used, which differ with regard to medical aspects, liability and drug regulations:

- Non-conventional treatment
- Curative trial = Therapeutic trial
  - scientific trial (experiment on humans)
    - scientific clinical trials on healthy subjects
    - therapeutic clinical trials on patients
  - testing of therapy concepts
    - observations on drug/therapeutic strategy application
    - drug monitoring studies

These definitions differentiate according to the purpose of the action (scientific/therapeutic), the methods, the number of trial subjects and the object of the trial (drugs/other diagnostic or therapeutic strategies).

The legal valuations of medical actions are based on the prerequisites for authorization, on the requirements for conducting the trials and on the subsequent duties in connection with different trial types. The most important parameter is the risk potential for the individual subject.

The protective regulations do not strictly follow the definitions of the different trial types but cover all types.

LEGAL BACKGROUND

In the U.S., the conducting of clinical studies in adherence to "GCP-guidelines" of the FDA has been initiated in 1977, and has meanwhile been laid down in the form of guidelines or, in some cases, only in recommendations.

These are regularly updated and documented in a so-called "Code of Federal Regulations" (CFR). The relevant regulation for GCP-Basic Formulations is the subject of Regulation #21. These guidelines have meanwhile gained considerable international acceptance.

In Europe, the "Committee for Proprietory Medicinal Products" (CPMP), a special committee of the European Union, gave final approval to the "Note for guidance – Good clinical practice for trials on Medicinal Products in the European Community" on July 11th, 1990. The EC note on GCP has been in operation since July 1st, 1991. The primary aim of these guidelines is to establish basic principles for standards of GCP to be adhered to when conducting medicinal studies on human beings. Correspondingly, the GCP-guideline is directed primarily towards the pharmaceutical industry. The GCP guidelines must also be followed when data obtained from other sources, e.g. from the clinic, are to be used for the application for approval. It is important to note that the principles mentioned are pertinent to all four phases of the clinical investigation, including bioavailability and bioequivalence studies. According to actual jurisdiction the GCP guidelines will also have to be applied by analogy to cases where, for example, a new therapy concept is tested outside of clinical medicinal trials.

Even the *therapeutic attempt* (novelty treatment) which consists of an individual treatment differing from the standard therapy, can be involved. It is able to generate hypotheses for research and can therefore constitute a preliminary stage for a clinical experiment designed to examine the hypothesis, followed by a research and treatment oriented clinical trial on patients ("research treatment").

The definition of a therapeutic attempt may be of special importance within the assessment of oncological therapy concepts because of its significance for the refundability of drugs. Combination studies in the area of oncology often do not fit into the legal pattern of clinical trials. Oncology has therefore been accorded a special status by means of the following statement:

"In oncology, drugs which are licensed for a specific field of use are often administered in different combinations, also in connection with radiotherapy and/or surgery, with the aim of working out new therapeutic concepts. These are to be treated as therapeutic attempts".

"Licensed for a specific field of use" also refers to drugs of which a higher or lower dosage is being tested (see Deutsches Arzneimittelgesetz §29 Abs. 3, Abs. 2a).

A legal requirement that is important for the clinician is the stipulation that the trial protocol must be in keeping with the latest scientific developments. Consequently, the GCP guidelines will also have to be applied in countries which have not yet incorporated them into their national law.

When the GCP guidelines are implemented in national law, there are several points of special importance:

- the alteration and adaptation of national law concerning the necessity of hearing an ethics committee;
- the appointment of a principal investigator and a monitor;

- the alteration of the operating instructions of pharmaceutical entrepreneurs;
- the description of the tasks assigned to the monitor, the investigator and the principal investigator;
- the adjustment of the "Rules for the proper conducting of clinical trials";
- the alteration of the profession profile for physicians, e.g. with respect to the ethics committees, the arbitration proceedings, the requirement profiles for monitors, investigators, and principal investigators, as well as to the rules for recompensation of investigators, trial subjects, and patients; and
- the revision of national guidelines for the monitoring of clinical trials.

These measures are aimed at improving the ethical, scientific and technical quality of clinical studies and of the collected data, as well as at obtaining an internationally comparable standard. The GCP note covers these topics in 5 chapters.

Chapter 1 deals with the protection of participants in the trial, foremost the patients. In this context, the 1964 Helsinki Declaration of the World Medical Association in the current revision passed in Hong Kong in 1989, has to be mentioned. This declaration must be fully known to and followed by all engaged in research on human beings. According to it, the personal integrity and welfare of the trial subjects is the ultimate responsibility of the investigator.

Before the trials are conducted, the sponsor and/or the investigator has to submit a comprehensive trial protocol to an independent ethics committee which must declare its consent. In case of a change in the protocol, a new consent of the ethics committee must be obtained before the trials may be continued.

The principal investigator has a right to demand opinions and advice from the ethics committee in writing within a reasonable time limit. These committees are considerably more active than before and are equipped with extensive authorities.

The consent of a trial subject/patient may only be obtained after comprehensive information in both oral and written form. His/her consent to participate in the trial should be declared in written form. Oral consent is acceptable if documented by the signature of an independent witness recording the subject's assent.

Consent must always be given by the signature of the subject in case of a non-therapeutical study.

Relevant new insights gained during the trials necessitate the renewal of the consent. Subjects who are incapable of giving personal consent may only be included in a study after formal approval from the ethics committee.

The subject must be made aware that he/she is under no obligation to participate in the trial, and that a refusal to participate or a premature withdrawal from the trial will be without any disadvantages for his/her subsequent care.

Subjects as well as their relatives, guardians, or legal representatives must be given ample opportunity to enquire about the details of the trial. The subject has to be informed that his/her personal data will be scrutinized during audits or inspections as well as in the course of a centralized evaluation of data gathered in multi-centre trials, but that all data will be treated as strictly confidential.

Chapter 2 covers the responsibilities of the persons conducting the trial. The different responsibilities of the sponsor, the monitor and the investigator are defined and set off against each other.

The new regulations assign important tasks and responsiblity not only to the principal investigator and the investigator, but also to the *monitor*. The monitor has to pay a so-called "pre-study visit" to the investigator before the trial is begun, as well as a "study initiative visit" at the start of the trial. Further visits have to take place while the trials are being conducted as well as after their termination, e.g. for the recording of late events.

The monitor has to check the infrastructure of the trial site and the number of trial subjects available. This includes the obligation to ensure adequate information of all staff as well as the supervision of the procedures on location. The tasks of the monitor also include controlling the recording of data and comparing the data with the original results, taking into account the protection of data privacy. Furthermore, the monitor must assist the investigator in the administrative procedures as well as in the gathering of data. It is his/her duty to control that informed consent is being obtained from all subjects prior to their participation in the trial.

The *sponsor's* tasks include, among others, the duty to provide satisfactory insurance for the trial subjects as well as indemnity for the principal investigator. He also has to prepare a final report, and, in addition, intermediate reports, if need be. In the case of clinical oncological trials, which are conducted without an industrial sponsor, these tasks fall upon the person initiating the trial, i.e. the principal investigator.

The *investigator* must thoroughly familiarize himself with the trial protocol and with the properties of the investigational medicinal product as described in the investigator's brochure.

He/she must ensure sufficient time for conducting and completing the trial. He/she also has to provide retrospective data on numbers of patients in order to ensure an adequate recruitment rate for the trial. Furthermore, he/she has to submit an up-to-date curriculum vitae as well as other current credentials. Finally, he/she has to declare in writing that he/she has read, understands and will work according to the protocol and the rules of GCP, and accepts the supervision of the monitor as well as the control procedures and the agreed publication policy.

Chapter 3 contains new, detailed regulations for the handling of trial data. Future clinical trials will be submitted to a permanent internal and external quality control. Severe consequences can be incurred in the case of deviation from the system of GCP, of organizational faults and of any other procedure not properly adhered to. In the case of drug studies this may even lead to the refusal of the study by the authority. For the investigator, this may lead to recourse claims by the sponsor. It has to be noted that the discontinuation of a trial due to organizational faults is ethically unacceptable. Not only the ethics committees but also the supervising bodies have been given new, more powerful authorization for the surveillance of clinical trials, pertaining especially to the investigator and his trial site. The inspectors are already increasingly inspecting clinical trials and their investigators on the job.

Special attention is given to the adherence to GCP guidelines. Drastic fines can be imposed for violations of these rules, e.g. in cases where the written consent of the patient has been obtained too late or not at all.

The investigator must make all data and documents available to the relevant authorities immediately upon request. The producer must do so within a period of 2 days maximum (regulation in Germany). After completion of the trial, the data has to be retained for 15 years. Document safety of data files must be guaranteed. There are no corresponding regulations for comparative oncological studies with licensed drugs for indications stated in the protocol.

The biometry listed in Chapter 4 is an integral part of any clinical investigation or study. It must in advance be thoroughly examined and stipulated in detail. The GCP guidelines state extensive and detailed demands pertaining to the trial planning and the trial protocol. According to GCP, a well designed trial relies primarily on a thoroughly considered, well structured and complete protocol. This protocol must contain:

- the title of the project;
- the name of the principal investigator and his *locum tenens*;
- the registration number, if any;
- a definition and description of the trial's aim;
- the present state of data available;
- an exhaustive list of criteria for inclusion or exclusion of patients;
- detailed information on the methods, including the recording and the evaluation of data;
- samples of the forms used for the declaration of consent and for the gathering of data;
- a list of relevant literature.

The regulations pertaining to quality control, which are the topic of Chapter 5, have not yet been finalized.

Subsequently, the conducting of studies in four phases and the concept of *observations on application* as well as other trial types will be covered.

PHASES OF DRUG EVALUATION

Trials of drugs are carried out gradually in four phases; their aim is the launching of the licensed drug. Oncological studies follow the same pattern even though the object of the investigation is not a drug.

In Phase 1, a method or a trial substance is used on human beings for the first time. These can be healthy volunteers or patients, depending on the problem to be investigated. Typically, small groups of 10–20 trial subjects are used to determine the appropriate dose range and to test the drug tolerance.

The following Phase 2 consists of limited therapeutic pilot studies on patients. On groups of typically between 50 and 300 patients, the principal activity of a substance or a method is tested prospectively and the provisional indications, the appropriate therapeutic dose range as well as the adverse effects are determined. The majority of clinical studies in the past belonged to this Phase 2 type.

After the successful completion of Phase 2, Phase 3 covers the broad-range administration of the method or drug in the clinic and/or under practical conditions. *Phase 3a* consists of validating the method or the drug by way of comparison to other drugs or to placeboes or by way of a control group. The procedures to be followed in each individual case depend on the respective conditions and problems. The study is conducted in a prospectively randomized manner. Its aim is the validation and the fixing of definite indications as well as the discovery of rare adverse reactions and contra-indications.

On the base of the data thus gathered, the medical scientific data base can be enlarged and the launching of the product, in case of a licensing study, can be prepared in *Phase 3b*.

Phase 4 is dedicated to determining long term effects. In the case of oncological studies, which are not aimed at obtaining licensing for a drug, Phase 4 has so far been of no importance. At best, the patients recruited in Phase 3 trials are monitored on a long term basis, e.g. to determine the progress of a tumor or the survival rate. The American GCP regulations do not contain a Phase 4.

All phases of the study have to take the GCP guidelines into account.

For day-to-day clinical work, the therapeutic trial and the observation of application are of special importance.

In therapeutic trials, a method or a substance is administered to an individual as part of the physician's therapeutic freedom, for the purpose of treatment only. It is only in this case that the GCP guidelines do not have to be adhered to, and that the notification of the ethics committee and the supervisory body is dispensable, but nevertheless recommended for practical reasons. The supervisory body should be informed. Only then the trial subjects do not have to be provided with insurance cover (German regulation). The gathering of data, even in individual cases, for the evaluation of the drug's administration brings the GCP guidelines into operation; *in praxi*, this applies especially to the clinical oncological studies conducted to optimize therapeutic patterns.

For post-marketing surveillance, no consent of the patient and no special insurance is needed. It must be reported to the supervisory body prior to its commencement.

The clinical evaluation of photodynamic methods will have to take these guidelines into account. Otherwise, the rank of photodynamics will be as uncertain in the future as it has been during the past 20 years.

INDEX